rolfing

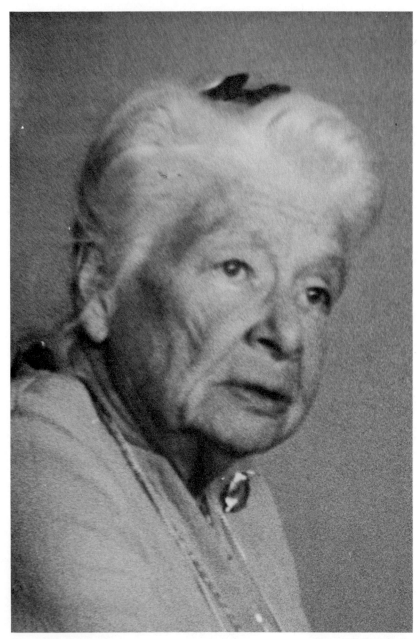

Ida P. Rolf

rolfing:

The Integration of Human Structures

Ida P. Rolf, Ph.D.

Illustrations by John Lodge, M.A.
Photographs by Ron Thompson

Harper & Row, Publishers
New York, Hagerstown, San Francisco, London

First BARNES & NOBLE BOOKS edition published 1978

ISBN: 0-06-465096-0

82 10 9 8 7 6 5 4

To the many people who helped carry the load,
and to Marianne McDonald, who made the load
so much easier to carry.

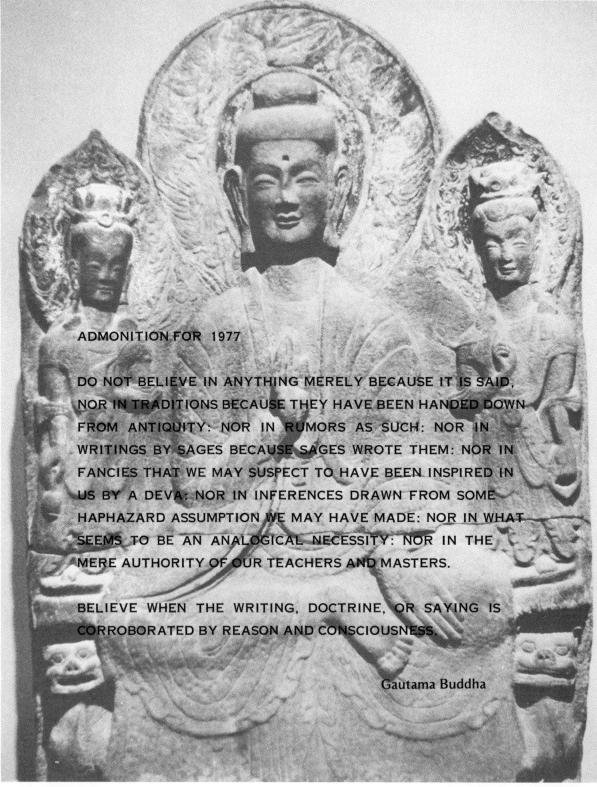

ADMONITION FOR 1977

DO NOT BELIEVE IN ANYTHING MERELY BECAUSE IT IS SAID,
NOR IN TRADITIONS BECAUSE THEY HAVE BEEN HANDED DOWN
FROM ANTIQUITY: NOR IN RUMORS AS SUCH: NOR IN
WRITINGS BY SAGES BECAUSE SAGES WROTE THEM: NOR IN
FANCIES THAT WE MAY SUSPECT TO HAVE BEEN INSPIRED IN
US BY A DEVA: NOR IN INFERENCES DRAWN FROM SOME
HAPHAZARD ASSUMPTION WE MAY HAVE MADE: NOR IN WHAT
SEEMS TO BE AN ANALOGICAL NECESSITY: NOR IN THE
MERE AUTHORITY OF OUR TEACHERS AND MASTERS.

BELIEVE WHEN THE WRITING, DOCTRINE, OR SAYING IS
CORROBORATED BY REASON AND CONSCIOUSNESS.

Gautama Buddha

Photo by George Connelly

Contents

Foreword

The writing of this book has extended over four years—four years of the odd weekend, the in-between couple of months stolen from a heavy schedule of teaching and lecturing, traveling and treatments. The perceptive will notice that it changes pace and level from time to time, the influence of time and discussions as the circle of rolfing has widened, the result of reflection on the questions of students. The book is intended for two types of readers: the interested but untrained layman and the professional wanting technical information. We have attempted to marry these two levels of complexity, chiefly through the medium of the illustrations and their captions, which often have more technical information than the text.

Structural Integration is a statement of a point of view. Although we have tried to retain a sense of how Structural Integration fits with traditional ways of seeing the body, the main effort has been to unfold its ideas and implications in the light of our experience. The technique of Structural Integration deals primarily with the physical man; in practice, considerations of the physical are inseparable from considerations of the psychological.

Many will read this book hoping that it will answer the question, What is rolfing? It does, of course, answer that question, but perhaps not in the expected form. The book is a demonstration of the principles of the body, the manner in which it is made, and how this creature can change. The technique of Structural Integration is a conversion of these ideas into a therapeutic tool. The technique itself involves a ten-hour cycle of deep manual intervention in the elastic soft tissue structure (myofascia) of the body. The goal of this treatment is balance of the body in the gravity field; the principle of the treatment is, in brief, that if tissue is restrained, and balanced movement demanded at a nearby joint, tissue and joint will relocate in a more appropriate equilibrium.

This is a simplified statement; the reality is more complex both in practice and in effect. We have made an effort to give *no* helpful hints to those who would enjoy a little home experimentation. The technique of Structural Integration is powerful, and the resultant changes are far-reaching. As practitioners, we do not aim for change alone; we wish to induce change toward balance. Change without balance can be destructive. Experience has taught us that recognition of balance and understanding its many ramifications are subtle arts and long-term disciplines. Balance in the body does not reveal itself to the dilettante; it is a matter of intuition, experience, knowledge, and study.

Structural Integration does not "cure" symptoms. In fact, as practitioners we refuse to consider or diagnose symptoms except to investigate possible reasons for postponing our work (e.g., acute pain or illness of any kind, prolonged or massive medication or addiction). In addition to the obvious change in structure and stance, there are many other varied effects of rolfing. They are best summed up in the phrase "I feel better" (or "lighter" or "easier"). The added ease, the improved vitality are the result of greater balance; this does its own beneficial work on physical and psychological ills.

We are asked if rolfing is permanent. Rolfing enters into the body's process and changes its course. Unless an accident intervenes, the body will continue along its new course. The effects of rolfing are not simply permanent, they are progressive.

We have included about a thousand photographs and drawings. The photographs give at least a static impression of the changes resulting from Structural Integration and illustrate definitions and comments on average structure. It should be noted that, with two exceptions, all photographs are of individuals processed by students during training classes. The two exceptions are practitioners of Structural Integration who received additional processing in the course of their training.

The anatomical drawings presented an unexpected and difficult problem. What was needed were drawings that would make graphic the anatomical balances discussed in the text. We soon discovered that the illustrations in standard anatomical books show no balance. Presumably, this is because the models used for these drawings are mostly hospital dissections, usually of bodies that suffered from disease and privation. John Lodge's problem was to convert this textbook anatomy to balanced, living anatomy. A practitioner of Structural Integration, he accomplished this in drawings that are masterpieces of clarity and style, giving a new look at human anatomy and a new point of view for the student.

As we have discussed the ideas of this book with friends and associates, it has become obvious that one of its contributions will be to the concepts relating psyche and soma. It is an accepted truism that body and mind co-act, express each other, influence each other, yet there are few satisfying constructs defining the relation. Does psyche determine physiology, or is the opposite true? Where do the various schools of physical and psychological human improvement fit in? What could be called a valid definition of human improvement? We are adding to this discussion the evidence of experience with the ideas and the technique of Structural Integration. We hope the reader will gain objectivity from our experience and perhaps shift the level of his understanding.

Rosemary Feitis
New York, 1973

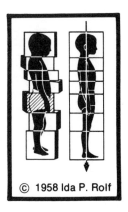

© 1958 Ida P. Rolf

Structural Integration is now more popularly called rolfing, which is a trademark of the Rolf Institute, Box 1868, Boulder, Colorado 80306.

R.F.
1978

Preface
Literal Thorns
in Literal Flesh

We are not stuff that abides,
but patterns that perpetuate themselves.
—NORBERT WIENER

As in all matter organized into biological units, there is a pattern, an order, in human bodies. Humans can change toward orderliness, or they can change away from it. Human bodies do change—your body can, any body can. We do not mean deteriorate or age in the commonly accepted sense. We mean that bodies—average physical bodies of flesh and blood—are amazingly plastic media, which can change quickly toward a structure that is more orderly and thus more economical in terms of energy.

Structural Integration is a system that induces change toward an ordered pattern. In general, it is a basic ten-hour cycle of treatment that balances myofascial* relationships. The key to all life experience is movement; in the segmented human structure, movement is expressed through the joints. In humans, the myofascial component determines the adequacy of the joint. Thus, by changing the myofascia and bringing it toward the normal, the practitioner of Structural Integration evokes a more normal (in our sense of the word) movement. This book sets forth the mechanics of this process and, in our laboratory photographs, records its effects.

*Fascia, in combination with the muscle it enwraps, is called myofascia. Structural Integration relies on one outstanding property of myofascia, its elasticity. See also the discussion in Chapter 3.

The possibility for this change derives from the structure of the body and its inherent message. It depends on the fact that a body is an entity, but not a unitary entity. Although the illusion of unity, of elementality, is created by the enwrapping fascia and skin, a human body is actually a complex, a consolidation of segments, the keystone of which is the pelvis. The perceptions, the responses, and the behavior of the integrated complex depend not on the individual units within the wrapping but on their relationship. An effective human being is a whole that is greater than the sum of its parts. Successful, meaningful integration depends on appropriate relationships in space among the components of the body.

The message of this medium—the body—is energy. To the worker in Structural Integration, energy is something so apparent in the body he processes that it is virtually palpable. To the subject who receives the work, the resultant energy change is even more dramatic; when he works or when he plays, he uses up less of his vital reserve. This happens within all bodies as a degree of balance is called forth.

Form and function are a unity, two sides of one coin. In order to enhance function, appropriate form must exist or be created. A joyous radiance of health is attained only as the body conforms more nearly to its inherent pattern. This pattern, this form, this Platonic Idea, is the blueprint for structure. In turn, the function of this more appropriate structure is vitality, vitality of a degree unknown to the average person.

In *The Human Use of Human Beings* Norbert Wiener has said, "We are not stuff that abides, but patterns that perpetuate themselves." For most people in the real world, the pattern body has been lost or is no longer visible. Therefore, in our culture, there is little or no recognition of what this ideal pattern body looks like. The purpose of this book is to unveil, for those who wish to see, the pattern underlying the random human body, to help them understand that the random body is deviant, how it became aberrated, and why more joyous function can result from more appropriate form.

When practitioners of Structural Integration say that the pattern has become random, what do they mean? In the average person, the pattern has become submerged under layers of fleshy disorder. (I do not mean fat—that is a different problem). When people come to us for what we call processing, we take the kind of photographs shown in this book. Such pictures show clearly a lack of symmetry and balance. Legs seem too large (or too small) for the torso; arms are similarly misfit. The upper half of the body may look much too small (or too large) for the lower half; the abdomen may seem too big (or occasionally too small) for the chest. The torso is not balanced over the legs; lagging along behind, it has to work to keep up with them as they walk. The abdomen may lead the body, and the legs scurry along trying to fit themselves underneath. The neck and head may well be six inches in front of the position that gravity and common sense dictate as appropriate. We are describing travesties of the body, you say? No, sadly enough; these are average bodies, and we challenge you to disprove it in any gathering of people, of any age selection.

If function and form are really one, and if physiology really reflects structural form, this picture of disordered structure is a sad commentary on the well-being of humans. We need look no further to recognize that the "reality" of life for these people is a bit grim. They are, they say, "healthy," in token of which they sleep to sleeping pills and waken to pep pills. When the going gets rough, they drink alcohol or smoke "pot" to drown the anxiety. They look in their mirrors and do not like what they see. It does not occur to them that their real dissatisfaction is with their physical, corporeal structure, with the way they are put together. This lack of recognition is understandable. Twentieth-century medicine, which has worked so many miracles, has been chemically, not structurally, oriented. Hence, the lay mind thinks of chemistry as the only outstanding healing medium—a drug for this, a shot for that. But any mirror or photograph would reveal that a great many problems are matters of structure, of physics—of a three-dimensional body fitting very badly into a greater material universe (the earth), which has its own energy field (gravity). Help must be sought in the terms of the problem—in the physics of spatial relations, of man in his environment, of man-as-a-whole in the energy field of the earth, gravity. And help can be found. The war within can end in a lasting peace.

At this point, doubt intervenes, whispering that we are miserable because of our emotions—chronic depression, frustration, anger, resentment, grief, greed, irritability. The backache, the neckache, and the shoulder tension seem to us secondary. What of this? The answer is that as structure becomes more appropriate, emotional turmoil can and does settle.

Emotional response is behavior, is function. All behavior is expressed through the musculoskeletal system. All function is an expression of structure and form and correlates directly with material structure. A man crying the blues is in reality bewailing his structural limitations and failures. He is, of course, unconscious of this. To him, his emotional response is a primary, independent condition.

The premise of modern psychotherapy is that man's outer circumstances are the projection of his inner, often hidden, self. This premise may be looked at from a different angle: a man's emotional state may be seen as the projection of his structural imbalances. No doubt this formula, too, is an oversimplification, and there are unknowns that time and the psychotherapists will uncover. But a man who undergoes integration of his corporeal structure experiences the basic link that exists between structure and emotion. As he moves toward structural balance, he knows that his psychological make-up has changed as well. He can experience to his own satisfaction that his psychological hang-ups are literal thorns hooked in literal flesh. They can disappear only as the flesh changes, as the barriers within the flesh are disengaged, and as the free flow of body energy and fluids is established. Whether the change is induced by a psychological or by a somatic therapy, change in the flesh must occur in order for there to be a successful therapeutic outcome. Looking at bodies that have been organized according to these premises, you can almost see the lines of force defining the energy field that is a man. You sense the hidden pattern revealed, and intuitively you know that this is "right."

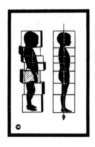

1
Twentieth-Century Monism

New times, they say, require new remedies. New times also demand and consequently receive new forms, new ideas, perhaps a new man. One of the pregnant ideas of this decade is that human behavior is basically an outward and visible functional response of structural organization (or lack of it). This idea (traditionally called *monism*) is not making its bow for the first time. One modern reincarnation of monism is psychosomatic medicine. Within this particular framework, psychotherapy again postulates that our external circumstances are projections of our internal being.

Personality and the increase in human potential dependent on its well-being have inspired many words and much soul-searching. New impetus has been given to man's age-old quest for self-understanding, and old solutions are being re-examined. In general, personality is considered a wraithlike, mischief-making phantom, either strong and determined or weak and imbecilic. We assume we all have one. It may be intangible, invisible, immeasurable, and occasionally intolerable, but there it is. Speak of personality, and people nod sagely. Speak of changing personality, and a nest of hornets rises at once, buzzing about: psychiatrists, psychologists, psychoanalysts—Freud, Jung, Reich, Perls, an endless stream. It seems that each man has his favorite "cure," or else declares for gloom and doom and loudly states there is no help anywhere.

Such chaotic controversy suggests that a basic factor is still hidden, still unexplored. The people most involved in the problem are, of course, the psychotherapists. They have sought, and to some degree have found, understanding and therapeutic value in various psychological approaches to the inner man. It is logical to expect that a successful approach to a psychological phenomenon such as personality could be made through an exclusively psychological approach. However, many psychotherapists would concede that, as of the mid-seventies, they are not really satisfied with the results of this logic.

A new approach to man and his personality is therefore receiving at least a tentative welcome. Instead of examining the psyche, the newer insight looks at the physical aspect as a more practical, economical, down-to-earth approach to man. The idea that we have something that can be called a physical personality is unconsciously held by most of us. Although not universally credited in all details, the classification by William H. Sheldon in *Atlas of Man* of types and personalities has had a pervasive if subliminal influence on our thinking. His assumptions in correlating behavior patterns with different types of physical structures have become valuable informational maps. We may accept these assumptions intellectually, but find it harder to recognize their implications. Physical personality is not something separate, strange, or different from psychological personality, but part of an internally covarying psychophysical entity.

We have trouble in wholeheartedly accepting the physical personality as a mirror image of the psychological person; the "I" seen in three-dimensional form. We resist the idea that a random and disordered corporeal being must reflect disorder in the psychological being. This nonacceptance is understandable. The two aspects unify only at the subliminal level. By definition, the subliminal exists outside conscious awareness. But as the body changes in structural processing, we can observe psychological changes paralleling physical improvement.

We are dealing with the idea that not only his physical body but also his environment is a projection of man's psychological personality. Essentially, this is monism, the belief that all manifestation is the expression of one substance. This idea has been the basis of yoga, especially Tantric yoga, for many centuries. Monistic ideas have come to the forefront repeatedly in many cultures, but invariably have receded again in deference to dualistic concepts of body and soul. Since it locates the origin of a problem outside its victim, the logic of dualism is much simpler and more appealing, in that it implies diminished personal responsibility. In dualistic thinking, the ills and accidents of our bodies may be blamed on circumstance, on a god (vengeful or otherwise), or a least on a *deus ex machina* (colds are the result of germs). Monism permits us no such escape; here, the cause of a problem lies within the problem itself.

The unresolved conflict between monism and dualism, as in other perennial confusions, suggests the presence of a hidden factor. For thousands of years, human beings have tried to change their personalities through a variety of practices. Archaic rites of totemism (e.g., eating a lion's heart to acquire courage) bear witness to the antiquity of these practices. Most of the people who have succeeded in making a fundamental change have attributed their success not to rational methods but to supernatural accidents, religious conversion, magic, prayer, et cetera. (We refer here to the kind of change that operates at the depth where somatic and psychic components mingle. This is not to be confused with more superficial levels of behavioral change.)

Man's struggle with his physical limitations is just as ancient. In the earliest cultures, physical vigor meant the difference between survival and nonsurvival. Today, we recognize the drastic changes that overtake us through disease or aging, but success in reversing such trends usually eludes us. We may try physical training, with its emphasis on the body beautiful, but eventually we recognize that it cannot change the basic underlying patterns that govern our being.

As a result of our failures, monism today is discredited. We might be able to accept the notion that our philosophy is wrong, but we cannot conceive that our best efforts at self-improvement may be misdirected. In spite of all this, many thinkers still see reconciliation of the monism-dualism conflict as possible, and the modern cultural climate nurtures new developments of both ideas.

Modern thinking focuses on process, and the hope of reconciliation lies in this new point of view. We moderns do not want to catch, hold, and define the wraith "personality"; we only want to change it. The new approach postulates that you change the personality by changing the body and the structure of the body. Psychosomatic medicine seeks to change the psychological person in order to reach the physical symptom. Both imply a rough equivalence of emotional personality with corporeal body. Change initiated from either direction should solve the problem equally well. Within limits, this is true. It comes to a question of which is the approach of choice.

On the basis of their experience, practitioners of Structural Integration have concluded that the easiest, quickest, and most economical method of changing the coarse matter of the physical body is by direct intervention in the body. Change in the coarser medium alters the less palpable emotional person and his projections.

Some people find it difficult to envisage an interaction through which body structure can decisively influence the emotional person. For them, the actual experience can prove the point. The physiological fact is that responses of nerves and glands in the physical body underlie emotional states, and in fact *are* the emotional states. It is only our denial of the implications of this statement that makes it seem unlikely.

For too many of us, a vast, willful ignorance of our own processes keeps us in the dark. This ignorance has been compounded by many factors, not the least of which is a teaching called by the misnomer physical education. The assumption in most Phys. Ed. school departments is that endless "doing"—calisthenics, acrobatics, gymnastics, violent sports—builds "good bodies." The ideal, they think, is the body beautiful of the newsstand magazines. A modicum of truth baits this trap and makes it attractive. It is clear that heavy, repetitious exercise, by bringing blood and fluid to local muscles, does cause them to enlarge and, up to a point, improves their functioning. After this point, however, the body becomes rigid and muscle-bound. Certainly, there are individuals who get themselves looking like cover boys, but only those young and innocent would fail to say, "Who wants it?" A more experienced critic recognizes this type as rigid, limited in outlook, preoccupied with himself and his physical beauty, lacking in perception and sensitivity, and, even more damning, unable to do a really good day's work in either a mental or a physical field.

This line of evaluation may lead the sophisticated critic to a flash of perception. He is suddenly aware that in fact he has been using the physical personality of the cover boy as an index for evaluating the man's emotional person. He has been equating physical and psychological personalities. He asks himself whether this is legitimate. As he gains experience of this "model" man, he is apt to realize that his intuitive evaluation holds up fairly well. To say the least, this beautiful man is probably mentally rigid as well as physically immobile. Fortunately, this type of personality, which is the logical end product of orthodox methods of physical training, is not reached by too many. Is it rejection—subconscious, perhaps—of this type that makes many of us shy away from Phys. Ed. in our youth? We remember with embarrassment the depths of perfidy to which we descended in our high-school days to escape the hated "gym."

There may well be other more rational factors involved in the dislike some students feel for Phys. Ed. Orthodox physical-fitness methods often fail to take into account that differences in the structures of young people are vitally significant and should be a central determinant of any Phys. Ed. program. A program that fails to differentiate fails to give effective help. This statement refers not only to children with gross aberrations such as spinal curvature (scoliosis), but to the innumerable less apparent but very real structural deviations—results, for example, of childhood accidents.

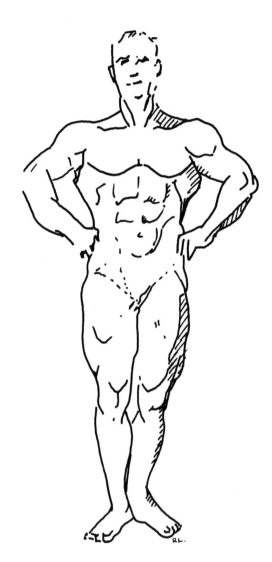

At the age of ten, Johnny roller-skated down a flight of concrete steps, bumping down the last six on his derrière. Since he broke no bones, Mama thought no damage was done. But at eleven, Johnny could no longer keep up with his contemporaries in athletics. He couldn't even sit cross-legged. By fifteen, his knees were hurting; by sixteen, he was getting very heavy-hipped; by seventeen, he was sent to a doctor to find out what "disease" was affecting his knees and his walking. Eventually, the doctor obliged and gave it a name. At thirty-five, Johnny was trying to get rid of the "disease" by psychotherapy. Pity the poor psychotherapist.

In the meantime, what has happened to Johnny's personality? When a boy can no longer challenge his peers physically, as became obvious in Johnny's physical-training program, what happens to his self-image? When he feels inadequate and insecure, both consciously and unconsciously, what kind of compensation does he make down through the years?

Endless psychological problems have been blamed on insecurity. Unnumbered mothers have wept on being told, "Johnny feels insecure; you didn't give him enough love as a baby." This means that Mama must shoulder the guilt. But Johnnies without number have felt insecure because they *were* insecure, and no mama appeared in the picture at all, nor did any guilt. To Johnny, one leg felt longer than the other, not because the bones were longer. but because the time he fell down the stairs (or off the bicycle, or off the roof), he rotated his pelvis. One hipbone therefore is slightly forward of the other and/or slightly higher; one leg seems longer. In addition to the primary problem, compensatory distortions have occurred throughout the body—he is round-shouldered and, perhaps, knock-kneed. Papa's communications to him are predominantly "For god's sake, boy, can't you stand up straight?" In point of fact, Johnny can't. He only knows that he doesn't feel right. The psychiatrist will call him insecure, and that's precisely what he is. For when your two legs are not properly under your body, you are insecure, and you'll act like it and feel like it.

Inevitably, the bedeviled individual will cope with this insecurity by some kind of compensation. Whether he becomes brash, loud-mouthed, and resentful, or apathetic. withdrawn, and timid depends on other factors. In either case, the family may well send him to a gym or in some way try to build up his body. And he does get sturdier. He weighs more; quite possibly he can wrestle or box, though not very well. Perhaps the weight settles around his hips, as though the flesh wanted to splint the insecurity at the joint. Nonetheless, gym or no gym, at the deep level the joint is still no more secure than it was. Johnny's dividend from the hated gym—his new potential for wrestling another kid down—does not change his subconscious realization of his own insecure stance. On many planes, his "I" senses this.

Is the remedy for this particular Johnny to be found in psychotherapy? No, not at this time. The remedy can be found only at the level of the insecurity, namely in the structural deviation of the pelvis. New security accompanies a restored balance in the pelvis. Nothing else does the job. When this has been done, Johnny within minutes reports, "Gee, I feel different." And within hours, the relaxation of his emotional personality becomes apparent even to the neighbors.

How many people who seek help from psychotherapists fall into the above category? In how many psychotherapeutic patients are the symptoms really manifestations of physical aberrations of which they are unaware? It's a hard question to answer. Certainly, the number of people coming under this somatopsychic (rather than a psychosomatic) category is higher than most people realize.

Another large class of patients seek help from psychotherapists even though their symptoms seem to them to be physical. Like Johnny, they would describe themselves as psychosomatic sufferers. But the route by which they arrived at their condition was very different. Their ills stem from an emotional rather than a physical trauma. For example, the person who as a child was chronically angry will, as a young adult, have literally embodied this personal history. His head sits forward on his neck, he "leads with his chin," his head is drawn down into his shoulders in a permanently defensive position, and even his walk bespeaks twenty-four-hour-a-day tension and aggression. If you put your hands on his shoulders, you feel a hard, unyielding mass. If you approach the man psychologically, you are apt to find him equally tense, equally unyielding, equally hard. Inside himself he is having a hard time, too. Perhaps his wife or his girl friend, perceiving his psychological misery, has managed to lead him to a psychotherapist. Even so, the going is rough and slow. Meantime, he is getting older and developing symptoms that alarm him: Is he going to have a heart attack? Can he be getting an ulcer? Why does his head ache so much? Why does the doctor say his blood pressure is so high? Should he join a health club?

Does the psychotherapist have the answer for this man? Yes, but again, not at this point. The man's emotional problems are literally anchored in the concrete of deviated muscular and structural patterns that are the projections, still alive in the adult man, of the angry five-year-old. Until the physical situation can somehow be changed, the psychotherapist can make very little headway. "You do not run because you are afraid, you are afraid because you run," said William James at the turn of this century, and nothing since has changed the validity of his observation. Our angry friend is chronically angry because his body is still fixed in a physical attitude of anger. Until he can change this, until the muscles can relax and become mobile, until the fluid supply can respond appropriately to here-and-now emotional variation, he is going to be wedded to his problem. When this man can stand up straighter, when his neck can lift out of his shoulders and he can see the light of an emotional day, the psychotherapist's task will become simpler.

How would you characterize your own problem? If it is physical, it will have arisen from, or at least been accompanied by, a deviation of your muscles from the position of structural balance. If it is emotional, you will express this seemingly very different problem in a fixation of structural elements similar to that of your brother whose trauma was physical in origin. In both cases, the fixation of the flesh interferes with the energy flow that is the essence of life. Our experience in Structural Integration underscores the fact that this is the story of much illness and also of the average aging progression that we all dread.

It is certainly true that genetic endowment exists; so does genetic misendowment. But much of what is blamed on genetic misendowment is simply progressive deterioration. Much, if not all, chronic organic disease starts as functional inversion or perversion. Something physical or emotional interferes with the flow of body fluids or body energy to an organ; slowly the organ deteriorates, is unable to carry on, and stops functioning. Some other organ tries to compensate, but its load is too heavy to handle the extra work. Eventually the compensating organ also gives up.

Aging moves in a similar pattern. As people live longer, they have more time to accumulate the falls, the accidents, the whiplash injuries, or the emotional traumata that finally produce the relative immobility and apathy of age. Certainly, there is a phenomenon properly called aging. Glandular and functional changes are part of this. But if we could be sure that we would stay active, independent, busy, and spry right up to the last chapter and the last page, the terror of old age would fade to a chimerical ghost.

What is the key to these great goods? It is the reality behind the word *structure*—the observation of it, the understanding of it, the realization that it can be changed, and the learning of how the needed change can be induced. For it is not structure alone but the integration of structure that is the key. We seek to create a whole that is greater than the sum of its parts. We are searching for a method to foster the emergence of a man who can enjoy a human use of his human being.

2
Road Map
to Structure

Structure is the subject and substance of this book. It is a road map for a way of seeing which has led to the technique called Structural Integration. The system, like its name, underscores the need for patterned order in the human body. It is a physical method for producing better human functioning by aligning units of the body. Invariably, in matter, appropriate order is more economical of energy than disorder. Therefore, as man becomes aware of himself as a more patterned structure, he feels himself revitalized. He no longer wastes his vital capital. Comprehensive recognition of human structure includes not only the physical person but also, eventually, the psychological personality—behavior, attitudes, capacities.

Insight into body structure depends on sharpened perception. There is a pattern in the body, visible in its contours. We must learn to see it, to know with surety that a particular contour speaks of underlying elements fitting together in a certain way. Or, just as significantly, a body contour may reveal that underlying elements have failed to mesh in accordance with structural demands. A structural pattern exists; work in Structural Integration is not so much creating this pattern as uncovering it.

We may well ask, What is structure? What does it look like? What am I looking for when I look for structure, and how do I recognize it? Structure in general, structure in human bodies in particular—what is its function? What is its mechanism? To what extent can it be modified in humans? If you modify the physical structure of a body, what have you modified, and what can you hope to influence?

The first question is, What is structure? What is structure in anything? In humans, it is decidedly *not* posture, although most people seem to think the two words are synonymous. Etymologically, the word *posture* contains an element of placement. The root of the word is the Latin *ponere,* "to place." The past participle, *positum,* means "it has been placed." Applied to humans, posture implies that something has been placed, or for the most part forced, into a space where properly and structurally it does not belong.

"Shoulders back, guts in," says the top sergeant, meaning you must *do* it, it doesn't come naturally. The minute you force yourself to maintain a posture of this sort, you betray that all is not well with your world. You show the world that your structure and your posture are at war.

In any plane, physical or nonphysical, structure implies relationship. Living bodies are such forceful and intimate expressions of vital energy or its lack that the fact that they are also material manifestations in a three-dimensional world often disappears. Men are subject to the laws of the material world as well as to the laws of energy. Human bodies, houses, automobiles, airplanes, and all things in the three-dimensional world are structured in accordance with mechanics. This primary subdivision of physics concerns itself with the effect of the earth's energy envelope (its gravitational field) on so-called "material particles" and their aggregates. For these particles are not merely "material"; they, too, are energy fields. All aggregates of matter manifest energy at some level. Living, organic matter results from a stronger or more apparent energy field than its inorganic counterpart. The vastly greater energy field of the earth's gravitation can reinforce the smaller organic unit or destroy it, depending on the reciprocal interaction of the two in space. *Symmetrical, balanced pattern in a man's segmented aggregate of material units allows his lesser field to be reinforced by the greater field of the earth.* "The flow of energy through a system acts to organize that system," says the *Whole Earth Catalog*. Stable equipoise is the outward and visible projection of this positive energy reinforcement.

Balance reveals the flow of gravitational energy through the body. Asymmetry and randomness betray lack of support by the gravitational field. All these considerations are inherent in the word *structure* as it is applied to any three-dimensional system, be it human, vegetable, or inorganic. In no world can the flow of gravity reinforce imbalanced, asymmetric structure. Since it is segmented, the human unit is more plastic than the inorganic unit and succumbs more quickly to the unequal torques of everyday life. But thanks to this same plasticity, it can be repatterned.

The gravitational field of the earth is easily the most potent physical influence in any human life. When human energy field and gravity are at war, needless to say gravity wins every time. It may be a man's friend and reinforce his activity; it may be his bitter enemy and drag him to physical destruction. His structure holds the answer. Gravity is

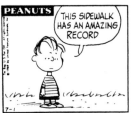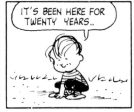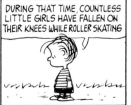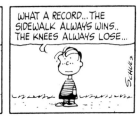

2-1 © 1969 by United Feature Syndicate

30

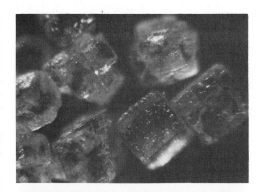

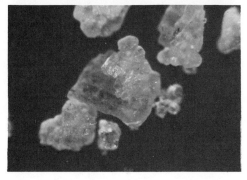

2-2 Chemists examine the material settling out from their solutions under a microscope. Is the material crystalline, that is, do all the emergent forms present one pattern (or at least a very limited range of two or three)? Do the lines limiting adjacent faces present well-defined angles and show the same typical angle measurements at interfaces? If the material has these characteristics, they are satisfied that they are approaching a "pure" substance (top). On the other hand, if angles are not sharp, show only sporadically, while the bulk of the material is ill-defined or amorphous, the chemist is warned that his substance needs further purification, that the qualities and measurements exhibited by these "random" forms are not accepted as those of the "pure" substance (bottom). The photos are of salt crystals.

with us from the time of our conception to the moment of death. It is so all-pervading that we cannot sense it, for humans perceive sensory stimulation only as it varies. (We recognize light because there are periods of darkness, sound because we know quiet.) We do not sense gravity, but we do adjust to it. We must.

In its most elemental physical aspect, the human body differs little from other aggregations of matter, even the inorganic. Thus, the behavior of an inorganic substance such as salt, originally thought of as a molecule (a union between two atoms), can be more reliably evaluated if the atoms are seen as energy fields, patterned miniature solar systems whirling in balanced orbits. When the chemist postulates that salt is the externalized manifestation of polar attractions binding negative charges to a positive core, the behavior of the substance becomes more predictable to him. To the biologist, the significant aspect is that a pattern of energy can be recognized in a real world.

For example, salt is a white crystalline substance with well-defined, specific properties—a given melting point, a known capacity for conducting electricity, a definite solubility in water of a given temperature, et cetera. Examination under a microscope shows crystals with sharply defined edges and with plane surfaces that meet at definite angles. Deviation from these specifics is evidence of an admixture of some other material, a so-called impurity. Significantly, any deviation makes chemical behavior less predictable. Thus, even in this relatively simple situation, behavior bears witness to a given structure.

In this system, in salt, structure is a relationship among atoms. In any energy system, however complicated, structure (relationship of units of any size in space) is experienced as behavior. *Structure is behavior.* In humans, conflicts resulting from gravity cannot be understood by seeing man as unitary and unchanging. The hypothesis of man as unitary has retarded understanding of his physical being. As an aggregate of weight-integrals, man is plastic, segmented, and movable. Subtle and sophisticated changes of relationship, voluntary or induced, can take place within him.

The conflict of man versus gravity involves his structure as an aggregate of units. Individual units must be heavy enough to have significant gravitational existence—e.g., head, thorax, pelvis, legs. These larger blocks are, in turn, composed of smaller elements—skull, vertebrae, pelvic bones. Because of differences in the way they occupy space as well as in their mass, the larger blocks are significant with respect to gravity. These differences have been recognized for a long time; anatomists as well as physiologists talk of the cervicothoracic junction, the lumbothoracic junction, et cetera. This nomenclature points up the assumption that movement at these levels is qualitatively different from movement at the ordinary individual vertebral joint. And, indeed, it is different.

A set of blocks offers some interesting analogies—more particularly, a set of blocks totally enclosed in a very thin elastic sack. In this metaphor, local variations in stretch on the elastic sack can serve as a measure of the strain and displacement of the weight blocks. Any child knows that only if he stacks the blocks vertically (the center of gravity of each block being vertically above the center of gravity of its neighbor below) will he have a stable arrangement. In our imaginary example, this stability would be evidenced in lack of strain on the enclosing elastic envelope. Any deviation from a stable arrangement will be registered by the elastic surface. There is only one strain-free arrangement: perfect vertical alignment of the centers of gravity of the blocks.

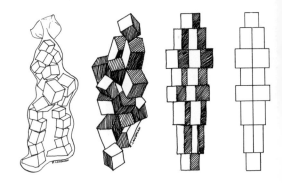

2-3 "Blocks in a sack." Common sense a well as scientific investigation dictates that order in structure allows better-defined and more appropriate function. This is true of simple inorganic forms as well as of complicated living organisms. The greater the order in the structure, the lower its entropy and the greater its energy content.

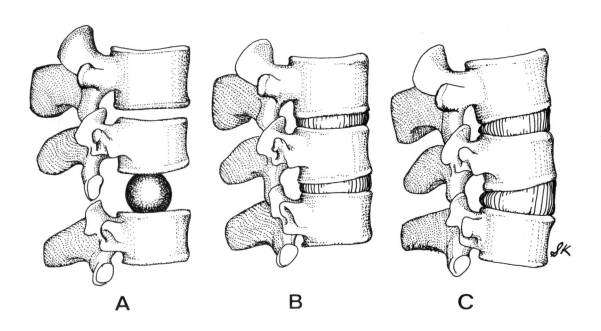

A   B   C

2-4 These are the smaller physiological counterparts (in the spine) of our "blocks." Vertebrae and discs form a compound unit. The disc component, by its elasticity, allows displacement of the vertebrae. To illustrate the function of the intervertebral disc, we may imagine a ball of gummy substance placed between two vertebrae (A). This ball becomes compressed between the vertebrae (B). Because of the resilience and elasticity of the discs, the vertebral column is able to bend

(C) and return to the vertical. It must be remembered that A is a purely metaphorical representation. At no time in history of the individual are the bony tissues of vertebrae and the cartilaginous tissue of the disc separate. As discussed in Chapter Three, they are laid down together in the embryo and are parts of a unitary system. B represents a relatively normal arrangement of spinal tissue. C shows the way tissue distributes in a lordosed or bending lumbar spine. Here are the anterior aspect bending lumbar spine. Here the anterior aspect of the disc becomes thicker than the posterior.

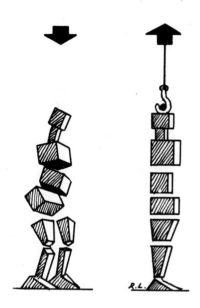

2-5 Weight drooping downward characterizes the random body, talks of a losing battle with gravity. A body in equipoise seems to lift, not droop. Somehow it seems to have an imaginary "skyhook " lifting it heavenward. The flesh-and-blood reality of the skyhook is the co-operating balances of myofascial spans.

Man's arrangement is not quite so simple. His larger blocks are in turn groupings of smaller components. These lesser units may be positioned in their own strain-free stacking, or they may be in some variation. Any variation from the vertical and horizontal grid will show strain. In the spine, for example, vertebral aggregates, both large and small, are joined by resilient cushions that permit tipping as well as rotating in various directions. Thereby the problem becomes even more complex. Remember that our blocks as well as our man are enclosed in an elastic sack. Strain spreads to all areas of the encompassing sack. It is possible to punch or pull one block into line with its neighbor above or below, but the telltale sack will still show residual strain in other places. It will continue to do so until all the blocks are aligned with their neighbors. For a strain-free system, as we have said, there must be a vertical alignment of each block's gravitational center; there must also be no rotation or tipping of the segments (Fig. 2-5).

Any and all human bodies can be analyzed by this metaphor (Fig. 2-7). Such analysis uncovers the aberration and distortion in structures. When you start to look at your fellow man in these terms, a new world opens to you. It is not necessarily a comfortable one.

Critical analysis of man's structural elements uncovers another facet that lends complication. The metaphor of neatly stacked blocks is unfinished. The human body, when

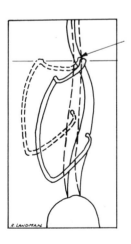

2-6 Lateral view: Rib position is determined by spinal structure. This schema shows how straightening of the spine allows the plane of the ribs to change. In a normal ribcage (dotted line), the top of the sternum lies approximately horizontal with the first dorsal vertebra.

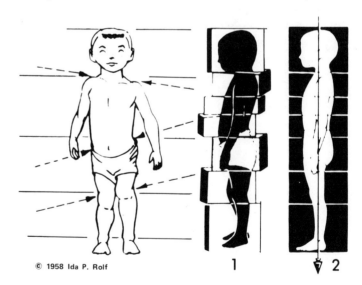

© 1958 Ida P. Rolf

1   2

2-7 All bodies may be analyzed by seeing them as aggregates of blocks. The blocks here direct attention to the levels of rotation and therefore greatest strain in the body. To transform Johnny 1 into Johnny II, whole blocks, not merely individual vertebral segments, must be realigned.

schematized to a set of blocks, shows wider, heavier, bulkier blocks at the shoulder level than nearer the ground.
Because their center of gravity is so high (the lumbar level)
in humans with long legs, the pelvis tends to rotate about
the axis connecting the heads of femurs. Our simpler system of blocks did not take this problem into account (Fig.
2-8). In human bodies, symmetry along all three major axes
is the only ultimate answer, not merely alignment in a
vertical dimension (Fig. 2-10). Achievement of this three-
dimensional symmetry requires a deep awareness of the
sum total of body elements. It also calls for recognition of
the mechanics of individual underlying units. Each segment
is characterized by its own elements of outstanding structural significance.

In terms of the over-all gravity problem, the pelvis has a
unique place. The weight of the torso transmits downward
through the hip joint to thigh, leg, and foot, and thence to
the ground. Since the earth's surface cannot adjust itself to
human movement, man must solve his gravity problem by
making a change in himself. The ball-and-socket joint of the
hip is by design best able to achieve this accommodation.
Problems and also possibilities in the hip depend on the
muscular elements of the pelvis and the connecting tissue
that joins thigh (from below) and torso (from above) to the
pelvis.

A body is not a simple sack filled with homogeneous pro-
toplasm. The skin is a sack, in a sense, but only to the extent
that it is a protective casing. Within this casing lies a complex of specifically oriented, precisely directional fibers.

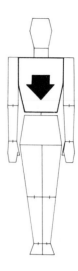

2-8 The simple metaphor of the body as a set
of blocks becomes more complicated as we see
that man is top-heavy; his shoulder width is
greater and bulkier than his legs.

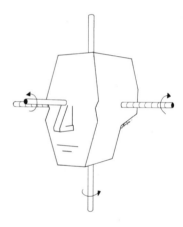

2-10 Schema of skull with three rotational axes.
Ideally, all of the blocks of the body would offer
a symmetrical balance that allows rotation around
their three axes - horizontal, vertical (sagittal), and
coronal. The nearer the blocks approach this symmetry, the greater the well-being of the individual.

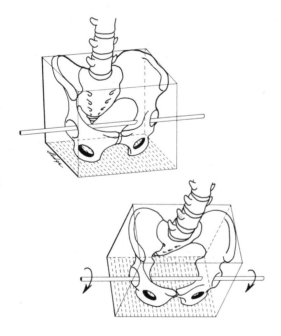

2-9 Anterior view: Balanced pelvis at top,
dumped pelvis at bottom, with anterior rotation
on horizontal axis. The ability of the body to
adjust to the earth's gravitational field lies in the
horizontal rotation of the pelvis around an imaginary line connecting the heads of the two femurs. In an ideal body (at standing rest), this
line would be horizontal and there would be no
tendency toward asymmetric rotation.

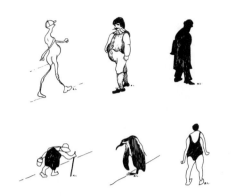

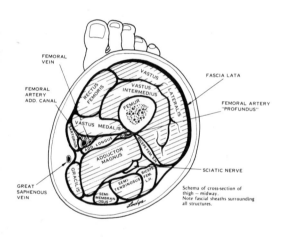

2-11 Many of our fellow citizens might be cartoons rather than patterned human energy fields. Their body language betrays their misuse of gravitational energy.

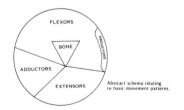

2-12 View from above: These pictures, taken from a later chapter, show the complex structures your hand can feel beneath the skin. They represent cross-sections of the thigh and hip about midway to the knee. Note fascial sheaths surrounding all structures. The circle is abstract, relating to basic movement patterns.

Each of these is a factory; each functions at optimum production or with lagging efficiency, depending upon many individual factors. Any factor can report as stress; not the least important is the unique directional pull of individual fibers. The schematic drawings in this book, drawn from living models, make this easy to envision. In a dissected body, it is not so obvious. In a living body, the anatomy talks to the seeing eye and to the probing hand. Recognizing the articulation of bones under the skin by palpation calls for visualization. Our schematic drawings can add specificity.

If you wish to explore a structure in your own body, place your hand on your thigh. If it has never experienced the orderly change that comes with Structural Integration, the flesh under your hand is apt to feel undifferentiated—overly dense, or too soft and lacking in solidity, or like large lumps held together loosely under the skin. These are extremes in the spectrum of spatial, material, and chemical disorganization. It is often difficult to recognize in such unpatterned flesh the model for the well-organized elements of our schematic drawings. If you are able to take advantage of Structural Integration, you will be thrilled by the changes. Areas of disorganization differentiate into the "picture in the book." You can feel the energy and tone flow into and through myofascial units. This type of processing dissolves the "glue" that, in holding fascial envelopes together, has given the feeling of bunched and undifferentiated flesh. Muscles themselves seem to come to form and life.

As for you, what can you feel? The cross section in Fig. 2-12 shows you (again, schematically) what is present in all legs, to be recognized by sensitive and inquiring fingers. In general, energy must be given to the muscles through manipulative work before your hand says to you, "Yes, of course, this is it. This is the picture in the book." What has happened? Your fingers are reporting that bunchings have separated into individual units, that these individual muscles seem to find themselves slightly relocated. This is the work, the energy that must be contributed by the hand of a practitioner before the chaotic undifferentiation gives way to orderly pattern.

As fascial tone improves, individual muscles glide over one another, and the flesh—no longer "too, too solid" —reminds the searching fingers of layers of silk that glide on one another with a suggestion of opulence. When the energy of tissue reaches this level, a muscle that moves can really lengthen and take on its individual appropriate function. Flexors flex, extensors extend. This is good function, and it is determined by good structure. The fascia takes on a tone level that makes separation and differentiation of muscles possible.

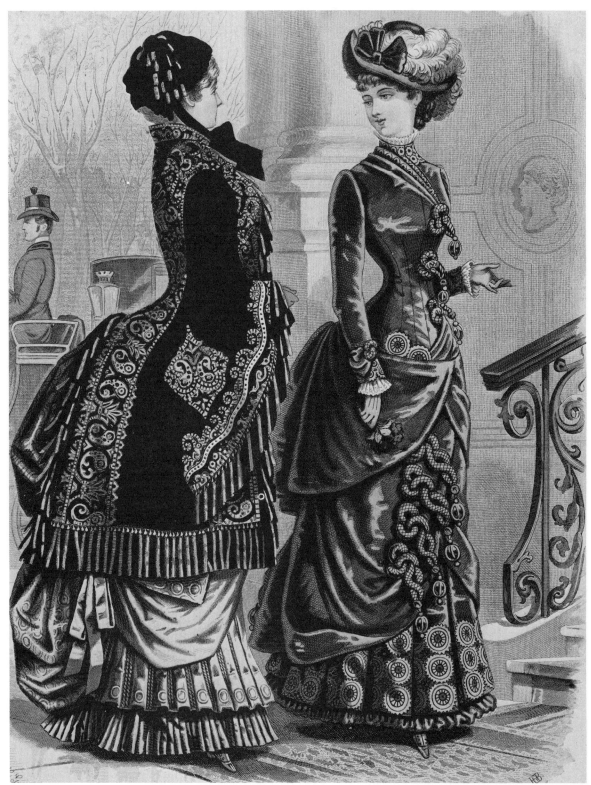

3-1 Clothes, through creating an image, create the self-image (and thereby the behavior) of the person.

3
Fascia–Organ
of Support

This book makes no pretense of being an anatomy book. Our goal is to establish a new point of view, a new way for a man to understand himself. His body is not only an instrument of man's self-expression, it is himself. The core of this new understanding is a different and more specific appreciation of the role played by the connective tissues, especially the fasciae, as a very significant working system of the physiological man.

We are in an age of cultural transition. We no longer honor the understanding of body structure developed by our Victorian forebears, with their emphasis on posture, nor have we found a satisfactory substitute. Our conscious understanding of structure is not yet sufficiently developed. As a result, our bodies tend to become physically random and mechanically disordered; the lawlessness of the body then seems to gain ascendance over the individual's life. Order or lack of it begins in the unconscious, the insidious level that is below man's awareness of what's going on. Awareness is impossible, for through his body man has become the dramatization of his unconscious image.

We hope to demonstrate here that the borders of this chaos can be pushed back. By structural organization of the body, specifically of its fasciae, we can lessen disorder at the unconscious level. We have evidence that we can bring the body to at least some degree of conscious order.

An individual in trouble unconsciously modifies his flesh, solidifies his mental attitude into biological concrete. When he does, the here-and-now goal of psychotherapy fails to have meaning for him. Within the physical boundary of his skin, what can account for the creation of this immobility? In the case of the hypermobile body (and psyche), on the other hand, what components are manifested in this lack of stability? Answers to these fundamental questions require a closer examination of the whole biological unit we call a body.

37

The genesis of each of us, as we all know, is from the fertilized ovum. This seemingly simple unit quickly differentiates into three functional systems—ectoderm, endoderm, and mesoderm—in that order in time (Fig. 3-2). In Structural Integration, our concern is with deviations of structures deriving from the mesoderm. In any human body, position in physical three-dimensional space (in other words, physical structure) is determined by elements deriving from the mesenchyme (a subdivision of the mesoderm), namely bone, muscle, ligament, tendon, and fascia.

The primary elements—bone, ligament, and tendon—develop from cells as nuclei appearing in the mesenchymal substance. As the units take form, less differentiated residue forms casings, sheaths of areolar tissue around the developing centers. The early function of the sheath seems to be protection; later, it develops into support. This is fascia.

Fascia is one of a multimembered group of connective tissues. The specifications of the word are often unclear, especially to the layman. This is understandable, for compared with other systems, relatively little information of interest to the layman has been published on this very important mechanism of support. In general, the physiological systems that get the most attention from researchers are those that are most subject to disease or other problems. But in spite of the high incidence of collagen disfunctions such as arthritis and the rheumatoid diseases, much exploratory work remains to be done. The tough fascial planes of sheets, colorless (since virtually avascular) and translucent, have not been explored for their very important structural contributions.

Verbally, fascia is often confused with muscle. Muscle is enclosed within the fascia, as the pulp of an orange is contained within its separating cellular walls. Just as it is possible to extract the juice and pulp of an orange and still have a shell that retains its shape, so it would be possible (in theory, at least) to remove the muscular pulp in a body from its fascial envelope, leaving its external form relatively intact. Muscle is a highly contractile and responsive unit; fascia is less so. As a protective layer, it must be more stable. In the myofascial system as a whole, each muscle, each visceral organ, is encased in its own fascial wrapping. These wrappings in turn form part of a ubiquitous web that supports as well as enwraps, connects as well separates, all functional units of the body. Finally, these elastic, sturdy sheets also form a superficial wrapping serving as container and restraining support for the whole body—this is the so-called superficial fascia, lying just under the skin.

The superficial fascia is very elastic, thanks to its

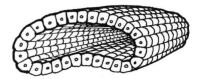

ECTODERM

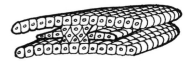

ENDODERM

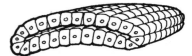

MESODERM

3-2 (After Kahn, Man in Structure and Function, Fig. 13)

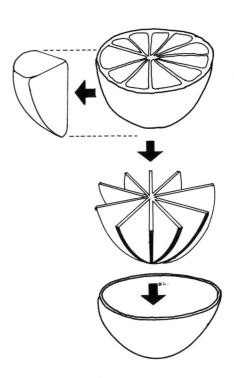

3-3

38

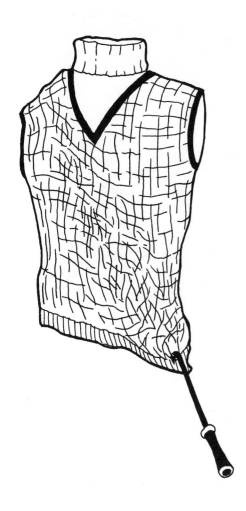

3-4 An elastic fabric, subjected to pull of any sort, transmits the strain in many directions over a wide area. If the displacement exceeds the elastic limits, an aberrant pattern remains.

crisscross network of fibers. It is clear that the tone of this tissue is a basic factor in well-being. It may be modified in many ways: the damage of an accident or surgical interference is often significant, for fascial tissue tends to become denser and shorter as it heals, as all of us can verify from old or new scars. As we shall see, this fascial web connects and communicates throughout the body; thickened areas transmit strain in many directions and make their influence felt at distant points, much as a snag in a sweater distorts the entire sweater (Fig. 3-4).

This is probably the mechanism through which reflex or pressure points become manifest. Here, congestion or malfunction of an internal organ will be felt as a limited spot of pain, sometimes quite intense under surface pressure, at a point very distant from its origin. For example, many women at certain times in the menstrual cycle report pain elicited by pressure on a circular area (perhaps an inch in diameter) at the very crown of the head. In other words, the uterine congestion of the menses sets up strain as far away as the top of the head.

Many people are aware that reflex points can be found on the sole of the foot. When individual visceral organs become congested, pressure on a specific point in the sole elicits pain, sometimes intense in quality. This happens in both chronic and acute congestions. In such reflex situations, fascial planes may be the route of mechanical transmission.

In the view of Structural Integration, fascia forms an intricate web coextensive with the body, central to the body, central to its well-being, central to its performance. Clearly, fascial tone, fascial span, is a basic contributing factor to bodily well-being. The more usual definition of tone refers to muscular readiness to respond to nervous stimuli. J. V. Basmajian* calls attention to the factor of tissue resilience as a significant part of tone: "The general tone of a muscle is determined most by the passive elasticity or turgor of muscular (and fibrous) tissues and by the active (though not continuous) contraction of muscles in response to the reaction of the nervous system to stimuli. Thus, at complete rest, muscle has not lost its tone even though there is no neuromuscular activity in it."

To some people, the words *tone* or *span* give rise to a feeling of ignorance. What is tone, what is span? Experientially, they know. Every adult human has felt the tension characteristic of hypertoned fascia. This is frequently a sign of high blood pressure, either temporary or chronic. On the

*J. V. Basmajian, *Muscles Alive* (Baltimore: Williams & Wilkins Company, 1967), p. 71.

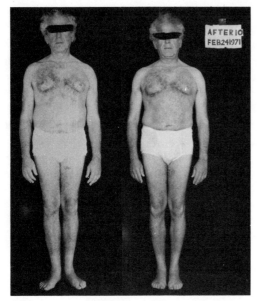
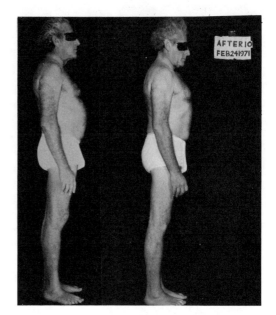

3-5

other hand, at one time or another everyone has been aware of the listless apathy of both flesh and spirit when fascia is hypotoned. The hypotoned are apt to have a low blood pressure. Poor tone is apparent in gross external contour as well as in subjective internal perception. Certain parts of the body are especially likely victims. The abdomen, for example, will tell the tale (Fig. 3-5). Do its contents sag into the pelvis? Are the pelvic contents restrained only by a toneless pelvic floor? This may keep them from spilling but adds nothing to the vital lift of a healthy individual. Tonelessness is never merely local. Since in these cases no additional floor or support is available for the upper half of the body, the gravity drag spreads upward. No help comes from the diaphragm either; through its involvement with the recti abdominis and the obliques, the diaphragm is sagging too.

The body economy requires the use of several types of connective tissue. All are basically structured from collagen and are constructed from the same units, but in different proportions. Of these, areolar (or loose) connective tissue is the most extensible, the most elastic, and the most widely distributed. Its fibers interlace in all directions. Body fat is deposited and stored in this kind of tissue. It is a fundamental part of the body's water metabolism and the mechanism through which the body guides and distributes fluids. It may even be used as packing material between organs.

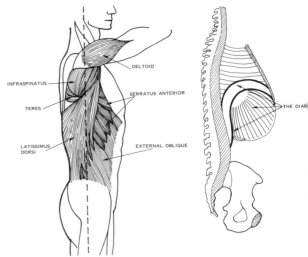

3-6 Lateral view: These diagrams show the lateral muscle structures affecting respiration and arm movement and the very powerful, dome-shaped muscle, the diaphragm, connecting the upper and lower torso. It determines the position and tension of the rib structure. In turn, rib structure defines and supports the space occupied by the diaphragm. Abdominal muscles and fascia support such a balance. Their myofascial sheaths encase the overlay of muscles and thus support the deeper core. Movement of the individual components of this overlay is determined by the direction and the freedom of individual fascial sheaths. Balance in the underlying structure is necessary to assure the grace and beauty of equipoise in the overlying wrappings.

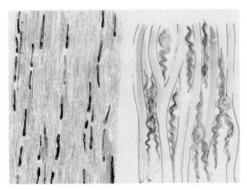

3-7 Left: Flattened nucleii are enwrapped within closely packed fibers of a tendon. Right: Bundles of collagen fibers.

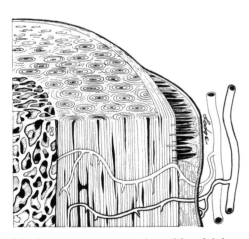

3-8 Bone structure seems unitary although it is a patterned aggregate whose elements are unified only by their collective derivation from connective tissue. This is impregnated with deposits of calcareous salts that qualitatively and quantitatively vary according to age, mobility, exercise, etc.

White fibrous tissue develops where situations involve tensile strain. Therefore it is necessarily more rigid, less extensible. The greater rigidity develops from the arrangement of fibers, which in this tissue lie in parallel bundles. When it binds bones together and limits movements, we call it ligament; when it connects muscle to bone or cartilage, it is named aponeurosis or tendon. White fibrous tissue may also form heavy fascial sheets such as the fascia lata. Aponeurosis differs from tendon in being thin. All these are connective tissues, derivatives of the mesoderm.

Whenever greater stability is required, as in the sclerous tissues (bone or cartilage), the organic collagenous matrix becomes impregnated with other substances that can contribute to this purpose. In cartilage, the matrix is modified by chondroatin sulfate; in bone, it is modified by mineral salts, predominantly calcium phosphate, though magnesium and many other trace minerals are also present (Fig. 3-8). For proper development of a sturdy bone matrix, the presence of vitamins C and D is also necessary. It is of practical interest here to note that adequate vitamin C (ascorbic acid) in the diet is very important to the health of all connective tissue. Serious absence of vitamin C causes scurvy, a connective-tissue disease. A wide range of chemical compounds may affect the health of connective tissues. For example, cortisone has an inhibiting effect, depressing the formation of both ground substance and fibers; somatotropin stimulates and favors their growth. Many hormones affect connective tissues, as do diverse other agents such as heat and cold, toxins and traumas, which change the tissues' chemistry and can give rise to disease.

Connective tissues, particularly the fasciae, are in a never-ending state of reorganization. The continuous metabolic interchange made possible through the intimate relation of fascia with water metabolism allows structural reorganization. While fascia is characteristically a tissue of collagen fibers, these must be visualized as embedded in ground substance. For the most part, the latter is an amorphous semifluid gel. The collagen fibers are demonstrably slow to change and are a definite chemical entity. Therefore, the speed so clearly apparent in fascial change must be a property of its complex ground substance. The universal distribution of connective tissue calls attention to the likelihood that this colloidal gel is the universal internal environment. Every living cell seems to be in contact with it, and its modification under changes of pressure would account for the wide spectrum of effects seen in Structural Integration. The observable speed of the changes that are induced supports this hypothesis in the light of what we know about the action of colloids and the physical laws governing them. The application of pressure is, in fact, the addition of energy to the tissue colloid. (It is well known in physics that the addition of energy can turn colloid gel into sol.) It is probably this more energized colloid that accounts for the different physical properties of the body undergoing Structural Integration.

There are different kinds of fascial layers. The superficial fascia is a fibroareolar tissue that houses much of the body fats (said to be about 30 per cent of body weight in women). It can stretch in any direction and adjust quickly to strains of all kinds. The deep fascia is a denser layer. In the healthy body, its smooth coating permits neighboring structures to slide over one another. However, following inflammatory illnesses or traumatic injury, layers adhere one to another —they seem to be "glued" together.* They no longer slide, but cause adjacent structures to tug on each other, thus contributing to general weariness and tension. The collagen of deep fascia forms bundles of parallel fibers, since this is the form best suited to resist tensile strain. For example, there is great tensile strain on the retinacula, which are bands of thicker fascia that restrain tendons or form pulleys against which muscles can pull. They occur above and below major joints—ankles, knees, wrists, and elbows.

Deep fascia has become identified with muscle in the lay person's mind. Indeed, while fascial sheaths can be split apart from other fascial sheaths very easily, it is not so easy to separate them from the enclosed muscle. This was probably the origin of the confusion between the two. Muscle is a colloquial term for a multidimensional unit that is difficult to separate into its component parts. In general, our use of the word is colloquial. However, most of our discussions here focus on the fascial component, the fascial envelope of the muscle. At this point, we would like to add a quote from Nobel Laureate Albert Szent-Gyorgyi, the head of the Institute for Muscle Research in Woods Hole, Massachusetts, and the greatest living authority on muscles:

A muscle is one of these everyday things which seem simple unless looked at closely. The closer the look, the more complex muscle and its function become. There is no other tissue whose functions involve such sweeping changes in chemistry, physical state, energy and dimensions. In their contractions and relaxations, muscles control the very pulse of life in man and animal. As a rule, new knowledge leads to better understanding. With muscles, things go in the opposite direction.*

*See page 129 for a discussion of "glue."

*In Leroy G. Augenstein, ed., *Bioenergetics* (New York: Academy Press, 1960).

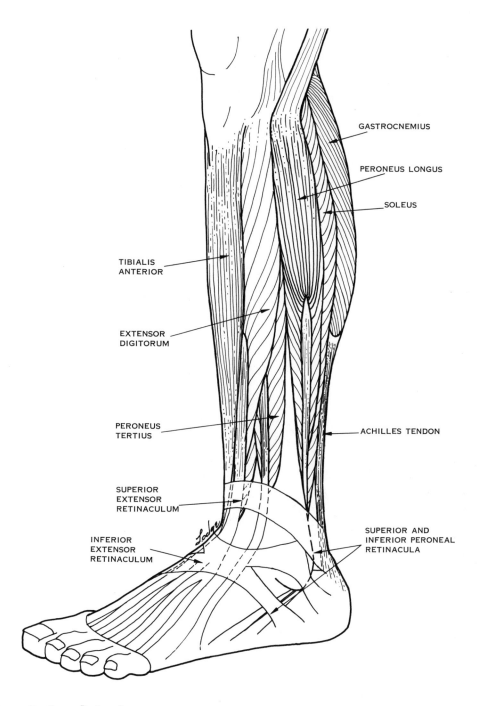

GASTROCNEMIUS

PERONEUS LONGUS

SOLEUS

TIBIALIS
ANTERIOR

EXTENSOR
DIGITORUM

PERONEUS
TERTIUS

ACHILLES TENDON

SUPERIOR
EXTENSOR
RETINACULUM

INFERIOR
EXTENSOR
RETINACULUM

SUPERIOR AND
INFERIOR PERONEAL
RETINACULA

3-9 Lateral views: Connective tissue. Protean in manifestation, it develops patterns according to the physiological function it is expected to perform, but it always defines and supports its structure. As long muscles cross the major joints, they are restrained and held in place by bands of tough, fibrous connective tissue called retinacula. The schema shows those at the ankle.

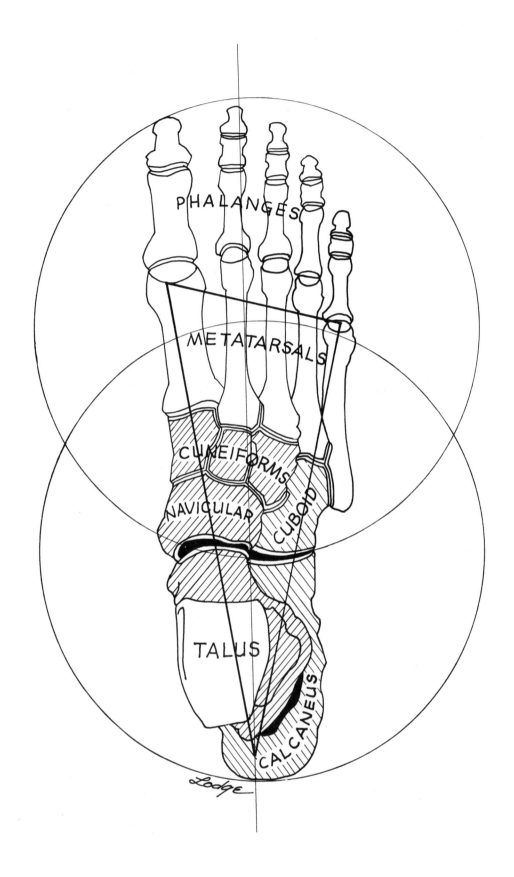

PHALANGES

METATARSALS

CUNEIFORMS

NAVICULAR

CUBOID

TALUS

CALCANEUS

Lodge

4-1

4
Feet: The First Challenge

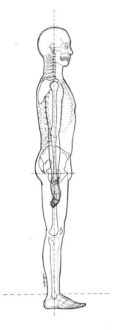

4-2 Only by bringing peace "from the ground up" can problems higher in the body be "under-stood."

Balance in the body begins with feet, for the basic work of foot and ankle is to offer a reliable base by which the upper body can relate to the horizontal plane of the earth. Competent feet and ankles must offer a mechanism for continual shifting and adjustment by the overlying body. Only by bringing peace "from the gound up" can problems higher in the body be "under-stood" (Fig. 4-2). Very often we find that the abstractions of language are metaphors expressive of physical fact—body language: it is literally true that problems in the upper body vanish as the feet "understand" them.

Conversely, feet are tattletales. Every imbalance at higher levels shows unmistakably in feet and ankles. As higher imbalances are released and approach an equipoise, changes can be seen in the feet and in the way lines of mechanical force are transmitted from feet through ankles and legs. Before aberrations in the upper body can disappear, ankles must be reconstructed, their lines of transmission freed, and structures made sturdy for their job of transmitting weight. This is our first challenge.

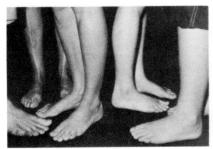
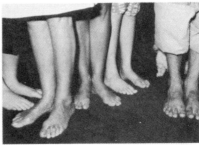
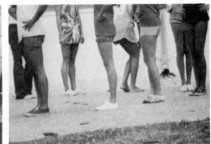

4-3 Random feet and legs.

Walking and standing have been systematized in many ways, but all systems originate in an attempt to make the use of feet more orderly and graceful. We have here a circular situation. Gait allows you to deduce structure; physical constitutents (muscles, bones, etc.) and the way they are put together predict the pattern of walking. Function reveals structure, structure determines function. A thorough understanding of components allows you to change their relations and thereby change the stride.

Have you ever watched feet at the beach? Have you seen the patterns they make? Have you looked at the prints feet like those in Fig. 4-4 make? When you watch footprints, do you observe how they track? How do yours track? Have you ever thought about tracking? Cars as well as feet make tracks. What kind of tracks would the car in Fig. 4-5 make? The answer of the three-dimensional world is the same concerning all material, be it feet or car wheels. Wheels that track like those illustrated cannot develop any real speed in their line of movement because they are not balanced with respect to the direction of their movement. Every turn of an unbalanced wheel erodes its axle and necessarily limits the useful life of the whole system. Much the same is true of feet. First and foremost, feet are material structures. They change in accordance with the laws of material structures.

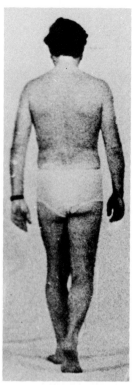

4-4 Can anything but strain be transmitted to this body as these feet move?

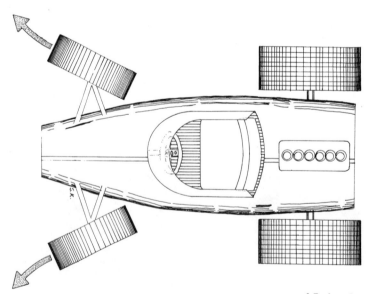

4-5 Imagine what will happen when this car tries to move.

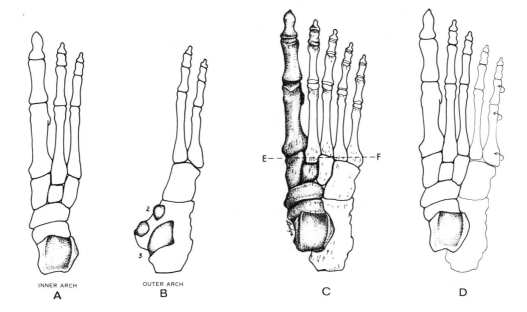

INNER ARCH
A

OUTER ARCH
B

C

D

4-6 Most people think of the foot as having three arches — lateral, medial and transverse. Few recognize the internal construction that directs the transmitted weight across these arcs, which we call arches. A competent foot (C) integrates two relatively independent units. The bony basis of the medial portion of the foot (defined by the three larger toes) (A) lies on top of the more lateral unit (B). It articulates with the latter at 1, 2, and 3.

The two units manifest quite different functions. By construction, the medial (A) accepts the weight of the leg (and the overlying body) at the talus (4). From there, logical and economical function demands that it be forwarded to, and distributed by, the three medial toes. The lateral portion (B) is not basically weight-bearing or weight-distributing. Its function is lifting and balancing. In the random, unorganized foot, weight is transmitted outward. Thus the medial portion of the foot is denied its responsibility and deteriorates from a lively, working unit to a static and relatively non-functioning part.

A foot in equipoise (D) automatically lifts the outer arch very slightly as it walks. The footprint of such a foot records that the lateral margin does not touch the ground. Instead, in its slight lift it affects weight transmission along its twin, the medial unit, directing weight in a straight line from talus to the big toes. This calls for a greater participation of the adductor muscles higher in the leg.

The arrangement of its twenty-six bones is a clue to one of the foot's vital functions: to spread the weight of the body over an area large enough so that the pressure of standing, walking, or running may be adequately distributed. It is generally assumed that a foot should somehow "have an arch." Actually, each foot does its work not by one arch, but by three (Fig. 4-6). An inner longitudinal arch *(A)* rides on top of an outer longitudinal arch *(B)*. These transmit weight as well as distribute it. There is also a transverse arch *(EF)* across the front of the foot. In any competent arch, contour is created and preserved not only by the configuration of the bones themselves but by tough connective tissue. This holds the two ends of the arch like a bowstring connecting the ends of a bow, thus allowing the weight of the body to be spread as on the base of a triangle (Fig. 4-7).

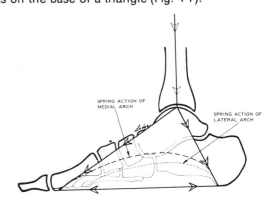

SPRING ACTION OF MEDIAL ARCH

SPRING ACTION OF LATERAL ARCH

4-7 Schema showing distribution of weight in foot and spring action of medial and lateral arches.

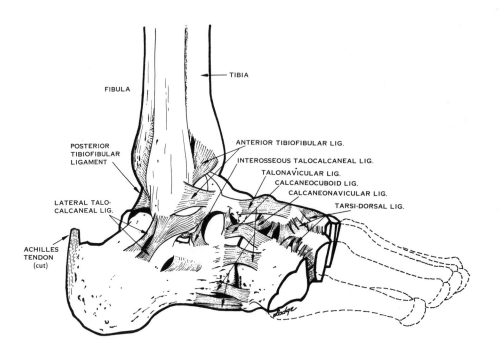

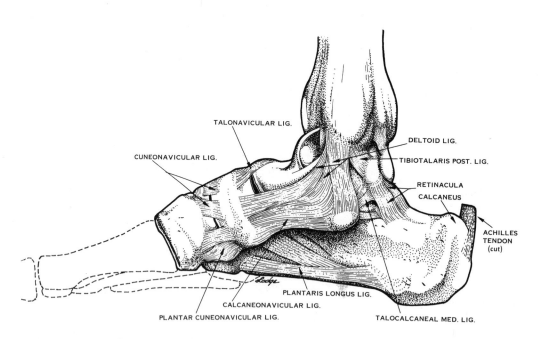

4-8 The deepest myofascial elements of the foot are tough, ligamentous bands binding bony surfaces together. They are held in place by overlying retinacula. Injury to any member of this complex pattern causes strain and distortion in many, if not all, of the others. The immediate result is an unbalanced ankle as well as foot.

Like all "elements" of the body, foot and ankle may be talked about separately, as they are in anatomy. Physiologically, however, they work as a unit, as a system. Our introduction to the foot must therefore include the ankle, for the weight of the upper body comes to the foot by transmission through the ankle. If body weight is to be balanced, the ankle must move freely and adjust competently. An ankle is a hinge joint. The construction of its moving surfaces indicates that its operation is most economical only if primary movement is limited to one directional line—fore and aft. True fore-and-aft movement is possible only in a symmetrically balanced joint. Within the wider range of possible movement, there is one position and direction of least effort: "home." For its maintenance, no vital energy is wasted; no effort, conscious or unconscious, is needed.

Any joint is as much or more the connection and enwrapping tendons and fascia as it is the bones by which it is usually defined (Fig. 4-8). In a competent joint, these elements must be capable of sliding freely on one another; individual members must be elastic in order to adjust to the demand made by related tendons. The drawings of the ankle in Fig. 4-9 show how length and elasticity of individual tendons precisely determine the position of bones. Clearly, chronic shortening of any tendon will aberrate movement. In the case of a joint where the shortened tendon has deteriorated and become predominantly gristle, aberration of movement can be serious. In the normal ankle joint, tendons can and do adjust to permit the sole of the foot to adapt to the ground. The work of the ankle is to effect contact of the sole of the foot with the earth's surface. Where individual tendons are chronically shortened or sufficiently deteriorated that they are unavailable for movement, there must be consistent adaptation or compensation in many other fascial elements. In this way, modification of tendons not only stamps its signature on the individual's gait, it also tells the story of his general lacks and needs.

Secondary, side-to-side movement of the lower leg calls for flexibility among the bones of the feet rather than of the ankle. The relation within the small bones must change as side-to-side movement of the leg on the foot is induced. If the position of the tibia and fibula is chronically displaced, the pattern of the small bones of the foot will be chronically distorted. Conversely, persistent distortion originating in the foot changes the external contour of the leg as well as the internal relations of its two bones. Any local deterioration of muscle or tendon within the leg results in deteriorating function deep in the foot itself and may also involve loss of movement in the ankle. As the design of muscle and tendon grows more apparent to the eye and hand, this becomes more clear.

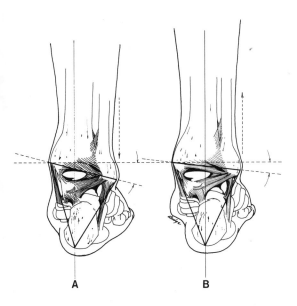

A   B

4-9 Posterior view: Here we show variation in weight transmission as deeper muscles in the leg are balanced. The deepest structures in the foot and leg are, of necessity, ligamentous. But ligaments, being basically collagenous, can and will alter as the other more superficial structures change toward balance. These deepest structures of the heel suggest how and why shoes wear out asymmetrically.

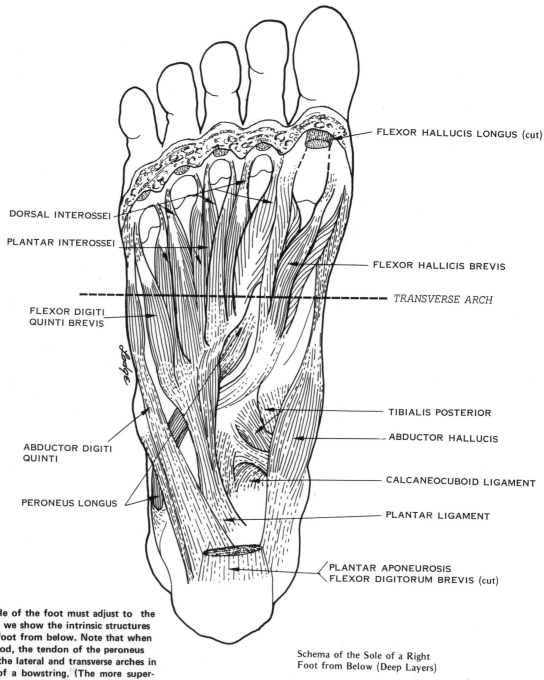

FLEXOR HALLUCIS LONGUS (cut)

DORSAL INTEROSSEI

PLANTAR INTEROSSEI

FLEXOR HALLICIS BREVIS

TRANSVERSE ARCH

FLEXOR DIGITI
QUINTI BREVIS

TIBIALIS POSTERIOR

ABDUCTOR HALLUCIS

ABDUCTOR DIGITI
QUINTI

CALCANEOCUBOID LIGAMENT

PERONEUS LONGUS

PLANTAR LIGAMENT

PLANTAR APONEUROSIS
FLEXOR DIGITORUM BREVIS (cut)

4-10 The sole of the foot must adjust to the ground. Here we show the intrinsic structures of the right foot from below. Note that when its tone is good, the tendon of the peroneus longus lifts the lateral and transverse arches in the manner of a bowstring. (The more superficial plantar aponeurosis has been cut, as have the abductors hallucis and digiti quinti and the flexor digitorum brevis.)

No part of the foot escapes its role of witness to anatomical and physiological balance. The foot that transmits weight primarily through the lateral arch will show rotation of the calcaneous and distortion of the line joining internal and external malleoli.

Schema of the Sole of a Right
Foot from Below (Deep Layers)

50

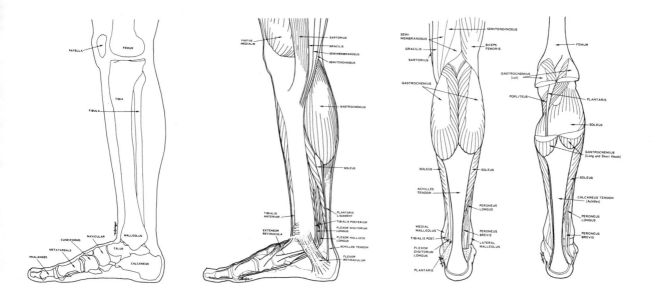

PATELLA · FEMUR · TIBIA · FIBULA · CUNEIFORMS · NAVICULAR · MALLEOLUS · TALUS · METATARSALS · PHALANGES · CALCANEUS

VASTUS MEDIALIS · SARTORIUS · GRACILIS · SEMIMEMBRANOSUS · SEMITENDINOSUS · GASTROCNEMIUS · SOLEUS · TIBIALIS ANTERIOR · PLANTARIS LIGAMENT · TIBIALIS POSTERIOR · FLEXOR DIGITORUM LONGUS · EXTENSOR RETINACULA · FLEXOR HALLUCIS LONGUS · ACHILLES TENDON · FLEXOR RETINACULUM

SEMI-MEMBRANOSUS · GRACILIS · SARTORIUS · GASTROCNEMIUS · SEMITENDINOSUS · BICEPS FEMORIS · SOLEUS · SOLEUS · ACHILLES TENDON · PERONEUS LONGUS · MEDIAL MALLEOLUS · TIBIALIS POST · FLEXOR DIGITORUM LONGUS · PERONEUS BREVIS · LATERAL MALLEOLUS · PLANTARIS

FEMUR · GASTROCNEMIUS (cut) · POPLITEUS · PLANTARIS · SOLEUS · GASTROCNEMIUS (Long and Short Heads) · SOLEUS · CALCANEUS TENDON (Achilles) · PERONEUS LONGUS · PERONEUS BREVIS

4-11 These three schema, picturing medial and posterior myofascial structures of the leg, give an idea of balance in the leg and foot. A competent arch must be stabilized by very strong muscles, located in the lower leg. The muscles pictured here are such. Capable of supporting an integrated body, they spell competent function in the foot as well as in the leg. This shows in the contour of the leg. Deep to balanced muscles, there must be well-balanced, well-nourished bones.

To carry the weight of the body, the foot's arches must be stabilized by very strong muscles. These muscles are far too large to be contained only within the foot itself. They are located in the lower leg; their force travels to the arches along strong tendons. Thus the ankle is not only a joint (hinge) but a pulley for these tendons in their path from leg to foot. Fig. 4-11 shows how individual muscles and tendons must be placed to create a structure that can walk.

The particular muscles pictured here are well-balanced, and so their pattern of local nutrition will of necessity be good. The concept of nutrition, or metabolism, is often oversimplified to *circulation.* Seen at this simplistic level, the process loses meaning. Properly, *metabolism* conveys the idea of basic underlying foodstuffs (metabolites) carried into the cell itself, and of waste products removed at the same depth. In any living body, a change in the metabolic efficiency, to be significant, must occur at the cellular level (in the ground substance of interstitial tissue), not merely in the chemical contents of the blood as it circulates. Muscles are important pumping mechanisms for this process. When their balance in space is appropriate, their capacity for their particular work is good; they will be resiliant and elastic, and their function in flooding and draining tissue will be effective. The owner of these effective muscles will not know he has them. In the case of feet, his feet "never give him any trouble." However, if one or several muscles become stringy, depleted, spatially displaced, or in any other way disorganized, the fluid flow and related metabolism will immediately deteriorate. If the barrier occurs in the leg, the function of related local areas of the foot necessarily also suffers.

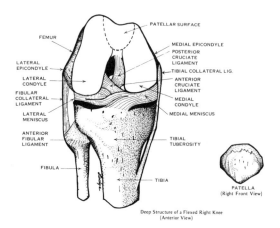

Deep Structure of a Flexed Right Knee
(Anterior View)

PATELLA
(Right Front View)

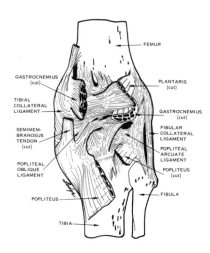

Knees, as well as ankles, function in accordance with this structure; like a door hinge, they work best and most economically in a single plane of movement—forward and backward (Fig. 4-12). Ideally, movement of knee and ankle joints should be parallel, and the joints themselves should be centered one above the other. Then movement of the individual is truly in a straightforward direction. His gait is economical, therefore his walk is graceful. He wastes no energy pulling or twisting any part of his leg to move it forward.

The more nearly their muscles and ligaments are in equipoise, the more nearly both knee and ankle joints can approach ideal hinge joints. In walking, true and economical movement demands that the line of movement of knee and ankle parallel the direction in which the entire body is moving. In other words, progression should be directed straight forward. If the foot does not track straight ahead (*A* and *B* in Fig. 4-13), balanced flexion cannot be provided by the ankle joint: its "hinge action" deviates from the direction required by the movement.

4-12 A balanced knee swings open much as does a well-oiled door hinge. "Creaking" is a sign that one or more members are out of balance, displaced or too short because of injury, etc. Even though a door hinge is apparently so much simpler, the basic principle is the same. At left (A) is anterior view of the deep structure of a flexed right knee. At right (B) is a posterior view of the right knee.

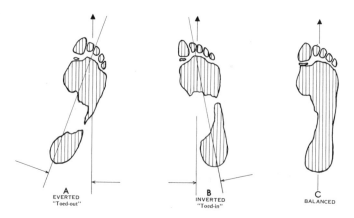

A
EVERTED
"Toed-out"

B
INVERTED
"Toed-in"

C
BALANCED

4-13 Footprints not only tell the story of myofascial and ligamentous organization of ankles, knees, and hip joint, but speak to the seeing eye of the amount of weight and the route by which it is transmitted in each leg. Thus a map of the anatomical well-being of an individual can be read in his footprints. Sadly, few people show either the straightforward directional tracking or the light, balanced weight transmission of equipoise.

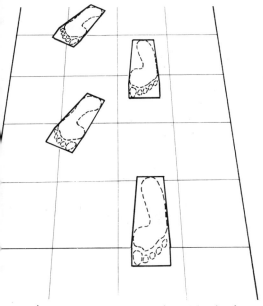

4-14 If the foot does not track straight ahead, hinge action deviates from the direction required by the movement.

Thus "tracking" can be very revealing (Fig. 4-14). Loud and clear it talks of the various joints and their competence. In our trip to the beach a few pages back, the majority of the tracks were "toed out." What does this say? Feet that make tracks like this will have legs like this (Fig. 4-15). The peroneal muscle on the lateral aspect of the leg will be thick and hard, since in consistently everting feet, the peroneals must become chronically shortened. Little sophisticated individual movement or muscle independence can be seen or felt in the leg when this individual walks. The muscles are practically glued together. Some benighted, well-meaning instructor taught the man this pattern of walking years ago. Now he "always" walks this way; in fact, he cannot walk any other way. His limited ankle movement is adjusted to, and determines, his gait.

4-15 Feet that make the tracks pictured will have legs like this: the weight will not be transmitted straight through the knees, but will undergo rotation at knees and ankles. This mechanism results as well in asymmetric function of calf muscles.

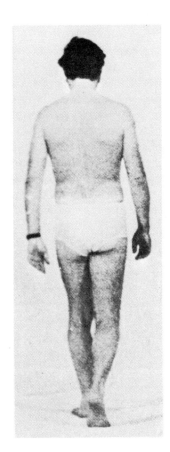

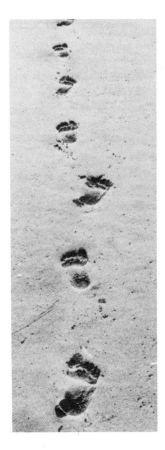

Free movement is unavailable in this ankle. When free fore-and-aft movement is no longer possible, the unused tendons in the joint slowly accumulate deposits that hinder free movement. Listen to such a man's tread. Since ankle movement is limited, he has to expend effort every time he flexes his ankle. He sounds heavy and slow. Often this is the man of the "body beautiful" pictures (Fig. 4-16). The sad part is that he likes it this way, to him it is the "right" way to walk. But then, at age thirty or thirty-five, he begins to realize that his body no longer functions as it once did. Even at this point, he would never suspect that his foot position had anything to do with it. "Toeing out" (technically called eversion) is the commonest of all the perverted patterns of foot usage; it is the saddest, really, because it is a learned method, not a natural structural failure. Our teachers, our parents, have taught us this stance and its gait.

Once his walking is secure, the young child does not naturally toe out, even when his body is temporarily unbalanced. The comfort within his untaught joints tells him that a straight-forward position of the foot is the one he prefers. It is the most comfortable position, and so to him it is right. Only after the motivation of school gym or army drill, a "charm-school" technique, or ballet school, does the young person succeed in modifying this straight-forward pattern of balance, forming what his elders happily, mistakenly, call a "good habit."

Balance at all points of the body is free flow. As legs and their joints approach equipoise, overlying muscular and weight patterns integrate. All body movement is dual action. At any given moment in time, movement is the result of the action of paired muscles: the moving muscle (agonist) and its balancing mate (antagonist). (It would be more realistic to look at these as cooperating rather than antagonistic units.) Balance results when agonist-antagonist pairs pull to an equal degree in their appropriate directions. Properly paired muscles are of similar strength and flexibility. In turn, proper "pairing" depends on precision of pull. The "good habit" of toeing out (which overbalances the tibialis groups by the peroneals) interferes with this type of anatomical, physiological balance. As a result, appropriate fore-and-aft movement is not possible at ankle or knee. In chronically everted feet, certain muscle groups cannot attain their full stretch and therefore lose range. When consistently shortened, one member of the pair gradually loses the ability to relax voluntarily. It is now chronically hypertoned—constricted. By this time, the man no longer perceives his chronic muscular contraction; tension is always present, but it fades into the background. To its possessor, it becomes normal, "himself."

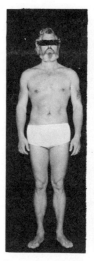
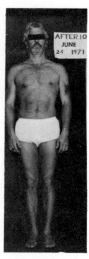

4-16 Since Charles Atlas established the idea of the "body beautiful" early in this century, it has become a goal for training programs of our young men. By the standards of Structural Integration, these bodies tend to be overly rigid, and many of their patterns aberrant. The photographs show how ten hours of processing in Structural Integration change such bodies, making them more resilient and more in tune with the balance inherent in the body. This is especially clear in the beautiful arc of the back bend.

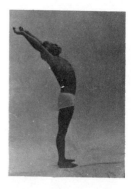

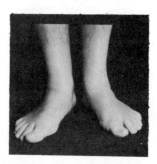

4-17 A close-up of Mr. L's feet before processing.

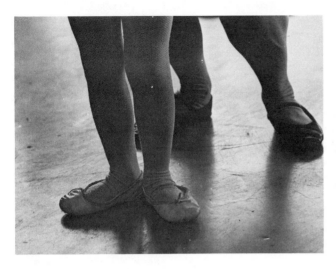

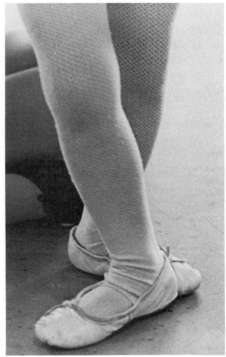

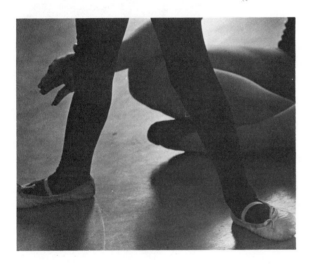

4-18 Consistant eversion of the feet in ballet positions can be accomplished only by continuous shortening of the muscles of the outside (lateral) leg - the peroneals. When this happens, knee and ankle must accommodate by rotating, and the leg as a whole loses its beautiful, well-defined contour.

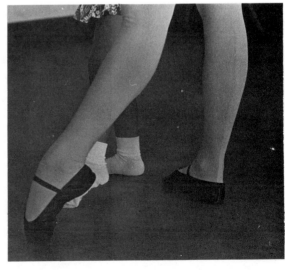

Clearly, a shortened myofascial unit can no longer play an appropriate role in balancing with an antagonist. Its movements are restricted in direction as well as in extent, as it compensates for the imbalance. The individual develops a pattern of walking and standing that becomes peculiar to himself. At a distance too great to distinguish his face, we say, "That must be Paul; that's his walk." Most famous of all everted gaits was, of course, the Charlie Chaplin walk. His was not so much a pattern of muscular imbalance at ankle and knee as it was of imbalance in the hip joint, a problem we will consider later. In playing the role he adopted as his, Chaplin needed this slovenly, unpatterned gait. A walk in a straight, balanced progression could not have carried conviction to his audience. People know intuitively that a fool, a "schlemiel" betrays himself by an unbalanced pattern of movement.

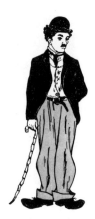

4-19

Not all foot problems are learned. There is the man who comes in and says boastfully (or ruefully, as the case may be), "Well, I have *pes planis,* flat feet. Of course, nothing can be done about that." No? Why not? Everyone recognizes the print of a flat foot. It is flat because the bones of the foot are too low; they are not upheld in an arch. Normal patterns do not appear; neither the medial nor the lateral border of the foot traces an arch. "But I was born this way," comes the answer. Yes, so was every child. The arch forms in response to demand. When the child begins to walk, the arch forms. It is created by the muscles of the lower leg, the peroneals, which we looked at in our first consideration of the ankle. By means of the strong tendons attached to the foot bones, these muscles literally hoist up the arches. To confirm this, look at the legs of flat-footed humans. Connected to archless feet are thick ankles and shins; the muscles of the lower leg do not interplay.

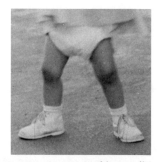

4-20 Our cultural pattern of heavy diapering is the origin of much disorganization later. It is apparent how this child has to walk "around" the thick barrier of cloth. In doing so, knee as well as hip take on an aberrated pattern of movement;

Any abnormally thickened part is the outward sign of lack of muscle movement. Thickening usually implies that fluids are collecting; immobile or toneless muscles mean that pumping action, the normal physiological work of muscles, cannot take place. When leg muscles do not expand and contract, fluid (lymph and interstitial fluid) collects through the pull of gravity, and the result is a characteristically patternless lower leg. You may have been born with a leg of that shape, yes, but you were not walking then, you were not calling for the interplay of leg muscles. Need you die with it? No, definitely not. Through manipulative patterning, these errant muscles can be organized to work together. Then the flat foot develops into an arched foot, as it should have when you were a tot.

A word of warning here, however. Time-honored treatments for flat feet have been either to build up the inner

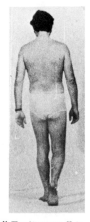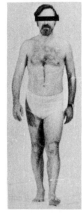

4-21 " Toeing out " is a pattern consistently taught to young people as desirable. But this "good" habit allows the peroneals to over-balance the tibiales, thereby interfering with anatomical and physiological balance. As a result, appropriate fore-and-aft movement is impossible at both knee and ankle.

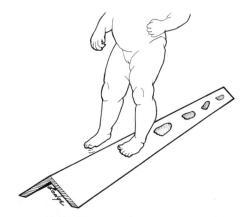

4-22 In the past, a standard correction for flat feet was to teach children to walk on inclined boards. Quite obviously, this in no way contributes to the balanced foot required in Structural Integration.

arch of the shoe or to subject the victim to exercises on boards set up on an incline (Fig. 4-22). These methods have never been satisfactory. Since they are based on two fallacies, they cannot be expected to reconstruct a leg. The first of these misinterpretations defines the problem as being basically in the foot. The fact is that the *result* of the problem is in the foot. The problem itself is in the inadequacy of the shin muscles that are supposed to be upholding the arch; the disorganization in the system as a whole can even include the thigh. The notion that the basic breakdown is in the medial longitudinal arch is the second fallacy. This misinterpretation also prevents therapists from successfully coming to grips with the flat foot. As we have observed, the inner arch rests on the outer arch. Contrary to the usual notion, it is the latter that breaks down first; the inner arch follows. Establishment of a normal foot demands a secure establishment of the outer and lateral arch first. As you look at average legs, you will note that the body weight seems to be transmitted down the outer edge of the foot. Much more weight flows through the outer arch. Put your hand under a random foot at the level of the arch; as the step goes over your hand, the outside of the foot is crushingly heavy. All is not well with any foot that crushes; the weight is not properly distributed.

In a foot well balanced by grace of structure (Fig. 4-24), the tone of the peroneals is good; they lend lift to the outer arch as well as to the heel and midfoot. The step of such a foot is springy. The foot transmits movement buoyantly and relatively weightlessly. When the step is balanced, the outer arch does not crush your hand as this foot steps on it, regardless of the body weight of the individual. A balanced foot will make a print like that in Fig. 4-25, indicating that both inner and outer arches are performing their tasks.

When all these structures function appropriately, balance is free to happen (it happens; it is uncovered, not created). The feet have spring, a sense of well-being that is infectious. In processing feet for Structural Integration, the first realization of change is an awareness of movement deep within the foot—muscles moving on muscles, bones free to adjust as necessary. A pebbly beach need no longer be avoided, for the foot adjusts internally to the rough surface. As the balanced foot walks, the fold in front of the ankle is horizontal and all is well with its underlying bony structure. Horizontal folds are outward and visible signs of symmetrical organization within. As processing continues, these folds are seen first in the soft tissue that overlies the related bones constituting the joints. Physiologically, the functioning of a "joint" depends on equipoise not only of the bony surfaces but of all its component parts—muscles, tendons,

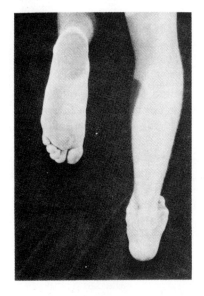

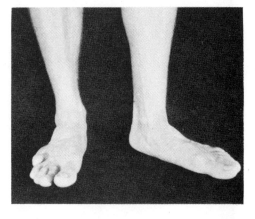

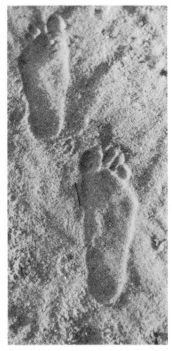

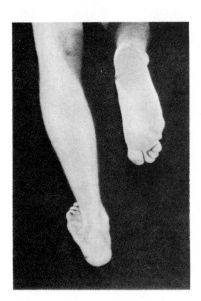

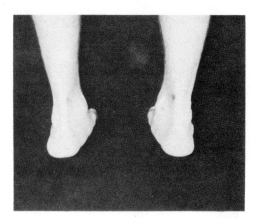

4-23 Random feet characterize random bodies.
Eversion of the feet, flat soles (which, in turn,
give flat footprints), weight transmitted along
the outer arch — all these are evidence of unpatterned disorder and potential, if not actual,
breakdown of the whole structure.

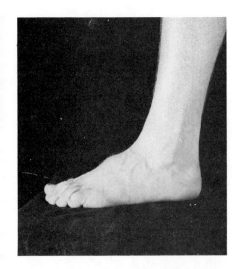

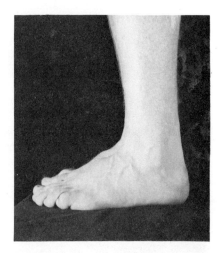

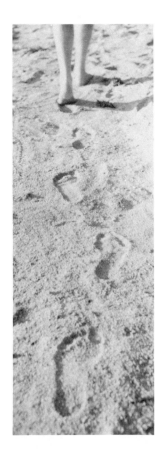

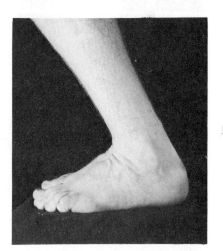

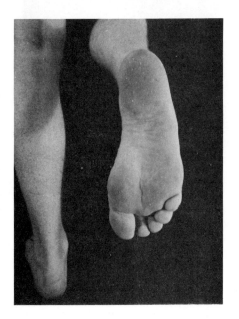

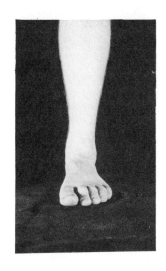

4-24 Myofascial balance can be seen not merely in the external contour of ankle and leg, but in the construction of the sole and the footprints it creates.

59

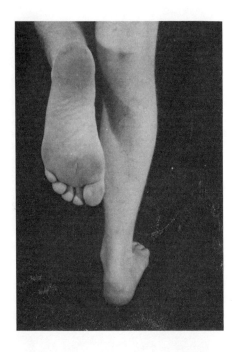

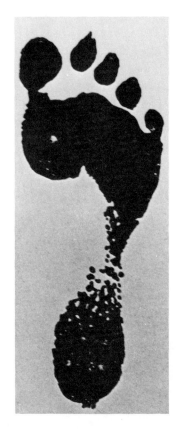

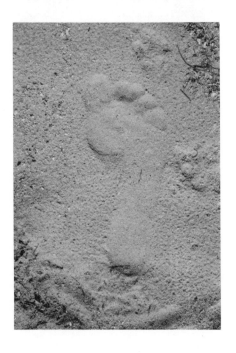

4-25

4-26 This footprint of an Australian aborigine, unshod since birth, sings of its joyous balance and directional ease. Comparison of this footprint with that of Mr. R (Fig. 4-25) shows the extent to which Structural Integration can evoke the pattern of the unshod foot.

(From R.D. Lockhart, G.F. Hamilton, and F.W. Fyfe, ANATOMY OF THE HUMAN BODY, Fig. 386. Reprinted by permission of Faber and Faber, Ltd., London, and J.B. Lippincott Company, Philadelphia)

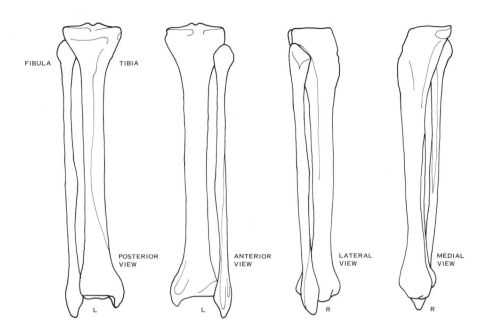

FIBULA   TIBIA

POSTERIOR VIEW   L

ANTERIOR VIEW   L

LATERAL VIEW   R

MEDIAL VIEW   R

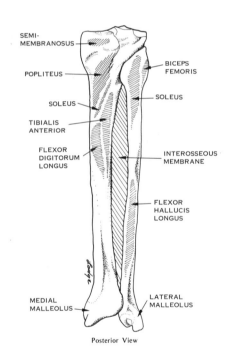

SEMI-MEMBRANOSUS

POPLITEUS

SOLEUS

TIBIALIS ANTERIOR

FLEXOR DIGITORUM LONGUS

MEDIAL MALLEOLUS

BICEPS FEMORIS

SOLEUS

INTEROSSEOUS MEMBRANE

FLEXOR HALLUCIS LONGUS

LATERAL MALLEOLUS

Posterior View

4-27 Tibia and fibula are the basic bony components of the leg. Appropriate relationship of these two bones ensures competence in the ankle joint. The fibula is very vulnerable to many types of trauma — a ski accident that twists the leg at the knee, a bicycle falling across the leg as its rider tumbles — that can seriously distort the tibia-fibula relationship. As a consequence, the alignment of knee, ankle and foot will be disturbed.

and cartilagenous structures as well as bones. Equipoise appears first in the soft tissue.

The term *leg,* anatomically speaking, applies to the lower limb below the knee. Above the knee, the lower limb is technically called the *thigh.* The leg is a system of soft tissue (muscles, tendons, fasciae, ligaments) related to two bones, tibia and fibula. The lower prominences of these bones form the internal (tibia) and external (fibula) malleoli—what we call the "ankle" bones. Following an accident or a consistent habit pattern, tone variations may occur in the muscles and the ligament holding these bones together, thus changing the contour of the ankle. Such changes in contour do not necessarily imply a shift in the actual position of the bony tibia or fibula; they may be the result of a shift in the position of the soft tissue or a buildup of tissue at the malleoli.

Resilient balance between tibia and fibula implies elasticity of the basic fibrous interosseous structure, permitting fine readjustments between the bones as called for by movement. Restoration of the normal design of muscles, tendons, and ligaments in the ankle manifests itself as a horizontal hinge as the ankle bends. In the surface contour, malleoli seem to be on a horizontal line, although anatomically the bones are not. Such an imaginary horizontal through the ankle is the sign of myofascial balance in the lower leg. When this occurs, the foot also shares the freedom. The sudden appearance of this sign of balance is not a miracle; it is merely the result of aid to a structure that has been losing the war with gravity.

A man's tracks tell quite a story. They inform quietly and discreetly about ankles and knees, but they shout the news about hips and pelvis. What is the message of the track in Fig. 4-28? Look at it. In flesh-and-blood legs, complete with muscles, skin, and connective tissue, this underlying structure is at first difficult to analyze. But a little practice makes it easy enough.

If only one foot is consistently everted, the ankle (1), the knee (2), or, perhaps more likely, the entire pelvic basin (3) must be rotated (Fig. 4-29). Occasionally, but very rarely, one leg is actually shorter than the other as a result of accident, disease, or congenital deformity. In this case, the foot of the shorter leg will be everted to compensate for the asymmetry above it; the knee itself may not show rotation, but the pelvic basin will.

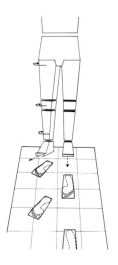

4-28 An unbalanced hip joint will show in a man's tracks.

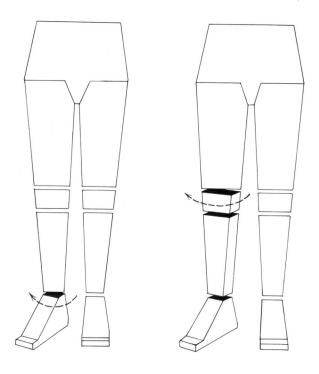

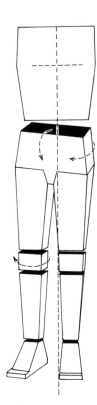

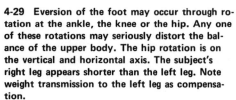

4-29 Eversion of the foot may occur through rotation at the ankle, the knee or the hip. Any one of these rotations may seriously distort the balance of the upper body. The hip rotation is on the vertical and horizontal axis. The subject's right leg appears shorter than the left leg. Note weight transmission to the left leg as compensation.

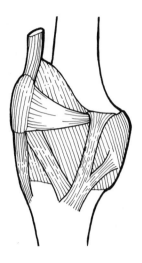

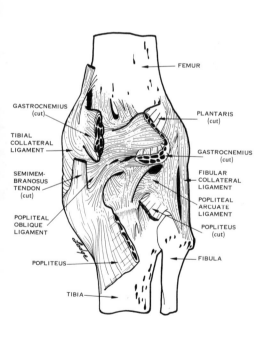

FEMUR

GASTROCNEMIUS
(cut)

PLANTARIS
(cut)

TIBIAL
COLLATERAL
LIGAMENT

GASTROCNEMIUS
(cut)

SEMIMEM-
BRANOSUS
TENDON
(cut)

FIBULAR
COLLATERAL
LIGAMENT

POPLITEAL
ARCUATE
LIGAMENT

POPLITEAL
OBLIQUE
LIGAMENT

POPLITEUS
(cut)

POPLITEUS

FIBULA

TIBIA

4-30 Posterior view: The underlying complexity of the knee may be disguised by the patterned overlying wrappings. Rotations of the knee occur in the very deep tissues, but will show in the surface contour.

The actual mechanical problems—the stresses and torques—may be best understood by considering the encapsulation of connective tissue surrounding the knee (Fig. 4-30). This is a simpler joint than the hip, both in its structure and in the movements it can perform. Therefore it is more tightly bound than the hip. Any disturbance—a torn ligament, a wrenched knee, a displaced kneecap—can be a serious matter. For a gait to be normal, softer tissue must confine the primary movement of the joint to a single direction—again, straight forward. When normal, straightforward movement is demanded of injured tissue, compliance is felt as pain. Pain and swelling in the soft tissue give rise to an aberrated gait, since the individual tries to escape the pain. This must modify the pattern of walking—in time, perhaps permanently.

Structural damage to the knee can come from apparently innocuous minor accidents. Have you ever fallen *up* stairs? "A mere nothing," you say. The blow comes below the joint, and one or both of the bones in the lower leg (tibia or fibula) are displaced backward. If the displacement exceeds the limit of elasticity of the soft tissue holding the bones in place, the various tissues will fail to return to position. Deterioration may then permanently limit the knee's full range of movement. More often, the damage is painful rather than permanent, but return to the normal pattern is slow. Rather than experience pain in the injured tissue, the victim will change his style of walking. He may evert the entire leg and foot from the hip (witness the walk of those who have had a cast on one lower leg). This gait, with its different degree of lateral rotation for each leg, in time evokes a new pattern in the muscles of thigh and pelvis. In this way, symmetry is unbalanced at the hips—but that is another chapter.

The psychological effect of foot problems of all kinds is remarkably consistent; a deep, unconscious feeling of insecurity. After all, on feet like yours, "you can't really have your feet on the ground, keep on your toes, or take a real foothold." Thus you rationalize. And as you become insecure in this one area, you go on to a progressive insecurity in others. Fortunately, none of these challenging problems is irremediable. Only those reflecting serious chemical deterioration (arthritis, polio degeneration, etc.) offer real resistance to improvement. Most leg (foot, ankle, and knee) problems are basically mechanical and therefore respond to the knowing hand and the guiding movement. Security moves back into the body.

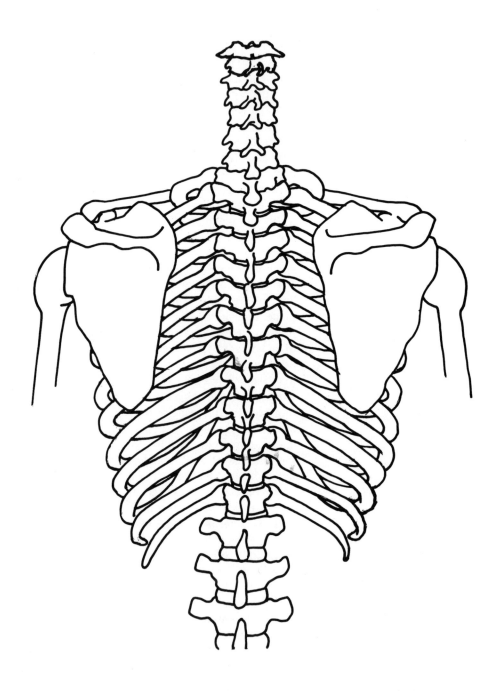

5
In a Balanced Body, When Flexors Flex, Extensors Extend

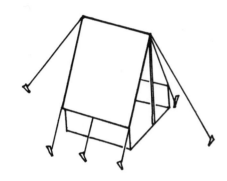

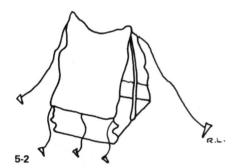

5-2

Our language calls the bony backbone the spinal "column," a misleading term. By common definition, a column supports a weight. A spine does not function in this way; by design, it does not and should not carry or support weight. The primary function of a balanced spine is to separate soft tissue and body parts. It is a lattice to which myofascial parts are attached. A tent demonstrates this difference. Ask a city man what holds a tent upright, and he answers, "Why, the tent pole, of course." But the woodsman knows that in a properly stretched tent, it is the downward pull of the left side that upholds the right side, and it is the right side that upholds the left (Fig. 5-2). The function of the tent pole is to ensure appropriate spatial balance for the two sides.

So it is with bodies. Bones determine spatial position of attached muscles and thereby also the efficacy of the agonist-antagonist balance. To a seeing eye, the surface contour of a body delineates the underlying structure. To the practitioner of Structural Integration, the problem becomes one of learning to see spatial masses and to sense their balance. He must see the ideal structural potential in the random body of the man on the street. He must work with the three-dimensional realities of geometry rather than the symbolic representations of algebra. The facts of physiological function support the assumption that structure determines function. In the musculoskeletal system, function is movement; in the cardiovascular system, it is circulation; in the intricate gut, digestion. All of these systems are embedded in the myofascial component, and physiologic activity in any one of them is directly related to spatial balance.

Any comparison of human with animal backbones demonstrates clearly that the human spine is a horizontal beam upended. Logically, therefore, tne spine should lie

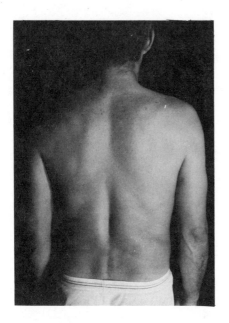
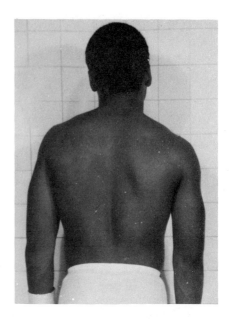

along the surface of the back, rather than in a deeply depressed groove (Fig. 5-3). Objective and subjective evidence demonstrates this. An overly deep spine, when released from abnormally short spinae erector muscles, can be induced to assume a place nearer the body surface. The individual then expresses his greater well-being in increased vigor and vitality, compelling indications of more appropriate structure.

Like a Christmas package, a body comes gift-wrapped —comes in several layers of gift wrapping, in fact. But the Christmas package contains a central nugget as an excuse for the wrapping, like an onion that in concentric wrappings hides its nugget—the tiny new plant that with time and care will unfold into a new organism. In the human body, the significant event is the relationship of component levels of wrapping, not the individual nugget. To paraphrase Mr. McLuhan, the medium itself is the message. A tour of the little-known country that lies inside the skin introduces a new world of these relationships and demonstrates their significance.

The surgeon or the anatomical dissector starts his work with an incision that, by its presence and in its infliction, violates the integrity of both function and form. There is another way to know a body and to understand its structural sense. This method, our method, recognizes that a body is organized in concentric layers, that body function can be understood only by realizing the interrelationship of these layers. In this type of analysis, our first concern is not with the skin (which derives from embryonic ectoderm) but with its underlying layers of fascia (derived from mesoderm).

5-3 Two examples of anteriority of the dorsal spine. In the picture of the young athlete at left, the anteriority is an aspect of the rotation in the dorsal spine. As he has specialized in shot-putting, his rotation is probably exacerbated by physical training. Note the compensatory strain at the sacrum. The photograph at right shows a pattern in which different areas of the spine have suffered from different degrees of impact. This man has been through several major automobile accidents. In both photographs, the position of the neck suggests a compensation to the aberrant dorsal spine.

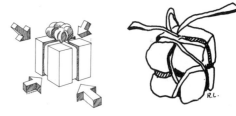

5-5

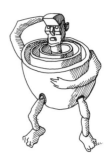

5-6 A man comes in concentric layers.

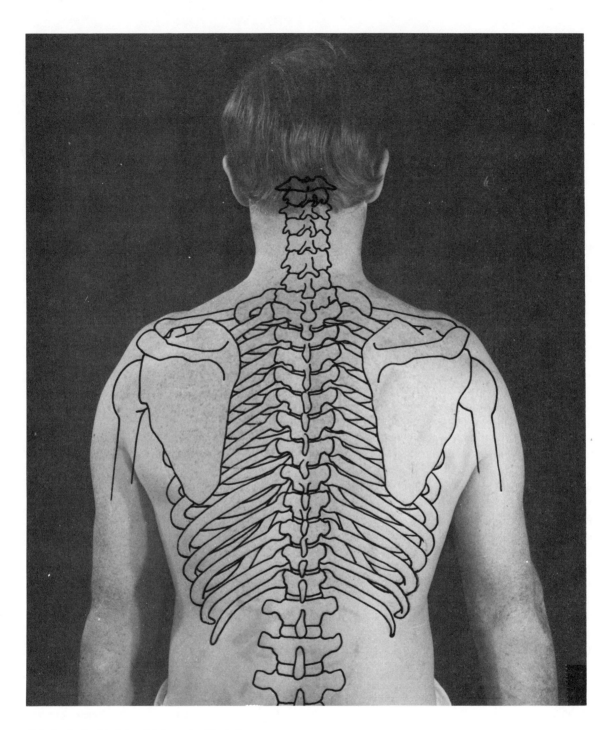

5-4 In the back of a well-balanced subject, the
spine is no longer too deep. As a child, this young
man had an anterior dorsal and a posterior lumbar
spine — at that time, a typical "soft body." This
photograph (and others of the same subject throughout the book) show the degree to which the aberrated
spine can be brought toward a "normal" position.

We have already looked at fascia as a body system and realized that it is a basic organ of structure. As we have said, the well-being or ill health of visceral organs and muscles is documented in the overlying fascia. The presence of surface fascial tension bears witness to congestion and blockage of blood and lymph flow in deeper tissue. Directional pressure on fascial envelopes, in changing both fascia and muscles, enhances lymphatic drainage and in this way affects local chemistry. This is one of the values of massage—the basic method, in fact, by which it does its beneficial work.

The schematic organization of muscles is in concentric levels. As a rule, the more superficial the level, the longer are the individual muscle fibers. Deeper levels, especially those very near the spine, may be only an inch or two in length. As muscles near their ends, their bellies are transformed into tightly woven but still elastic tendons and aponeuroses, which attach to bones by means of the overlying and attaching hyaline cartilage.

Certain more superficial body surfaces are of heavy protective layers, which do not and cannot collapse. For example, the band forming the outer aspect of the thigh (the iliotibial band, which is a thickened part of the fascia lata) contributes to the sturdiness of the leg; a large triangle (lumbar fascia) strengthens the lower back, covering deeper muscles. These local areas of thickened fascia should not be confused with the over-all thin but tough enclosing sack of superficial fascia, which is structurally different in fibrous design. In vibrant health, even very thick, tough local fascia is resilient and can shorten under stress or lengthen under relaxation.

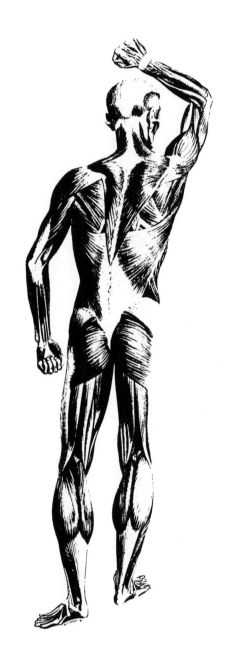

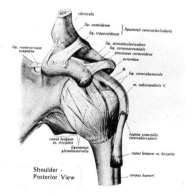

Shoulder - Posterior View

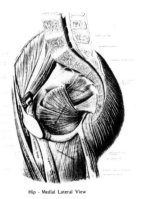

Hip - Medial Lateral View

5-7 These beautiful drawings emphasize the fascial wrapping of muscular units. They also demonstrate clearly the interdigitation that it so important to the appropriate function of major joints.

(Back view, from R.D. Lockhart, G.F. Hamilton, and F.W. Fyfe, ANATOMY OF THE HUMAN BODY, Fig. 258. Rerpinted by permission of Faber and Faber, Ltd., London, and J.B. Lippincott Company, Philadelphia. Shoulder and hip from Sobotta, ATLAS OF HUMAN ANATOMY, Vol. 1, Figs. 246 and 390.)

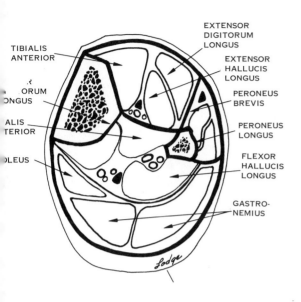

TIBIALIS
ANTERIOR

.ORUM
ONGUS

ALIS
TERIOR

OLEUS

EXTENSOR
DIGITORUM
LONGUS

EXTENSOR
HALLUCIS
LONGUS

PERONEUS
BREVIS

PERONEUS
LONGUS

FLEXOR
HALLUCIS
LONGUS

GASTRO-
NEMIUS

5-8 A cross-section of any limb shows how the fascia-enwrapped muscle bundles are fitted to make a whole. This is a section of the lower leg.

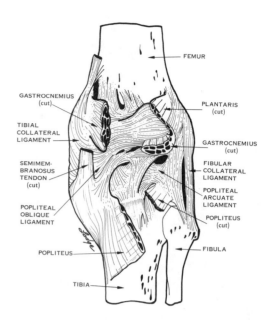

FEMUR

GASTROCNEMIUS
(cut)

PLANTARIS
(cut)

TIBIAL
COLLATERAL
LIGAMENT

GASTROCNEMIUS
(cut)

SEMIMEM-
BRANOSUS
TENDON
(cut)

FIBULAR
COLLATERAL
LIGAMENT

POPLITEAL
ARCUATE
LIGAMENT

POPLITEAL
OBLIQUE
LIGAMENT

POPLITEUS
(cut)

POPLITEUS

FIBULA

TIBIA

5-9 A "normal" right knee, seen from the rear. The joint is not compressed, and the span of the various ligaments is balanced.

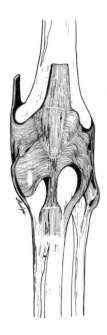

5-10 Aberrated ligamentous wrappings of a right knee joint, seen from the rear, showing the way compression can distort fascial patterns.

Shortening of a myofascial unit is as important and as legitimate a function as lengthening. It is only chronic shortening that causes concern. Such chronic, compulsive shortening is no longer referred to as contraction; it is called a contracture. Persistent contracture of very powerful tissue compresses the underlying joint (Figs. 5-9 and 5-10). In so doing, it imbalances other muscular structures whose integrity depends on precise balance in related joints. Such compression can enter awareness as pain or discomfort. The only permanent remedy is to balance the joint; frequently this requires balancing the entire body, for these various fascial links can elicit compensatory strain over wide areas. Compensations are simple to erase if the strain is recent. But thickening and deterioration of long-standing aberrations may require considerable time and work.

As you look at "random," compensated bodies, either in the flesh or photographs, consider what is involved in their "randomness." Often in your mind's eye you can see the development of the random body as it progresses from the four-legged position of the animal to the two-legged stance of the man. But the vertical development is incomplete. Few humans have reached the vertical of true humanness. Inevitably, you ask what could be added to permit better alignment. Space? Length? Why, of course, obviously the body is not long enough. Lengthen it; lengthen the spine.

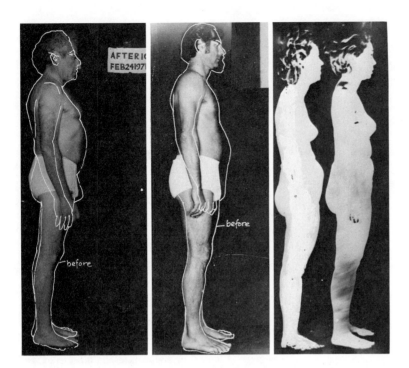

That is the answer. All these random bodies are too short, too compressed (Fig. 5-12). If you could just put a hook in the very top of their heads and lift them, they would be less "random."

But bodies are designed to contact the earth; of necessity, they must stand on feet, not be attached to the sky. So if you lift them by a skyhook and see their more slender, straighter beauty, you must put them down again, necessarily and sadly, and stand them on the earth. Then you recognize that lifting them by a skyhook will not basically change built-in structural compensations. These arose long ago in the body's adjustment to the earth's gravitational field. When gravity again takes over, when the feet are replaced on the ground, the old picture of thickening, shortening, compensating compression reemerges. *The inevitable action of gravity anywhere at any time on any soft, pliable mass is to bring it nearer to a formless, chaotic, spherical unit.* Thus in human bodies, gravity acts to shorten, thicken, and compress. Only the bones prevent bodies from becoming a thick, amoebalike ball.

Both form and function in any organism are differentiations from an original chaos. When the formal pattern is destroyed, any organic unit will lose energy and return toward the undifferentiated, formless, orderless world—a world of decreased energy, a universe where unique function dissolves into mass homogeneity. This lessening of

5-11 These are the first photos of a group of models whose progression through Structural Integration is documented throughout this book. We have drawn an outline on the male models of the contour before processing over the more balanced photograph of the man after ten hours of Structural Integration. For Miss T, we have included both before- and after-processing photographs for comparison.

We have identified our models by a name, such as "Miss T" as a convenience to the reader, to simplify identification throughout the book. The work of Structural Integration shown in these photographs has been done by students during training classes; the photographs were taken as records during the course of these classes. All models used in the book have had ten hours of Structural Integration processing, with the exception of Mr. D and Mr. J who, as practioners of Structural Integration, have had additional work during their training.

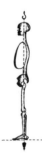

5-12

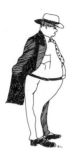

5-13 Middle age spread.

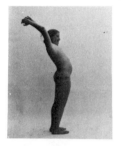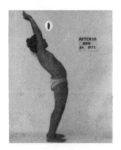

5-14 This twelve-year-old, in spite of her youth, shows the resistance of the spine to lengthening. This is especially apparent in the lumbar section, where the depth of the fold on the ventral surface measures the inability of the flexors (ventral) and extensors (dorsal) to work together in the Before picture. This lack is again underscored in the way in which the neck is drawn into the shoulders as she bends. The After photograph shows the body changes after ten hours of Structural Integration.

energy operates on many planes. The physical human being will slow up, get heavier from the waist down. His movement thickens and loses specialized differentiation and sophisticated control. The picture dramatized by our expression "middle-age spread" tells the story: vertically they shorten, laterally they widen. The increase of entropy, of formlessness, is limited only by the structure imposed by the bones. Psychologically, too, there is less energy. It is recorded in lowered alertness, withdrawal of attention from the outer environment, and increased preoccupation with real or imagined inner affairs. Compression is apparent in the static human. You long to get hold of that overcontracted figure and stretch it. But the real complaint of the body toward life and its own compression does not become apparent until the man is required to move.

In the conventions of physiology and kinesiology, the basic unit of movement is the paired flexor and extensor. The first member of the pair, the flexor, brings the ends of body parts closer together (flexes them). The second member separates the ends (extends them). A bent body is said to be in flexion; straightened, it is in extension. Straightened past the vertical reference line, it is said to be hyperextended. In a bending body, by definition, flexors have been activated and have "flexed" it—they have shortened and drawn extremities together. But what of the extensors, what have they been doing in the meantime? When you bend your back, what does it look like? Does it lengthen or shorten? Does it pull into your shoulders? A basic test of body structure is its pattern of flexion. If the body is balanced, not only do flexors flex, but the extensors simultaneously extend.

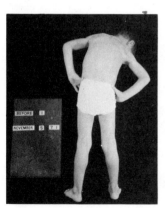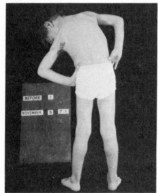

5-15 The bends of this six-year-old demonstrate the inability of his spine to lengthen appropriately. This is especially apparent at the level of the shoulders and neck. The legs compensate for the immobility higher up.

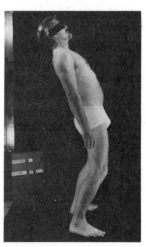

5-16 The limitations of a random body in backward bending are apparent here.

71

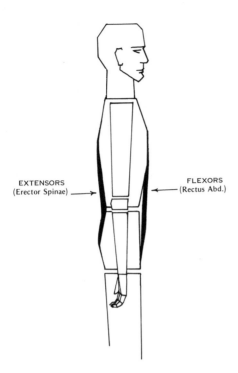

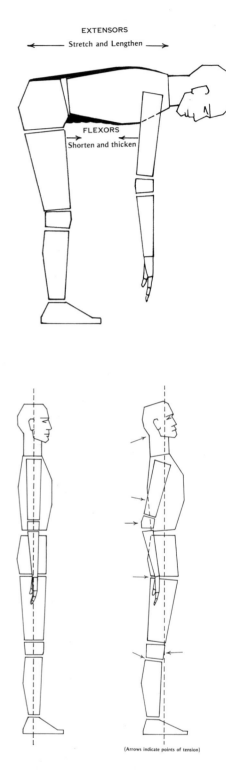

Lay a hand, a whole hand, palm down along an individual's backbone. Ask him to bend. Experience what your hand tells you is going on. Do you feel the back shorten as he bends, or does it lengthen? If it lengthens, the extensors have been activated; both flexors and extensors are participating. Does his back lift your hand as he bends? Then the flexors are flexing but the extensors are not able to follow. Does his back permit your hand to flatten further? If your hand is flattening, his extensors (erector spinae) are lengthening—extending. Be sure your pressure is strong enough so that your hand may feel through the top level of muscle and inform you of what is going on below. It is on the deeper levels that the significant action takes place.

If you will do this on many bodies, you will become aware of the very different character of each. Some seem to have no overlying flesh, and your hand feels as though it were right on the backbone. Some feel as though the flesh had dried out and become like catgut—stringy and knotted. Some have tough, steely, unyielding cables along the backbone, virtually incapable of stretching. These are usually backs that have been injured in some way, and the flesh, toughening, tries to compensate for the injury. Then, in your mind's eye, try to relate what your hand has felt to the posture of the man bending.

5-17 From left to right, flexor-extensor balance, flexed body, straight (or extended) body, and hyper-extended body.

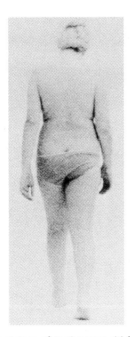

Not all backs are rigid; some are very soft (Fig. 5-18). The spine, which should be giving the necessary support to softer tissue, is failing in its job; some ribs seem too close together, some too wide apart. This kind of soft body usually belongs to a woman. As she puts her hand on her back, she exclaims in wonder, "Why, it feels as though there were a hole there!" Objectively, the woman's whole body feels too soft. She may say, "Oh, I'm just too fat. I should lose forty pounds." In reality, the situation has nothing to do with pounds. It has to do with structure. Areas of bony framework lie too deep to support the soft tissue efficiently. Women who complain of lower-back problems often have this type of spine. If your hand and imagination are in tune, you will feel this spine as somewhat like the accompanying figures, where local areas lie too deep.

Then there are people whose whole spine fails to give appropriate body stability. They have what looks like a deep vertical groove. The spine lies embedded in the groove, and the back bulges on either side. The bulges are the shortened, thickened spinae erector muscles—extensors lying to either side of the spine. When the vertebrae of the lumbar spine are as anterior as these in the two photographs in Fig. 5-20, the whole spine is effectively shorter and the fibers of the spinae erector are chronically thickened.

5-18 The picture of twelve-year-old Dee illustrates what we mean by a "soft back." Here the spine seems to lack ability to hold surface tissue apart. People are apt to mislabel this "fat." It is really a deficiency in structural balance.

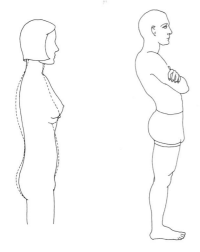

5-19 The dotted lines in the female figure outline a "random" body. As it becomes integrated, its contours are transformed to those indicated by the solid line. The influence of the lumbar spine (lower back) on the entire overstructure is clearly apparent. The male body offers another illustration of a spine that is unable to hold soft outer tissue apart. Here, as in practically all spines of this character, the major weakness is in the lumbar spine. If this can be put back in its proper place (and so strengthened), the entire body will be able to straighten.

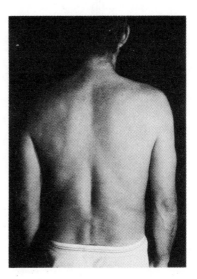

5-20 We repeat one of the men from page 66 here to emphasize the thickened muscular masses lying on either side of the spine, which are typical of many shortened spines. The muscles act as a splint to support the out-of-place vertebrae. The aberrated position of the bone prevents their "supporting" themselves through balance.

Sometimes the entire length of the spine, not merely a limited area, seems too far forward, too anterior (Fig. 5-21). This is the hypererect posture. Few people recognize this as a structural aberration; they are apt to say, "John (or Jane) has such a beautiful posture; so erect, so dignified." That it is a source of stiffness and immobility goes unrecognized until it becomes more supple through the change accompanying integration. Then its owner frequently becomes ecstatic over his new freedom.

Anterior displacement of the entire group of lumbar vertebrae is a very frequent spinal aberration. This may result from failure of the individual to grow out of (in other words, to stabilize) the weak, undeveloped lumbar spine natural in the very young child (Fig. 5-22). Anteriority in dorsal vertebrae, on the other hand, is often the result of an accident. This may have been relatively minor (a childhood fall downstairs), but without informed help, the wound or bruise of the injured segment heals in an aberrated position. Neighboring structures adapt as best they can to the strain of thickened scar tissue. In adapting to weakened balance, compensating vertebral segments may be displaced toward the dorsal surface; the segment is then said to be posterior. All of these problems can be spotted visually (Fig. 5-23).

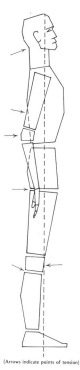

(Arrows indicate points of tension)

5-21 In a hyper-erect body, the spine as a whole is necessarily too far forward in the dorsal area.

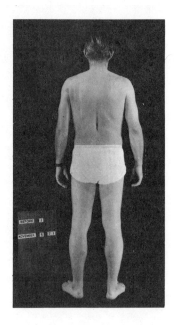
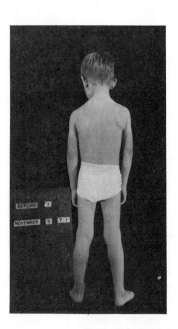

5-22 This father and son have similar spinal patterns. The child's is only a little immature for his present age, but if it fails to develop, then he will, as an adult, imitate his father's structure.

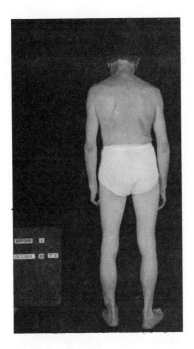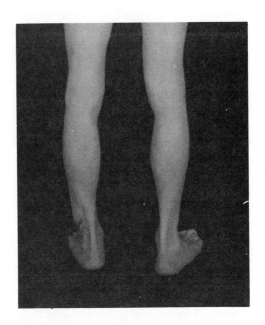

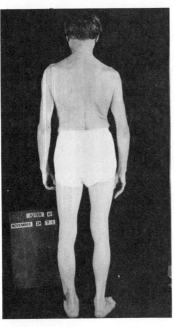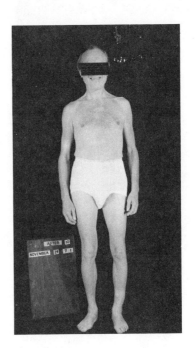

5-23 Early accidents can determine a man's later physical history. The shin pictured shows how this seventy-year-old man still carries the marks of a much earlier accident (in this case, in the leg). It is clear that a body carried over a leg as crooked as this cannot be in balance. This assumption is borne out by the photographs of the over-all person, showing a dramatic change during his progression in Structural Integration.

Rotation of the vertebrae, rather than simple lateral or anterior-posterior displacement, underlies the most dramatic of the spinal aberrations—scoliosis, or "curvature" (Fig. 5-24). This pattern often follows polio, though spontaneous (so-called idiopathic) curvatures are relatively common. A spine can be rotated as a whole, or it may be partially straight with an exaggerated rotation of a group of vertebrae or of a single vertebra. But all rotations exert compensating strains on neighboring and/or distant units.

The rotated or unbalanced spine shows very clearly under the strains of motion. Look at these random bodies in flexion; you can see—almost feel—their failure, feel where they are "hung up." You can sense the underlying structure and its flaws, sense that a smooth flow of energy or of movement is not possible. Try an experiment with a model of your own choice. How does he bend? Lay your hand on his bending back. As you feel through the superficial layers, try to have a clear picture of the bony adjustments as well as the muscular happenings. Can you feel areas that are lengthening, areas that are not? Are any areas actually shortening? Can you perhaps be aware that some of these tough vertical ropes of muscle have spread away from the spine rather than lengthened vertically? Would you guess that if they didn't spread, they might be able to lengthen?

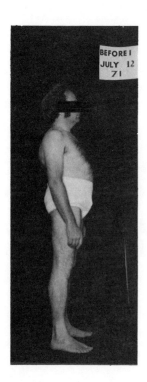 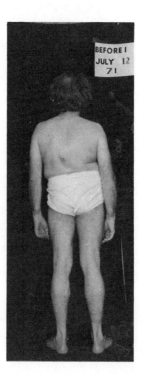

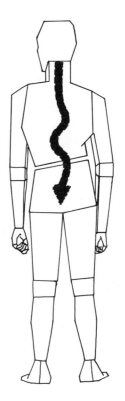 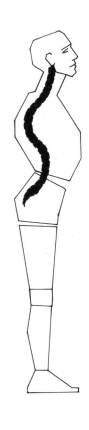

5-24 Scoliosis (lateral curvature of the spine) is the name given to this type of aberration — a severe rotation of the lower dorsal or upper lumbar spine around one of the vertebrae. This key vertebra has been forced anterior and rotated around its vertical axis. In a typical scoliosis, the lumbar spine is anterior, the dorsal is posterior.

Severe aberrations of this type result from poliomyelitis or a serious accident. There is also the so-called idiopathic scoliosis, which appears spontaneously in young people, usually at eight to ten years of age. There seems to be no identifiable trauma preceding onset — possibly it is linked to a genetic picture.

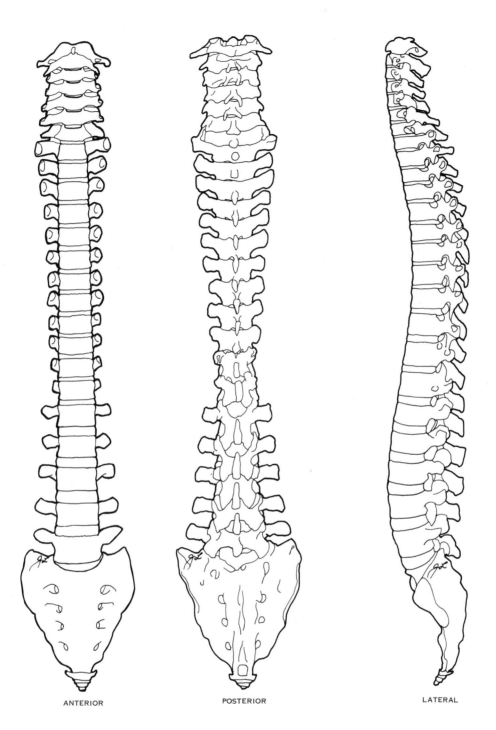

ANTERIOR   POSTERIOR   LATERAL

5-25 Three views, left to right, (anterior, posterior, and lateral) of the body core, the spine. This
is not the spine of a random body; the overlying
body is approaching equipoise. Note the variation
in width between dorsal and lumbar vertebrae. Observe (in the lateral view) the shallow angle of the
sacrum and coccyx in relation to the lumbar spine.

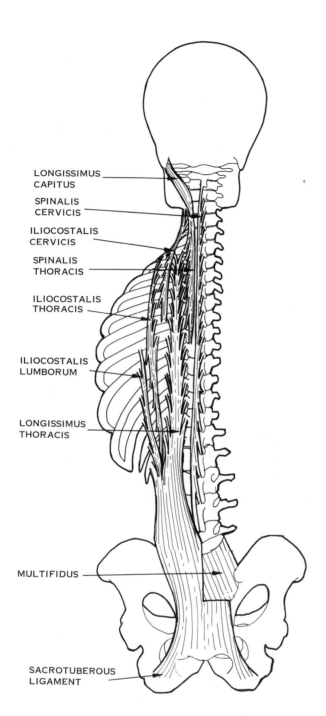

LONGISSIMUS
CAPITUS

SPINALIS
CERVICIS

ILIOCOSTALIS
CERVICIS

SPINALIS
THORACIS

ILIOCOSTALIS
THORACIS

ILIOCOSTALIS
LUMBORUM

LONGISSIMUS
THORACIS

MULTIFIDUS

SACROTUBEROUS
LIGAMENT

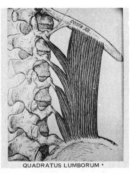

QUADRATUS LUMBORUM

(From Sobotta, ATLAS OF
HUMAN ANATOMY, Vol. 1,
Fig. 299)

5-26 Posterior views: The erector spinae are the
major antigravity muscles, the trunk of the tree that
branches into the antigravity extensors (spinalis,
longissimus, and iliocostalis) of the upper back.
Rooted in the dense fascia of the lower lack, these
muscles thin and branch as they ascend and the
weight they control lessens.

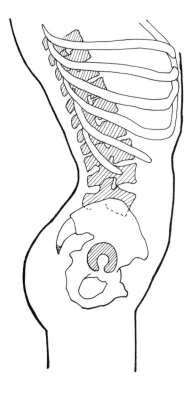

Mentally removing the more superficial layers under your hand uncovers a deep muscular trio generically called the erector spinae muscles. This is the basic extensor system of the backbone, and therefore of the body. Seen schematically, it consists of three ropes of interweaving vertical elements. Its design makes clear that any shortening of one of this trio must cause deviations within the entire complex. Distortions of individual elements or parts of elements shorten, thicken, and twist the body as a whole. If these muscles become displaced laterally through accident, repeated or sustained overeffort, or prolonged slump, the erect symmetrical pattern of the whole body must suffer. Any distortion in the human body, from any cause, is accompanied by shortening, loss of length. This is the effect of gravity. It is the collapse of the tent.

Can you see or feel that some of these backs twist as they bend? Two sides of a back are seldom evenly balanced. In any given place, one side is usually shorter than the other. This is often caused by a dominant "handedness" (consistent overuse of one hand), though differences of development may have many causes. The individual accommodates the shorter side by twisting (rotating). The rotation may seem like a twisting of the ribs on the pelvis. If you have trouble visualizing how the thorax (rib cage) is rotated on the lower spine, imagine how a cork can be turned in the neck of a bottle. Suddenly you can see the pattern of rotation clearly.

More commonly, however, rotations occur as twistings of the pelvis itself (or the sacrum, fifth lumbar, etc.) around a lower lumbar vertebra. The muscular strain enters awareness as chronic pain and weakness in the lower back, with strain on one or more intervertebral disc. Eventually, tissue deterioration ensues, then problems with the discs and/or sacroiliac articulation become chronic.

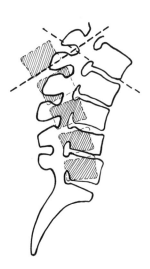

5-27 **Lateral view: A schematic representation of an anteroposterior lumbar lordosis and of its behavior in bending. Real life is not so schematically clear: a lumbar lordosis is always complicated by rotations of one or several spinal vertebrae around the vertical axis. (From Sobotta, ATLAS OF HUMAN ANATOMY, Vol. 1, Fig. 299)**

Deviations from symmetrical pattern may be seen in any public place. The gym, Turkish bath, swimming pool, and most of all the beach offer opportunities to observe human bodies, each with its own unique historical landmarks. Such observations translate into data about flesh. They also give you clues to problems of personality: strong points and weak ones, stresses and strains, energy limitations that must be overcome or allowed for before energy can be doled out for creative accomplishment. All bodies record the physical and emotional traumata of living—the happenings of a man's life. Here the "moving fingers writes" indelibly. For the average individual, episodes of many sorts have modified his structure and left their mark on whatever balance he may have had originally. There are measuring sticks that can assay these limitations: visible compression and the three-dimensional relations of the corporeal body are the indices. Unfortunately, though clear to his neighbors, they are usually invisible to the man himself.

Symmetrical patterns, those without accompanying aberrant compressions, testify to joyous living. But do not misinterpret—I am not saying that the man who is six foot two is more joyous or freer than the man who is five foot nine. Perhaps the structure of our six-two man calls for six-four, and the extra two inches measure the compressions within his body. Perhaps the genetic design of the five-nine man was just that—five-nine. In that case, Mr. Five-Nine is enjoying rare freedom from stress as well as freedom of movement. This will not be the man who is guarding his "disc problem" or nursing his sacroiliac. If his height is adequate to his pattern, his extensor muscles will be balanced and relatively symmetrical. His spine will be long and straight and adequate. Insecurity is not a word printed in boldface caps in his personal dictionary.

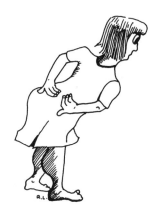

5-29 "Oh, my poor aching back!"

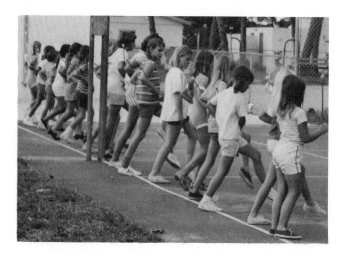

5-28 Pictures like this emphasize the differences in muscular response patterns of "random" bodies. All these girls think they are giving the same response to the same command, "Go!"

6
The Seat of the Soul
Is Physiological

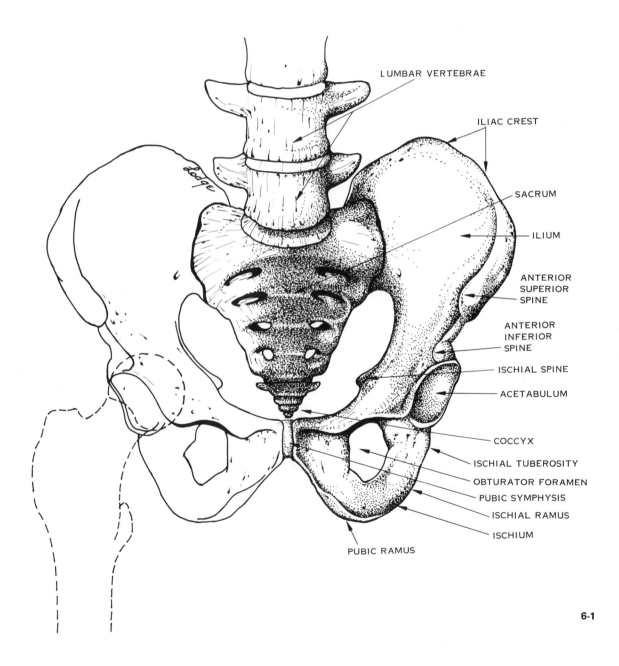

LUMBAR VERTEBRAE

ILIAC CREST

SACRUM

ILIUM

ANTERIOR
SUPERIOR
SPINE

ANTERIOR
INFERIOR
SPINE

ISCHIAL SPINE

ACETABULUM

COCCYX

ISCHIAL TUBEROSITY

OBTURATOR FORAMEN

PUBIC SYMPHYSIS

ISCHIAL RAMUS

ISCHIUM

PUBIC RAMUS

6-1

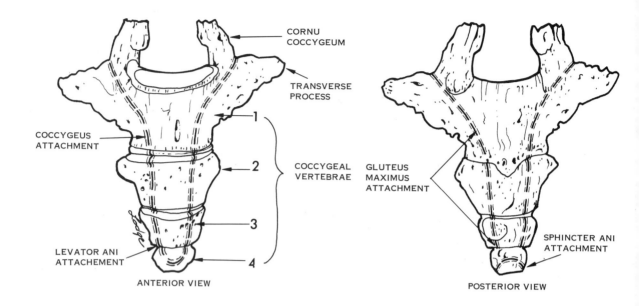

ANTERIOR VIEW

POSTERIOR VIEW

For countless years, men have known that the pelvis is of very special and vital importance. (The word *sacrum* means sacred bone.) It is the physiological locus for personal emotional factors of sexual satisfaction and fertility. Ancient Indian Tantric physiology recognized the pelvis as the area housing fundamental energy, the seat of the fabulous Kundalini. There were and still are sects who regard the ganglion of Impar (nerve plexus immediately adjoining the rectum) as the seat of the soul. Today, as well as two thousand years ago, they consider it central to the well-being of the individual and, consequently, of the race. In the light of present knowledge, with its emphasis on scientific and analytic concepts, can we accept this idea? What correlation of modern scientific thought would substantiate this pre-eminence?

The precise locus of the body's center of gravity is understandably controversial since it will vary with body type and carriage. It tends to center around the lumbosacral junction, and appropriate balance here is therefore of prime importance to bring about coordinated body movement as well as to act as a focus for the individual's kinesthetic sense. In addition to this integrative function, the pelvis performs service as a container. Anatomists recognize this: the word *pelvis* means basin. Clearly, in form and in function, the pelvis is basic.

6-2 The pelvis at its deepest level presents a bony basin. Its terminal segment, the coccyx, which is illustrated here, offers attachment for individual muscles of the pelvic floor.

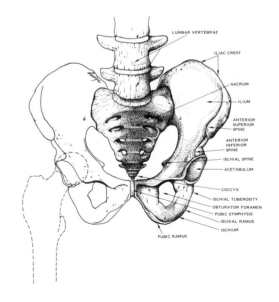

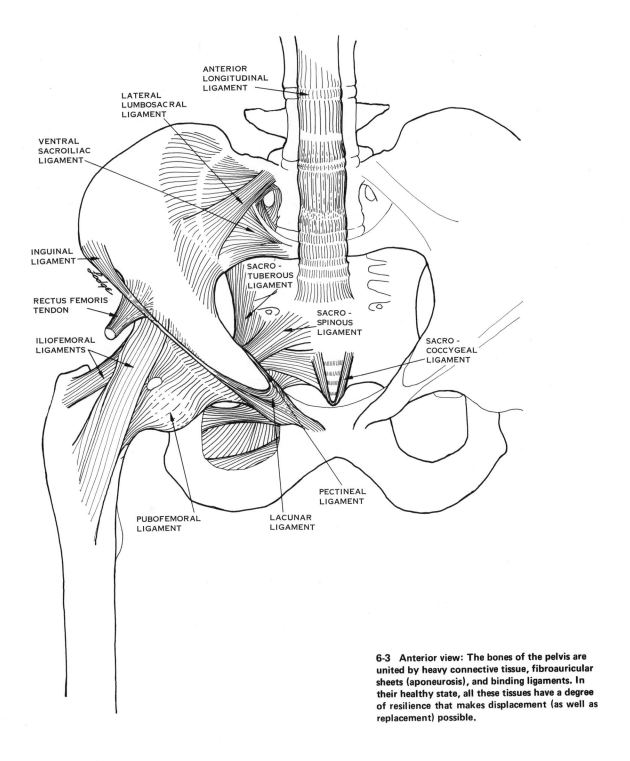

ANTERIOR
LONGITUDINAL
LIGAMENT

LATERAL
LUMBOSACRAL
LIGAMENT

VENTRAL
SACROILIAC
LIGAMENT

INGUINAL
LIGAMENT

RECTUS FEMORIS
TENDON

ILIOFEMORAL
LIGAMENTS

SACRO-
TUBEROUS
LIGAMENT

SACRO-
SPINOUS
LIGAMENT

SACRO-
COCCYGEAL
LIGAMENT

PUBOFEMORAL
LIGAMENT

LACUNAR
LIGAMENT

PECTINEAL
LIGAMENT

6-3 Anterior view: The bones of the pelvis are
united by heavy connective tissue, fibroauricular
sheets (aponeurosis), and binding ligaments. In
their healthy state, all these tissues have a degree
of resilience that makes displacement (as well as
replacement) possible.

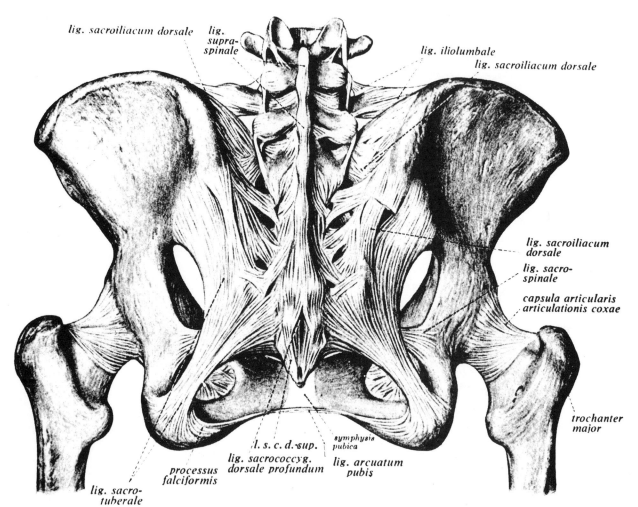

lig. sacroiliacum dorsale   lig. supra-spinale   lig. iliolumbale

lig. sacroiliacum dorsale

lig. sacroiliacum dorsale

lig. sacro-spinale

capsula articularis articulationis coxae

trochanter major

l. s. c. d. sup.

symphysis pubica

lig. sacrococcyg. dorsale profundum

lig. arcuatum pubis

processus falciformis

lig. sacro-tuberale

crista sacralis mediana

6-4 This evocative illustration depicts a pelvis seen from the back. It shows clearly how heavy connective tissue, ligaments, etc., unite with the surface of the bone, forming a structural union inseparable by ordinary accidents. If the ligaments should lose their elasticity, physical trauma could then cause the bone to break, for the bone is more frangible than the ligaments. When shortening and chemical deterioration set in at this deep level, it is hard to change the picture. As compensating areas open, however, these levels can and do change spontaneously, though months or even years may be necessary to permit this very deep change. (From Sobotta, ATLAS OF HUMAN ANATOMY, Vol.1, Fig.259)

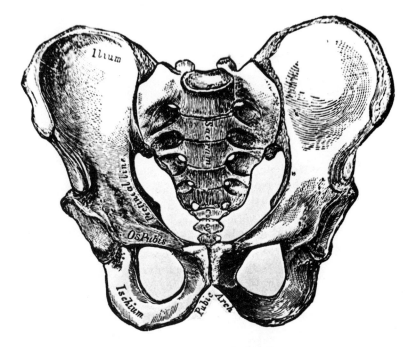

—Male pelvis.

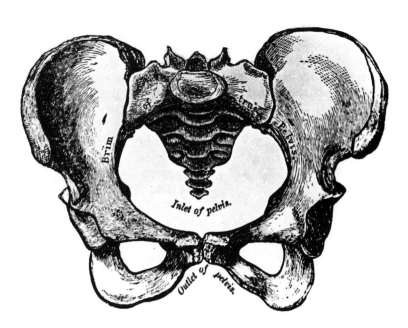

—Female pelvis.

6-5 Anterior views: A comparison of male and
female pelves. (From Goss, ed., GRAY'S
ANATOMY OF THE HUMAN BODY, Figs. 4-175
and 4-176)

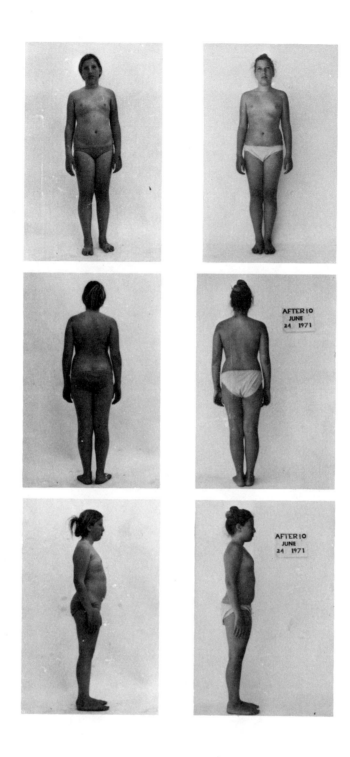

6-6 Most random bodies show a pelvis tipped forward. The contents are then restrained only by the superficial muscles and skin of the abdomen instead of being " contained " by the basin.

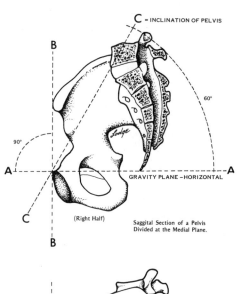

C = INCLINATION OF PELVIS

B

60°

90°

A ---- A

GRAVITY PLANE – HORIZONTAL

C

(Right Half)

B

Saggital Section of a Pelvis
Divided at the Medial Plane.

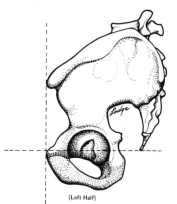

(Left Half)

Most people know that the proportions of male and female pelves differ. This does not alter the fact that certain functions are shared. Both serve as containers and, through the sacrolumbar junction, form a mechanical bearing on which the upper body balances. In its role as basin, the pelvis contains the abdominal viscera. This offers a clue as to how it must be balanced in space to perform effectively. In a random body, the abdominal contents too often are held up merely by the muscles and skin of the anterior abdominal wall. If the plane defined by line *A* (Fig. 6-7) deviates too widely from the horizontal, obviously the contained pelvic contents will spill. In a tipped pelvis, viscera may be restrained by the abdominal wall, but they cannot be housed snugly within the basin.

When the pelvic contents overflow, the overlying abdomen becomes either the little round "potbelly" or the more diffuse "bay window." Its owner bewails his fate—he is putting on too much weight, he must stop taking cream in his coffee, etc. Remedies that have nothing to do with the case are explored verbally. Sometimes he actually does progress as far as not taking cream in his coffee. If an activist, he goes on a low-calorie diet and takes up jogging. But the basic contour of the abdomen refuses to change, though the general figure may become more svelte. Calories have very little to do with this particular manifestation. The fact is that the man, ruefully looking at his bay window in the mirror, is experiencing the evidence that his pelvic basin is spilling its contents. The tilt of his pelvis makes it incapable of performing its function as a container.

Pelvic tilt is related directly to the position of the lumbar spine and the sacrum. As we have said, in a balanced pelvis, the line *A* is horizontal. To the extent that this is not so, strain is reflected into the sacrolumbar junction and movement is impeded. According to our observations, this is one of the most important joints of the body. We see that a very slight mobility at this joint stimulates the autonomic plexi of lumbar and sacral areas; pumping of vital body fluids also relates to some extent to it. In light of this, the seat of the soul—according to Edgar Cayce, the soul is the monitor of the unconscious functions of the body—is physiological and a function of the sacrolumbar junction.

6-7 Seen from the side, the pelvis presents this appearance. The horizontal between the coccyx and pubes and the vertical between pubes and anterior superior spine of the ilium are sensed as the definition of "balance" in the pelvis and the body as a whole.

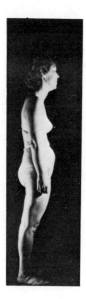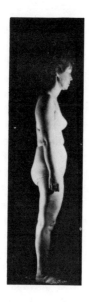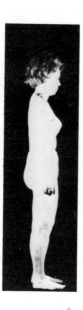

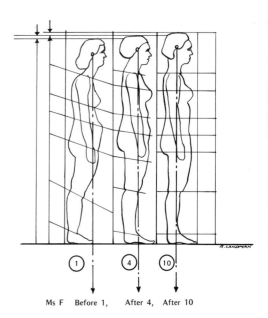

① ④ ⑩

Ms F   Before 1,   After 4,   After 10

If the lumbar spine is aligned as shown in Fig. 6-8, the pelvis must have tipped and the abdominal wall be loose and sagging. Can this woman straighten up? Indeed not. If she tries, after a minute or two she abandons the effort: "It's just too much to think about." The weight of abdominal contents is supported by willpower rather than by structure, and she quickly tires. As soon as her attention is diverted to something else, her configuration again reverts to the form dictated by the various shortenings and thickenings of fascial envelopes and by the ligamentous or tendinous deviations that characterize her particular physical problem.

6-8 These schema, developed from photographs of a woman during her ten hours of Structural Integration, show the progressive change of body planes during this period, before, after four hours and after ten hours. The transformation from oblique planes through major joints to horizontals is clear.

The next obvious question is, What controls and what changes these pelvic planes? As we have said, pelvic tilt correlates directly with the placement of the lumbar spine. In addition, the pelvis must conform to the leg. The head of the femur rests in the socket of the pelvis (acetabulum) (Fig. 6-9). The pelvis adjusts to the movement of the thigh by rotating in this joint. When a person is standing, his leg and foot are organized primarily to the ground, not to the pelvis. The pelvis adjusts to the movement by rotating slightly around the head of the femur.

The position of the lower limb is relatively fixed because the sole of the foot must be in appropriate contact with the ground. The bony ball-and-socket joint of the hip (acetabulum and head of the femur) is strong and simple, designed for easy rotation in virtually all directions. The femoral head inserts into the acetabulum and is encapsulated there and fixed by ligaments. Seen from the front, the deepest layers may be schematized as in the drawings. This joint permits the pelvis to adjust to thigh and leg.

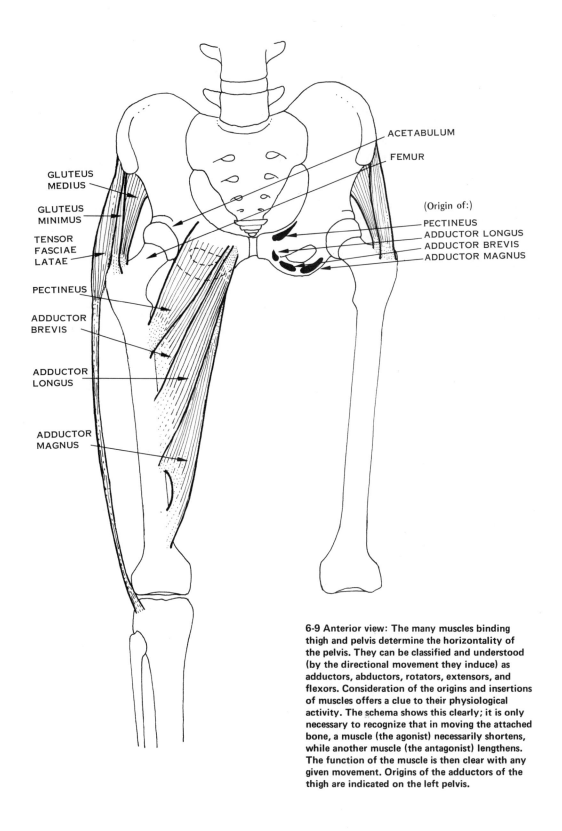

GLUTEUS
MEDIUS

GLUTEUS
MINIMUS

TENSOR
FASCIAE
LATAE

PECTINEUS

ADDUCTOR
BREVIS

ADDUCTOR
LONGUS

ADDUCTOR
MAGNUS

ACETABULUM

FEMUR

(Origin of:)

PECTINEUS
ADDUCTOR LONGUS
ADDUCTOR BREVIS
ADDUCTOR MAGNUS

6-9 Anterior view: The many muscles binding
thigh and pelvis determine the horizontality of
the pelvis. They can be classified and understood
(by the directional movement they induce) as
adductors, abductors, rotators, extensors, and
flexors. Consideration of the origins and insertions
of muscles offers a clue to their physiological
activity. The schema shows this clearly; it is only
necessary to recognize that in moving the attached
bone, a muscle (the agonist) necessarily shortens,
while another muscle (the antagonist) lengthens.
The function of the muscle is then clear with any
given movement. Origins of the adductors of the
thigh are indicated on the left pelvis.

However, the "joint" is much more than the bone of the ball-and-socket. All muscles and ligaments that weave or support its structure are part of it. This is true of any joint. Trouble in any one of the component parts—muscles, ligaments, bones—is apt to be interpreted or at least verbalized as being in the joint. Unnumbered casual, hasty diagnoses of "arthritis" reflect nothing more serious than a shortened or displaced muscle or ligament resulting from a recent or not-so-recent traumatic episode. True arthritis, on the other hand, is deterioration of the joint, characterized by chemical change in the blood and in joint tissue. Arthritic pain is the result of joint compression. Not all cases of true arthritis are painful; where there is adequate capsular space, the individual may well be pain-free. When your shoulder or your hip hurts, it is well to paraphrase an old adage: not only is all that glitters not gold, but, even more hopeful, all that hurts is not necessarily arthritis. It may be merely pseudoarthritis, a disorder in the tendons and ligaments. Not until your doctor has diagnosed it as an arthritis on the basis of chemical tests is it necessary for you to pre-empt that porch rocking chair because you are lame with "arthritis." Appropriate muscular organization can give the pseudoarthritic movement and render him pain-free.

Getting acquainted with a human body naturally and logically starts with the more superficial aspects. Contours can be seen as well as palpated; the eye is one of our most valued measuring sticks. Visual evaluation makes it clear that the position of the pelvis (and therefore the position of the integrated body) demands good operational balance in the thigh.

In addition to flexors and extensors, anatomists classify muscles functionally as abductors (those that in shortening draw a part away from the body's midline), adductors (those that bring the part toward the midline), and rotators. For symmetrical function and good operational balance in any part, all must balance in muscle tone as well as in length. However, in our cultural pattern, it is very common to see abductors, particularly those of the leg, that have become very tight and decidedly short (especially in males or in athletes of either sex). To the touch, such aberrated muscles seem unstructured and are sometimes painful. At times they are so tight they seem like bone rather than myofascia. In the thigh, rigidity or flaccidity in any of these myofascial elements transmits strain immediately to the pelvis and especially to the very important pelvic floor.

In its massive function of supporting and transmitting weight, the thigh needs powerful structuring. One of its strongest elements is a heavy protective fascia, the fascia lata. This important support has great responsibility in

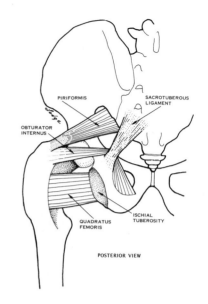

POSTERIOR VIEW

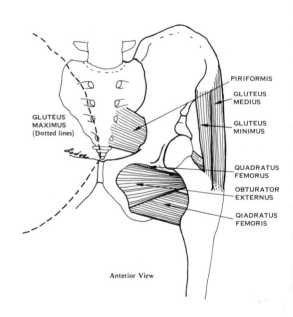

Anterior View

6-10 Rotators of the thigh (anterior and posterior views), in shortening, displace the relation of the thigh to the pelvis. Thus, even one chronically shortened individual rotator can induce highly aberrated movement, reflecting into the over-all gait. As time passes, the "one" shortened unit induces unpredictable compensations in its sister muscles, and a generally aberrated pattern appears.

90

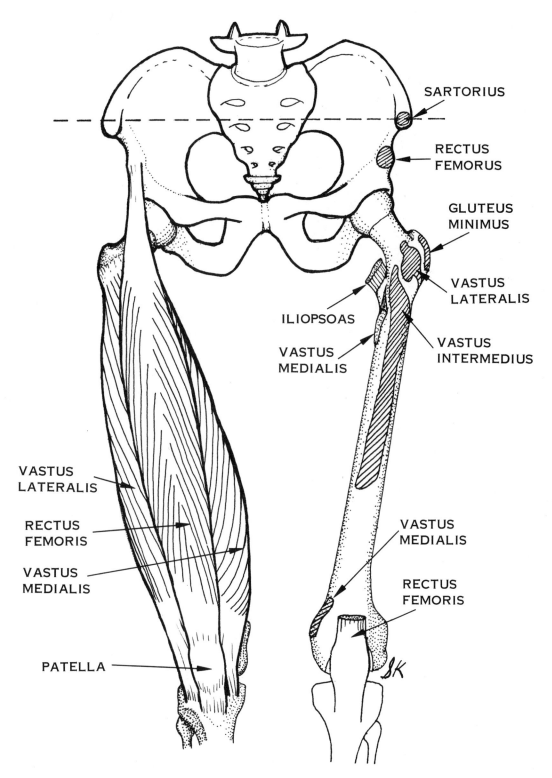

SARTORIUS

RECTUS FEMORUS

GLUTEUS MINIMUS

VASTUS LATERALIS

ILIOPSOAS

VASTUS MEDIALIS

VASTUS INTERMEDIUS

VASTUS LATERALIS

RECTUS FEMORIS

VASTUS MEDIALIS

VASTUS MEDIALIS

RECTUS FEMORIS

PATELLA

6-11 Anterior view: The quadriceps and related group act as flexors of the thigh. As such, they are antagonists of the hamstrings.

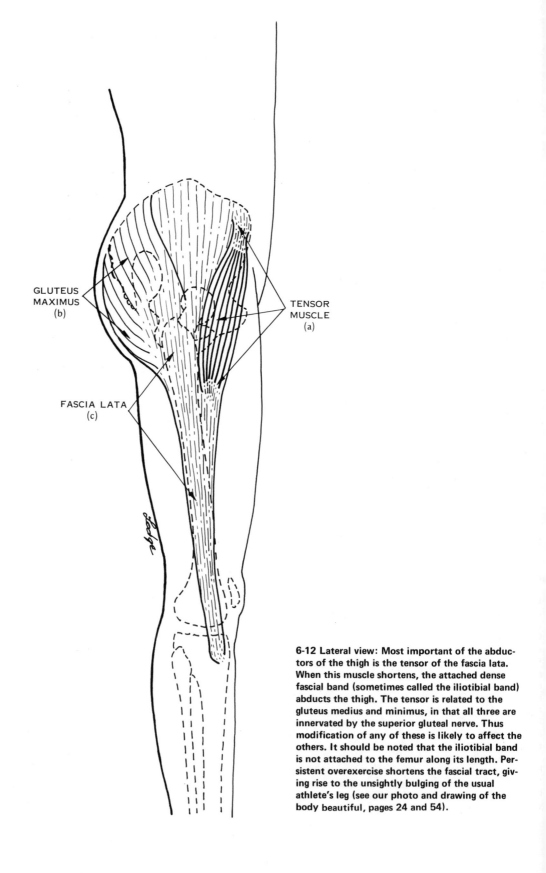

GLUTEUS
MAXIMUS
(b)

TENSOR
MUSCLE
(a)

FASCIA LATA
(c)

6-12 Lateral view: Most important of the abductors of the thigh is the tensor of the fascia lata. When this muscle shortens, the attached dense fascial band (sometimes called the iliotibial band) abducts the thigh. The tensor is related to the gluteus medius and minimus, in that all three are innervated by the superior gluteal nerve. Thus modification of any of these is likely to affect the others. It should be noted that the iliotibial band is not attached to the femur along its length. Persistent overexercise shortens the fascial tract, giving rise to the unsightly bulging of the usual athlete's leg (see our photo and drawing of the body beautiful, pages 24 and 54).

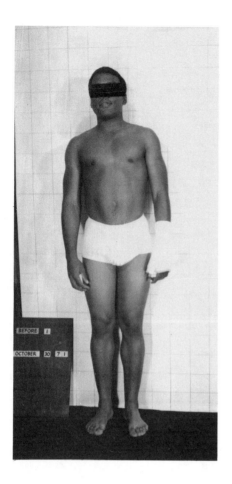
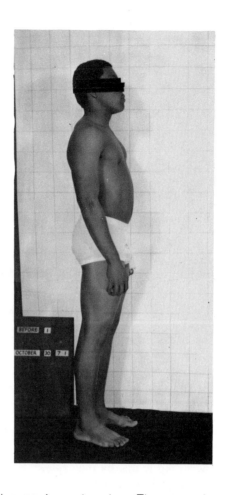

6-13 This successful young athlete carries with him the clues to his problems. In the next few years, they will become more troublesome and finally will remove him from his high place in competitive ranks. Can you see that his entire right leg is rotated? It is rotated not as a whole, but in terms of its segments: the right foot is rotated with respect to the shin. The rotation of the right leg on its thigh shows in the lack of freedom at the knee, and this restriction may be seen in the groin as well. He has tried to escape these restrictions by rotating his thorax on the pelvis. Note his right shoulder (the man is an expert in shot-putting) and see how asymmetric is the junction of neck and shoulder as well as head and neck. The effects of these rotations are strikingly clear in profile. (A photo of this young man after Structural Integration is included later in this book.

In attempting to strengthen his thighs, Mr. P has overdeveloped his abductors, especially the tensor fascia lata (which in turn shortens the fascia lata itself). The thigh then rotates externally, as you can see in the position of his left thigh.

maintaining man's erect posture. The gymnast proud of his muscular pattern may have lower limbs that look like those of athlete Mr. P (Fig. 6-13). This surface contour is the tracing of the underlying fascia lata; its tone is controlled by a muscle, the tensor fascia lata. Persistent exercise of this muscle shortens and toughens the fascial iliotibial tract until it is reminiscent of a steel cable. The tract crosses both knee and hip joints. Here spatial compression is possible and shortening of this band forces the bony joint surfaces closer. The first effect of this compression is to squeeze cartilaginous elements (medial and lateral menisci separating the bony surfaces). There is a space limitation to this compression response. Further shortening can occur only through a rotational displacement. The man now begins to feel himself muscle-bound, rigid, less free. He moves more slowly. Some types of compressive adjustment in the lower limb also transmit stress to the adductors and rotators. At this stage, pelvic balance is seriously threatened. This has been the story of the average athlete and of his progression from supple youth to musclebound, rigid adult.

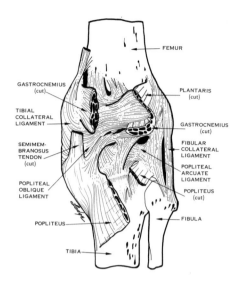

GASTROCNEMIUS (cut)
PLANTARIS (cut)
TIBIAL COLLATERAL LIGAMENT
GASTROCNEMIUS (cut)
FEMUR
FIBULAR COLLATERAL LIGAMENT
SEMIMEMBRANOSUS TENDON (cut)
POPLITEAL ARCUATE LIGAMENT
POPLITEUS (cut)
POPLITEAL OBLIQUE LIGAMENT
POPLITEUS
FIBULA
TIBIA

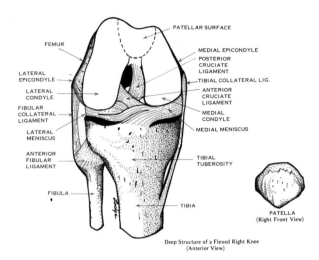

PATELLAR SURFACE
FEMUR
MEDIAL EPICONDYLE
POSTERIOR CRUCIATE LIGAMENT
LATERAL EPICONDYLE
TIBIAL COLLATERAL LIG.
LATERAL CONDYLE
ANTERIOR CRUCIATE LIGAMENT
FIBULAR COLLATERAL LIGAMENT
MEDIAL CONDYLE
LATERAL MENISCUS
MEDIAL MENISCUS
ANTERIOR FIBULAR LIGAMENT
TIBIAL TUBEROSITY
FIBULA
TIBIA
PATELLA (Right Front View)

Deep Structure of a Flexed Right Knee (Anterior View)

The extreme of the spectrum of joint competence is a different tale. The woman whose legs are flabby and soft is apparently the polar opposite of the athlete; in fact, she hates athletics and always has. She doesn't walk when she can ride, she doesn't stand when she can sit. In some respects, however, she is like an athlete. The movement of her legs lacks balance. Consequently, she feels no security as the pelvis rides on top of the legs.

Ball-and-socket hip joints, by their heavy, well-designed structure, should offer extensive range of movement to the overlying pelvis. Potentially free (but not too free) shifting of the plane of the pelvis is inherent in their superb design. But when the guy wires and supporting structures are no longer equal in length and tone, awareness (conscious or suppressed) of a basic insecurity is inevitable, be it in the athlete or in the activity-shunning soft man or woman. In man or woman, the original distortion of the thighs may have happened in many ways—by deliberate, persistent contortion, as in the athlete or dancer (see our photos of dancers in Chapter 3), by the disorganization caused by falls or accidents, or by the muscular distress of a difficult childbirth. If you wish to understand the pelvis, observe the legs and how they function with it. You will see individuals in whom the thighs are set too wide apart; you will see some whose thighs are too close for proper balance. But more clearly than any other single index, the slope of the gluteal structure tells the facts. As we've noted before, however, the body is a very plastic medium. The position of the pelvis is not immutable; it can be changed.

6-14 Sturdy, stable legs require sturdy, stable knees. In any structure, stability depends on a balance between deep structures and their superficial counterparts. This is especially true of knees. Looking at the following photographs, try to imagine the strain under which the knee joints of these girls must be working and the paths through which the strain is transmitted upward.

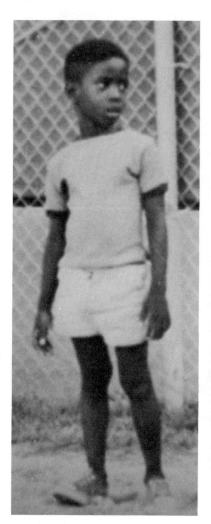 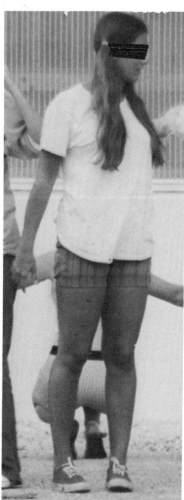 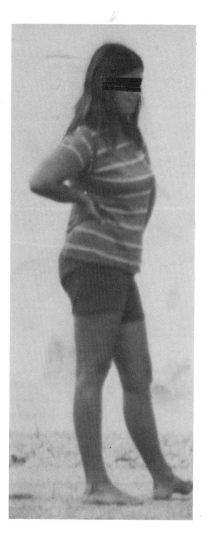

6-15 Three photos were picked at random from a large number taken of young people on a Florida beach. Note how every joint in these bodies shows rotational distortion. Each aberrated joint is compensating for some other. These are not the hard, compressed joints of the athlete. Here we see the compensatory pattern of the "soft, immature" bodies, where muscles and ligaments have insufficient tone to maintain structure.

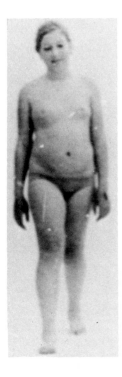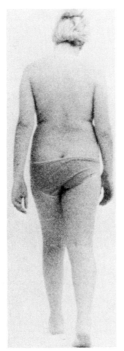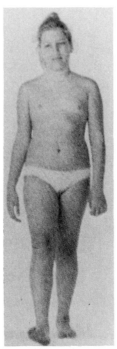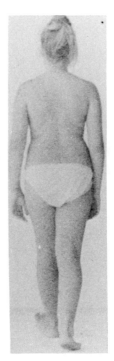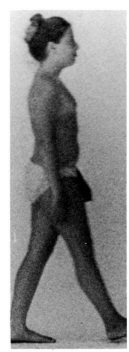

6-16 Dee, age twelve, is typical of what we think of as a "soft body." Fortunately, Dee is not as badly off as the girls in Fig. 6-15. Softness is one extreme in joint imbalance; it is not so much the result of softness as of imbalance in which inner muscles are too tight and short to balance outer muscles. People tend to think of such girls as fat, but diet won't cure this situation. The answer is to organize the structure.

Before processing, as she sits, Dee displays the rigidity of the deep muscles. Note the difficulty with which the thighs adjust to the sitting posture, and the distortion and backward thrust of her knees as she bends over. As Integration progresses, the constriction of thigh and knee eases, as shown in the position photographed after ten hours of work.

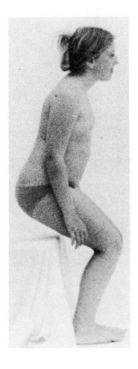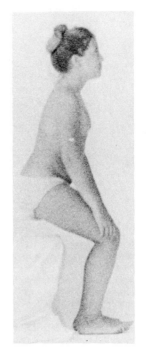

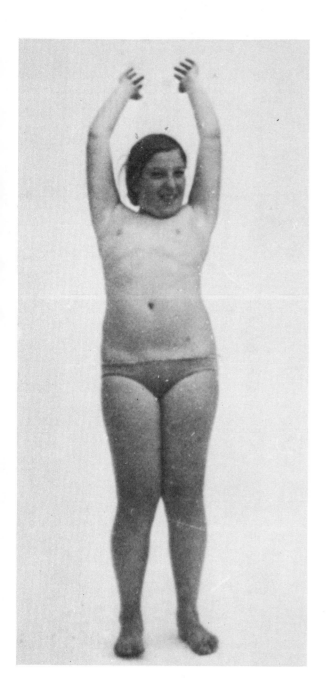
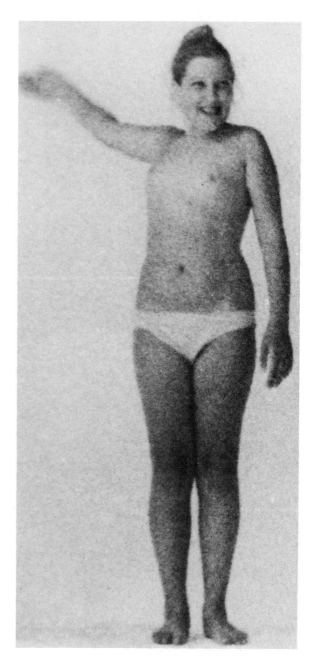

6-17 After ten hours of processing, the change in deep tissue and the release of joint compression is easy to see. As she lifts her arms, she no longer involves her whole body down to her knees. Note, too, how much more grown up Dee is, even though these pictures were taken only six weeks apart. This gives a new and different slant on the concept of maturity.

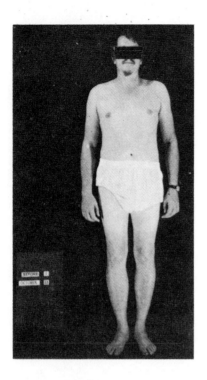 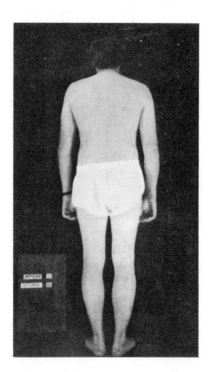

6-18   This man's pelvis seems too wide, but the apparent width is not always a matter of width of bone. The functioning of many muscles is involved, particularly the rotators and glutei. When unbalanced, they give an outward flaring to the thighs, creating the appearance of width.

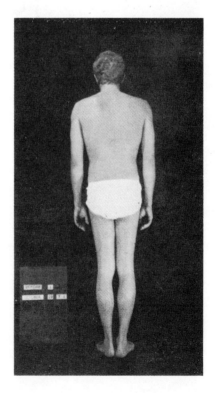

6-19   The ratio of the shoulder width to hip width characterizes the effectiveness of a body. Here the pelvis seems too small, glutei and rotators too constricted. The man at all times feels tense and physically insecure.

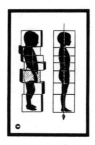

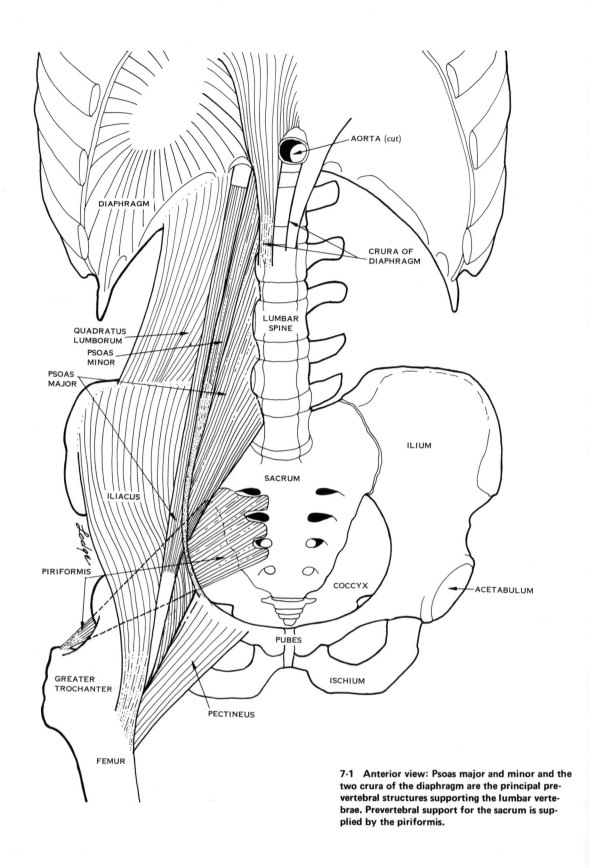

DIAPHRAGM

AORTA (cut)

CRURA OF
DIAPHRAGM

LUMBAR
SPINE

QUADRATUS
LUMBORUM

PSOAS
MINOR

PSOAS
MAJOR

ILIUM

ILIACUS

SACRUM

Lodge

PIRIFORMIS

COCCYX

ACETABULUM

GREATER
TROCHANTER

PUBES

ISCHIUM

PECTINEUS

FEMUR

**7-1 Anterior view: Psoas major and minor and the
two crura of the diaphragm are the principal prevertebral structures supporting the lumbar vertebrae. Prevertebral support for the sacrum is supplied by the piriformis.**

100

7
Your Psoas

Clearly a pelvis must be knit into the entire body fabric, above as well as below, ventral surface as well as dorsal. The dorsal surface helps establish and maintain the span of the lumbar fascia. The lumbar fascia, in turn, determines the placement of the erector spinae group, composed of three major antigravity muscles: spinalis, longissimus, and iliocostalis. (The deeper-lying quadratus lumborum, briefly touched on in Chapter 5, arises from the crest of the ilium rather than from the lumbar fascia.)

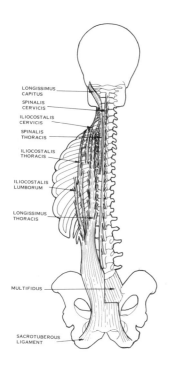

LONGISSIMUS CAPITUS
SPINALIS CERVICIS
ILIOCOSTALIS CERVICIS
SPINALIS THORACIS
ILIOCOSTALIS THORACIS
ILIOCOSTALIS LUMBORUM
LONGISSIMUS THORACIS
MULTIFIDUS
SACROTUBEROUS LIGAMENT

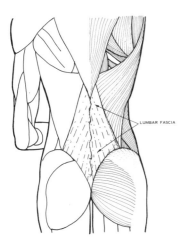

LUMBAR FASCIA

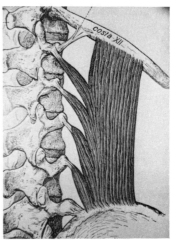

(From Sobotta, ATLAS OF HUMAN ANATOMY, Vol. 1, Fig. 299)

7-2 Posterior view: Postvertebral support for the lumbar spine is supplied by the extensors (erector spinae and to some extent the quadratus lumborum) and the outermost fascial wrappings (the lumbar fascial).

Greater length (and therefore greater elasticity) in the extensors offers resilience and span to upper and midback tissues. Then the back of the pelvic basin (the crest of the ilium) can seek a lower level. This change in pelvic plane allows the line *A* in Fig. 7-3 more nearly to approach the horizontal. The effect of such changes—although in themselves they are small (perhaps a quarter of an inch)—is

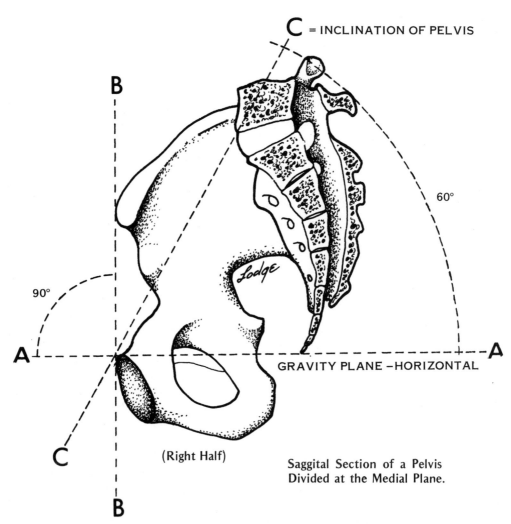

C = INCLINATION OF PELVIS

60°

90°

GRAVITY PLANE –HORIZONTAL

Lodge

(Right Half)

Saggital Section of a Pelvis
Divided at the Medial Plane.

7-3 Lateral views: The signature of the balanced body is the horizontal line that joins the tip of the coccyx and the pubes. When this primary horizontal is well established from above and below, the anterior surface of the anterior superior spines of the ilium can define a vertical plane with the pubes. Shortness in one of the muscles attaching to it rotates the pelvis and distorts and strains all these relations.

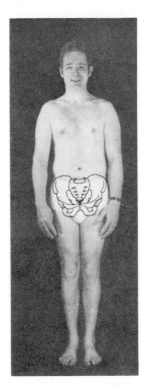

7-4 The position of the bony basin, its horizontals and its verticals, determines the competence of the overlying body. No human can approach equipoise until a substantial balance is present in the pelvis.

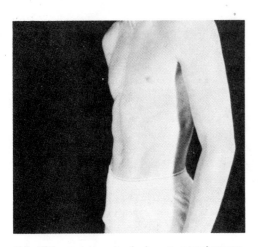

7-6 This young man has had no structural processing. The flat-chested contour of his upper ribcage is an index of shortened recti. If he tries to "develop his chest" through push-ups and/or pull-ups, he will further shorten the recti and put an additional drag on the ribs. It is clear that the shortened ventral surface will transmit considerable strain to his back.

greatly amplified in movement and balance. Reliable support from the lower limbs is another crucial factor in free pelvic movement.

It is impossible to overemphasize the importance of a free hip joint. As we have said, the general position of the leg itself is fixed by the foot. The plane of the sole must be horizontal to conform to the earth; when the body moves, it is the pelvis that must rotate. Therefore the hip joint must be free. First the pelvis must be able to rotate easily around the ball-and-socket joint. Then the question is, what muscular structure on the front of the body can be called on to stabilize the pelvis as it moves? What can counter the gravitational pull exerted on the body's anterior aspect by the flexors when the dorsal extensors have been lengthened? The rectus abdominis is the outstanding ventral flexor.

Physical-training programs are preoccupied with the rectus abdominis. Its importance in erect posture is universally recognized. All push-ups and sit-ups are specifically designed to "strengthen" it. In point of fact, however, the "strengthening" resulting from push-ups as they are usually practiced permanently shortens and hardens the recti. True strength is not hardening, it is resilience, adaptability, stability. It is characterized by elasticity, which allows quick recuperation from fatigue. Hardening of the rectus or any muscle means that muscular layers have adhered one to the other, are less able to accept the rapid lengthening and shortening essential to healthy metabolism and recovery in any tissue. Rapid alternation bears witness to reciprocal interplay of agonist and antagonist. In turn, this spells spontaneous (and almost instantaneous) recovery from weariness. This is health. This is strength.

Since muscles act as pumps moving food- and oxygen-carrying fluids (lymph, etc.) to and from cells, free alternation of extension and contraction constitutes an outstanding service. This is the rationale of exercise; it is the reason why all exercise is of some value. Unfortunately, the design of much exercise is built around popular misconceptions. The accepted myth is that if certain individual muscle groups need strengthening, repetitious specific movement patterns can be employed to accomplish this. This assumption fails to recognize that "strength" is a function of a reciprocal agonist-antagonist balance. Thus, according to the myth, recti can be "strengthened" by sit-ups or push-ups. Consistent indulgence in such specific exercise, however, shortens and hardens the frequently too short muscle and further upsets the agonist–antagonist balance; in random bodies, sit-ups and push-ups overdevelop and harden the rectus. In this way, they effectively weaken its hidden but very important counterbalance, the psoas.

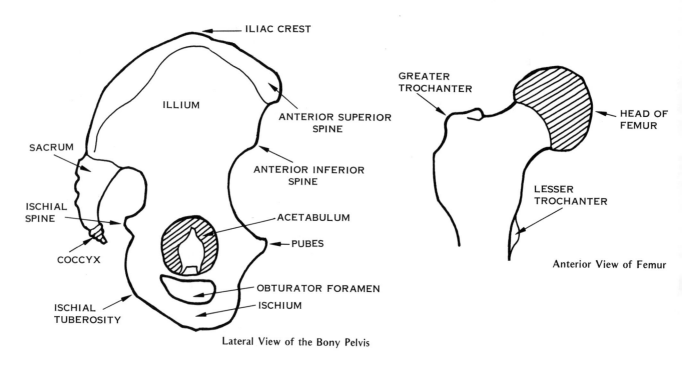

ILIAC CREST

ILLIUM

SACRUM

ISCHIAL
SPINE

COCCYX

ISCHIAL
TUBEROSITY

ANTERIOR SUPERIOR
SPINE

ANTERIOR INFERIOR
SPINE

ACETABULUM

PUBES

OBTURATOR FORAMEN

ISCHIUM

Lateral View of the Bony Pelvis

GREATER
TROCHANTER

HEAD OF
FEMUR

LESSER
TROCHANTER

Anterior View of Femur

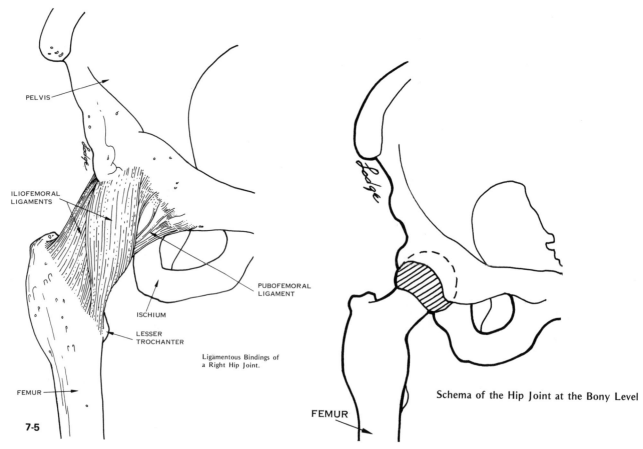

PELVIS

ILIOFEMORAL
LIGAMENTS

PUBOFEMORAL
LIGAMENT

ISCHIUM

LESSER
TROCHANTER

Ligamentous Bindings of
a Right Hip Joint.

FEMUR

7-5

FEMUR

Schema of the Hip Joint at the Bony Level

104

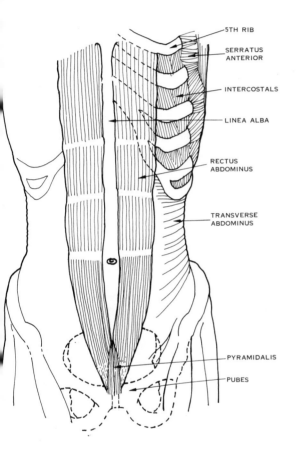

5TH RIB

SERRATUS ANTERIOR

INTERCOSTALS

LINEA ALBA

RECTUS ABDOMINUS

TRANSVERSE ABDOMINUS

PYRAMIDALIS

PUBES

7-7 Anterior view: These are the recti abdominis, the tough muscle pair forming the anterior wall of the abdomen. They arise from the pubes and insert on the fifth, sixth and seventh ribs. As this is too great a length for a single muscle to span for effective control, three tendinuous intersections interrupt the fibers; they reduce the effective length of the contractile segment and thus strengthen it. It is apparent that as the muscle chronically shortens or deteriorates, origin and insertion will be drawn toward each other. This means that the ribs (on which it originates) will be dragged downward, as illustrated in Fig. 7-6.

The recti insert, as shown in Fig. 7-7, into the pubes. In attaching to this center of the pelvic rim, they raise the anterior aspect of the pelvic basin and thus contribute to the horizontal position of the pelvis, which we see as all-important. If recti are shortened and thickened through repetitive flexing, complications arise. The most apparent distortion will be in the ribcage. The recti, arising from the ribcage, exert pull as far up as the fifth rib. Chronic shortening of these muscles drags down the rib structure as a whole, bringing the lower ribs too close to the pelvic brim. This chronic flexion strains the entire body, since neck and cervical spine are inevitably included in the compensation. The myofascial structures of the cervical spine become anteriorly shortened and therefore the head comes forward (Fig. 7-8).

This sag of the ribcage strains the three or four uppermost ribs as well. In equipoise, the anterior attachment of the first rib to the breastbone is very nearly horizontal with its posterior attachment to the vertebra. The more closely this approximates the horizontal, the more snugly the yoke of the shoulder girdle will fit and the more clearly the body will display a generally vertical-horizontal alignment. Random bodies cannot show this. Nor can bodies forcibly pulled away from the position of balance by ill-advised overexercise.

In turn, continued ventral sag in the first and second ribs displaces and raises the first dorsal vertebra in the back. This is the beginning of the so-called dowager's hump (Fig. 7-9), which many people find so offensive. Flesh and fat in any area of the body collect in response to biological laws. Wherever an insecure area is under consistent strain, flesh tries to ensure greater stability by enwrapping or splinting it. All unwanted and unwonted "humps," wherever found, have a similar cause and a similar remedy. (Of course, we are talking here about humps, not lumps—especially not the type of lumps that betoken tumors. These are in the domain of medicine, and if there is any doubt, however slight, let your doctor check it.) Structural humps yield to structural methods, and the hump at the seventh cervical vertebra is the most common. As the anterior ribcage is freed through greater length and greater elasticity in the recti, strain on the upper backbone lessens. The junction of cervical and dorsal vertebra then need no longer be splinted and protected by massed flesh. They form an easy juxtaposition, and the unbeautiful hump disappears.

Overexercise of the recti abdominis has consequences even more important than the structural implications of sagging ribcage and strained upper dorsal structures. All muscles, as we have noted, act in reciprocal pairs. Matched

105

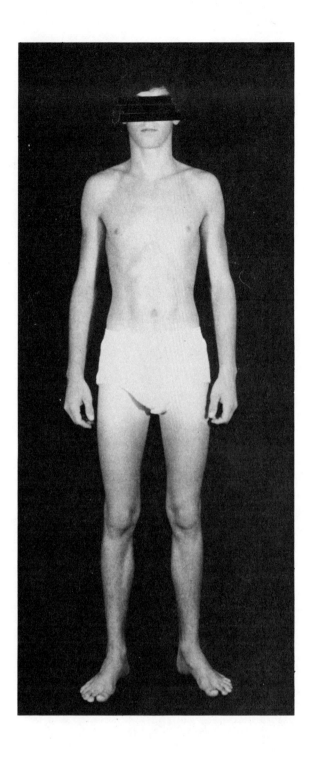

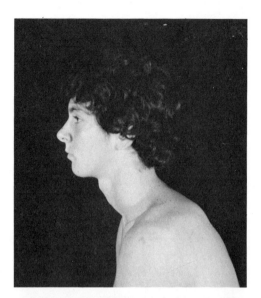

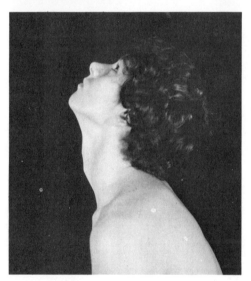

7-8 Note in the full-length view how the pull of the recti on the pubes has distorted the legs, and how the dragging ribcage has rotated the upper arms. Even the head and neck are seriously displaced by this downward pull, as evidenced by the close-up photos.

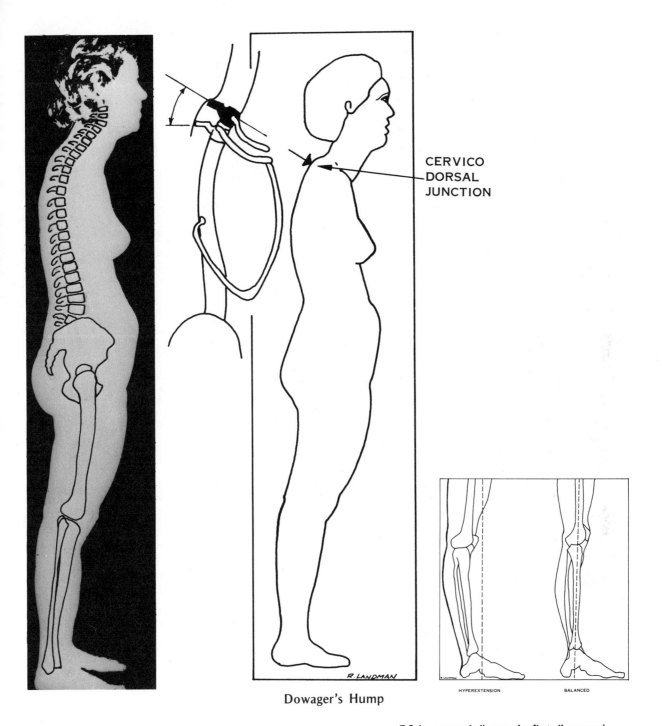

CERVICO
DORSAL
JUNCTION

Dowager's Hump

HYPEREXTENSION   BALANCED

7-9 In a normal ribcage, the first rib approximated a straight line from front to back. The "dowager's hump" is the result of a major sagging of the ribcage, tilting the first dorsal and seventh cervical vertebrae. The strain here reflects also into the lumbar spine. Note, too, how the distortion at the cervicodorsal junction requires that the leg compensates by hyperextending.

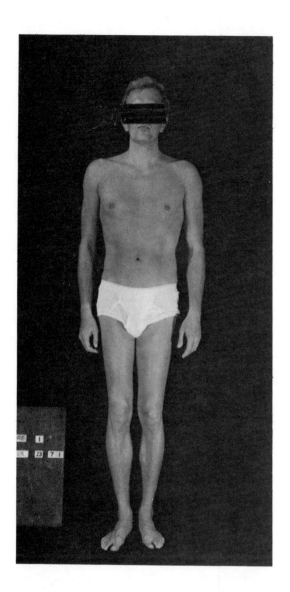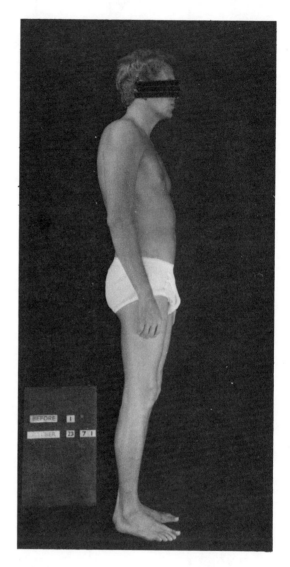

7-10 As in any random body, Mr. W displays mis-
mated agonist-antagonist pairs, particularly a serious imbalance between his very hypertoned (short)
psoas and non-resilient rectus. This tension is clearly apparent in the front view: notice the strained
implosion just below the diaphragm (the two ends
of the psoas) and at the groin. This transmits to
the adductors in the thigh, and indeed to all the
muscles of the thigh and leg. The lateral view tells
the same story.

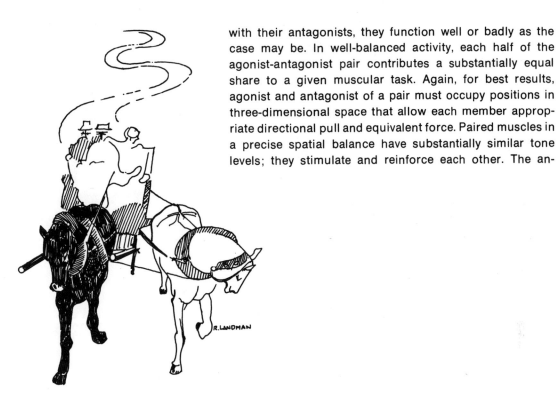

with their antagonists, they function well or badly as the case may be. In well-balanced activity, each half of the agonist-antagonist pair contributes a substantially equal share to a given muscular task. Again, for best results, agonist and antagonist of a pair must occupy positions in three-dimensional space that allow each member appropriate directional pull and equivalent force. Paired muscles in a precise spatial balance have substantially similar tone levels; they stimulate and reinforce each other. The an-

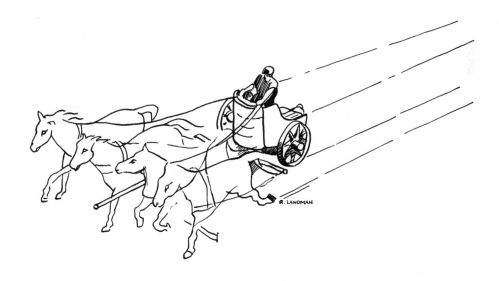

7-11

tagonist of a muscle consistently called on for unbalanced overactivity deteriorates very rapidly. The agonist then tries unsuccessfully to compensate for the weakened antagonist, and we thus have an additional factor making for progressive disorder and disorganization in the body.

The reciprocal agonist–antagonist relation between individual muscle groups is a prime factor in the health and tone of muscle tissue and of the organism in general. Certain of these paired units are of central importance; one of these is the psoas-rectus pair (Fig. 7-12). Though its name is unfamiliar to most laymen, in many respects the psoas is one of the most significant muscles of the body. The psoas unit is composed of two sections, the major and minor, which together can act as counterbalance to the recti. Like all important body elements, they have multiple functions. The psoas plays an important part in general body support; thus it maintains body structure and body relationships. But it is probably through its support of the autonomic lumbar plexus that it exerts its major impact; through the viscera innervated by this plexus, it can well exert a vital influence on bodily well-being.

The psoas takes its origin along the upper lumbar spine (the sides of the bodies and intervertebral discs of all lumbar vertebrae, the attachments extending backward to the transverse processes and forward to the sympathetic trunk). Thus for part of its length it runs along the anterior surface of the lumbar vertebrae. Its origin is in close proximity to the two tabs of the diaphragm called the crura; through these neighbors, the psoas can involve the respiratory pattern. The psoas tendon inserts at the head of the thigh bone, on the lesser trochanter (inner aspect) of the femur. Thus structurally it is a bridge between upper body and legs. The close proximity of the diaphragm to the psoas origin implies that imperfect psoas function will be reflected into the diaphragm and into the ribcage, for which the diaphragm forms the pliant, plastic base.

Having arisen from the sides of the lumbar vertebrae, the psoas pursues a somewhat devious, S-shaped route downward. It diagonally traverses the cavity of the pelvis, crosses the crest of the pubes, and continues obliquely downward across the capsule of the hip joint. It inserts by a tendon shared with the iliacus (the iliopsoas tendon) into the lesser trochanter of the femur. The iliacus lines the ilium, the large bone of the pelvic basin. (According to some anatomists, the psoas, part of a complex myofascial unit, is merely an upward extension of the iliacus.) Anything directly affecting psoas tone also affects, by way of the iliacus, the pelvis and its contents. Conversely, anything seriously influencing the iliacus affects psoas function.

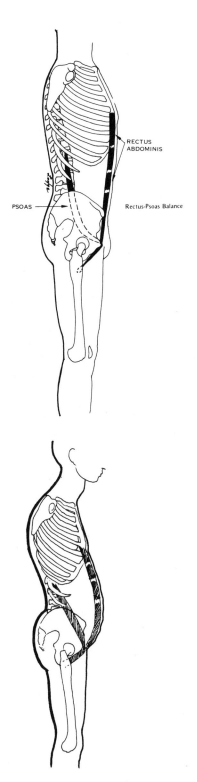

RECTUS ABDOMINIS

PSOAS

Rectus-Psoas Balance

7-12 Lateral view: Rectus-psoas balance (above) and imbalance (below). For clarity these schemata over-simplify the relation of psoas and rectus.

110

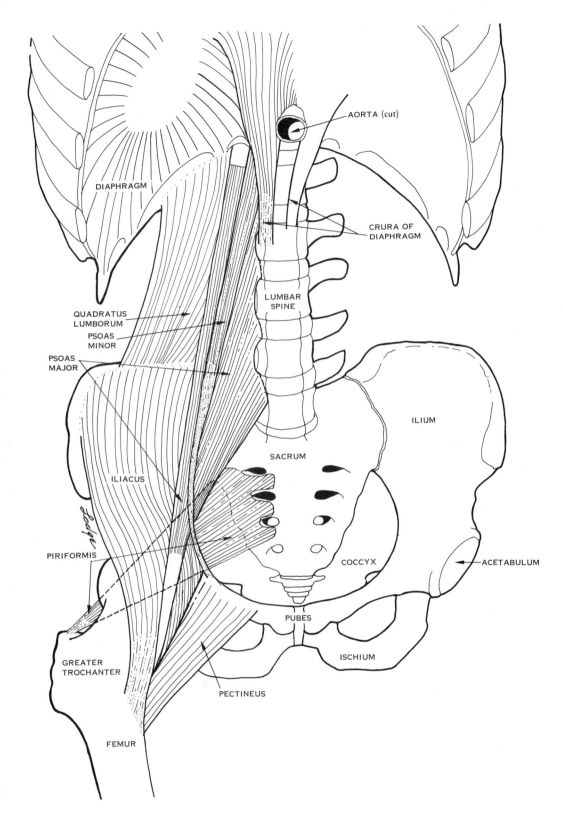

AORTA (cut)

DIAPHRAGM

CRURA OF
DIAPHRAGM

LUMBAR
SPINE

QUADRATUS
LUMBORUM

PSOAS
MINOR

PSOAS
MAJOR

ILIUM

SACRUM

ILIACUS

PIRIFORMIS

COCCYX

ACETABULUM

GREATER
TROCHANTER

PUBES

ISCHIUM

PECTINEUS

FEMUR

7-13

111

If a body is normal, the psoas should elongate during flexion and fall back toward the spine (Fig. 7-14). This seems illogical, but if your body has been integrated, you can verify it in yourself. By virtue of this, the normal psoas forms an important part of a supporting web holding the lumbar vertebrae appropriately spanned. By maintaining suitable distance between individual lumbar vertebrae, this prevertebral support assures length in the lumbar spine as a whole, irrespective of general body position. With the psoas functioning in this normal pattern, lengthening with every movement of flexion, the lumbar vertebrae cannot slip into the compression and misalignment that is the beginning of the "bad lower back." Serious anteriority of the lumbar spine must imply an incompetent or displaced psoas. The bulging anterior abdominal contour popularly referred to as a "bay window" tells the same story.

According to our observations, the psoas determines the structural position of the skeletal system. Through the latter, it must affect the physiological functioning of the viscera. The relation between the two nervous systems, the older autonomic and the newer spinal, is extremely complex and entails too much detail to be included in a book of this character. Stated in the simplest terms, the lumbar plexus is a spinal plexus embedded in the psoas, permitting intercommunication between the lumbar plexus and the spinal nerves which emerge from the spine where the psoas attaches (L1, 2, and 3 and portions of T12 and L4). Connections from the lumbar plexus to the autonomic system are extensive and intimate. Restricted movement or other mechanical interference in the psoas thus affects the general metabolic level, since this is monitored by the autonomic system as a whole.

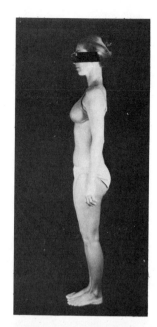

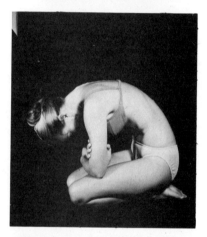

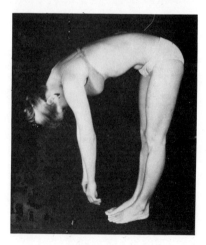

7-14 In an integrated body, the psoas falls back in flexion. This beautiful young woman, although well on her way, has not been fully aligned (as is evident in 1). Here it can be seen that a vertical defines the center of the head of the femur, shoulders and ears; the lower legs and feet do not fall on the line. It is clearly evident that the residual tension in this body is around the head of the femur and involves the rotators of the thigh, as indicated by the overlying glutei. In spite of this limitation, pictures 2 and 3 show the psoas falling back as the body flexes.

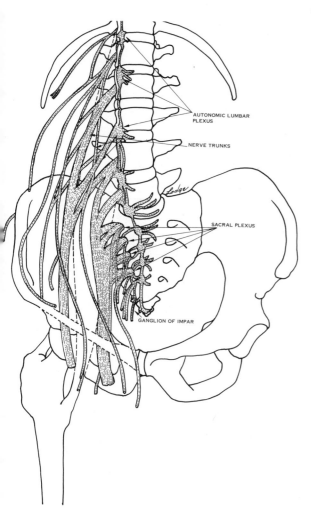

AUTONOMIC LUMBAR
PLEXUS

NERVE TRUNKS

Ledge

SACRAL PLEXUS

GANGLION OF IMPAR

7-15 Anterior view: Pictured here is part of the very important autonomic trunk and the lumbar plexus. The latter lies embedded in the surface of the psoas. It is clear that a change in vertebral relations or in psoas position will alter the location and tone of these nerve trunks and thereby affect their mechanism for physiological control. Structurally, the junction of lumbar and sacral areas is particularly vulnerable to distortion. Lumbago and sciatica are symptoms of structural disorganization of this area.

Along the anterior lateral surface of the entire spine lies the sympathetic trunk of the autonomic nervous system. This more archaic nerve unit is thought to be at a level below our voluntary control, although recent findings shed a certain doubt on this. It forms a series of ganglia that are centers integrating associated nervous elements. The great solar plexus, locus of the largest of these, is sometimes called the abdominal brain. It lies approximately at the level where psoas and diaphragm juxtapose. The lumbar plexus, with its network for visceral and muscular intercommunication, is the next lower neighbor and is embedded in the surface of the psoas itself. Structural weakness or metabolic insufficiency in the psoas thereby inevitably affects the lumbar plexus and its autonomic neighbors. If the psoas is inadequate, local nutritional exchange is disturbed, as is the metabolic rate in the lower digestive tract (specifically, basic elimination as well as food absorption). In other words, the message delivered by the common problem of constipation is a warning about the condition of the psoas and lumbar structure.

Good health in the lumbar plexus and its neighboring autonomic ganglia is basic to the well-being of man (Fig. 7-15). It contributes to adequate function in kidneys and adrenals through their nerve supply, and ensures effective metabolism in the reproductive system. The tone of the superficial muscles restraining the abdomen is controlled from this plexus (external oblique, internal oblique, transversus, rectus abdominis).

This is another circular situation. If the recti, through hyper- or hypotonicity, interfere with the optimal spatial position of the psoas, this reflects into the lumbar plexus and autonomic ganglia, affecting nutrition and tone of the abdominal muscles and viscera. Lowered muscular tone further shifts the psoas and, reciprocally, the rectus abdominis. Here we start a degenerating spiral, for under this spatial stress the psoas can no longer play its role of effectively supporting and guarding lumbar nervous structures. Psoas-recti balance is vital to the individual. Under Structural Integration a man himself recognizes this increasingly. As the tone of the psoas improves, the muscle can be felt objectively by palpation and subjectively through the individual's greater sense of sturdiness.

Psoas-recti balance is basic in the mechanics of walking as well as the idling activity of standing. As we said earlier, the psoas is a unique link between legs and upper torso. (The remaining portion of the link, psoas-rhomboid counterbalance across the lumbodorsal hinge, is discussed in connection with shoulder structure in Chapter 13. Effortless walking or standing implies a precise balance be-

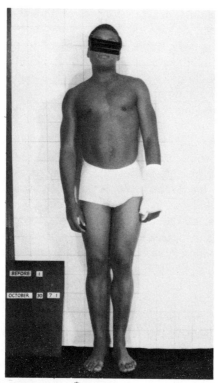
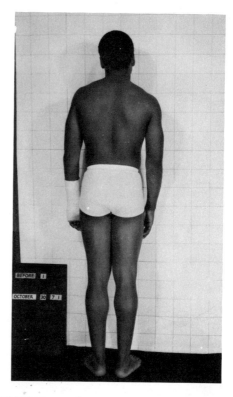

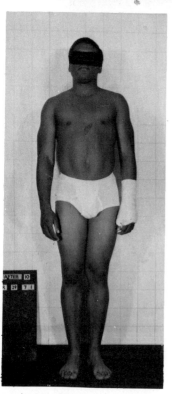
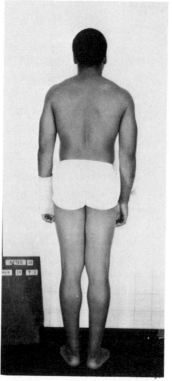

7-16 Mr. P's psoas revealed itself in moving, but an adequate psoas is also apparent in the standing man. Does re-examining the picture of this athlete suggest that his psoas may be shirking its job? In reality, the basic problem in this body is a distortion of the left psoas. His other body asymmetries are compensations.

If you do not see this at first, keep looking. You will soon notice (in the front view) the constriction and general lack of tone in the left groin. In the view of the back, you will see that his left hip seems forced back and that this shifts equilibrium throughout the body. Aberrative body patterns in the area of the groin always involve the psoas. Eventually, after ten hours of processing, the young man is very changed.

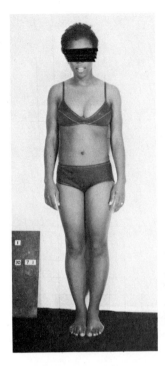
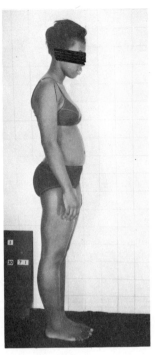
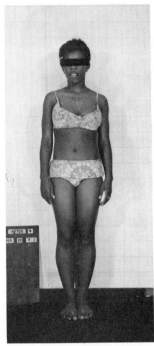
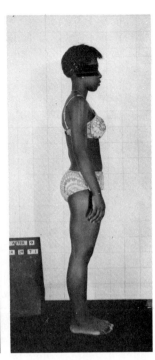

7-17 Here again, a beleaguered psoas cries its misery. This young woman's right psoas is obviously badly distorted. Her right lumbar spine lacks the supporting web of the psoas and has rotated, the transverse process is lying in a plane anterior to its left counterpart. Note especially the strain in the knees resulting from the more basic distortion in the groin.

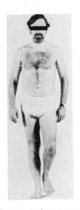
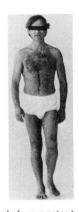

7-18 A man whose psoas is incompetent displays his problem in his gait. Mr. J here shows a wooden inflexibility over an area extending from waistline to midthigh. He seems to "carry" this area; it is not truly part of his walking. Instead, he walks with his shoulders and knees. The change as his body becomes better aligned is apparent in the second photograph, taken after processing (and after he shaved his beard).

tween legs and torso. Only a well-structured psoas can act effectively in this axis.

If the psoas lacks competence, its failure immediately becomes apparent in body contour and movement. A shortened psoas allows the ribcage to tip downward and forward under the pull of the recti, automatically making the rhomboids incompetent. There are two levels at which this is manifested most clearly. A deteriorated psoas, glued down as it crosses the pelvic brim, chronically flexes the body at the level of the groin, so that it prevents truly erect posture. Inappropriate span—too much or too little—in either psoas or rectus shows in a groin contour that seems inadequate—too compressed, and therefore insecure. This can be seen easily even through clothing. To the extent that the psoas tendon improves or its movement is freed, the groin broadens, becomes more solid. The iliacus, through the common tendon, also eases, lessening the inward drag on the pelvic basin and removing strain on muscles attaching to the anterior superior spine of the ilium. The upper trunk now fits into a more custom-made pelvic rocking chair. A beleaguered psoas cries aloud (Fig. 7-16). Its situation leaves clues throughout the lower body (Fig. 7-17). The individual's gait bears witness, since the psoas, together with the gluteals, determines primary leg movement (Fig. 7-18). (This is apparent from the illustrations and will be discussed in Chapter 9 at greater length.)

If psoas and recti are really sharing the load, any and all body movements involving flexion *allow the abdominal wall to fall back.* Although this seems illogical, it is nevertheless true. In normal, balanced flexion, the psoas does not shorten, does not bulge forward; it lengthens and falls back within the abdomen (Fig. 7-20). Because we see so few bodies with normal psoas function, we tend to think that in flexion the lower abdominal wall necessarily shortens and thickens. In fact, however, a normal psoas lengthens. The rectus abdominis—in other words, the abdominal wall—falls back.

You can test your own psoas by following these directions: Lie flat on your back on the floor. Now draw up your legs, preferably both together, dragging your heels and keeping them together (Fig. 7-21). Does the small of your back arch up? If it does, be aware that your psoas is not really able to take over its proper job.

Try this: Still lying on the floor, *just* turn the end of your spine under you. Now lift. Where is your abdominal wall? Heaping up into a mound? Now lie down with your lower back flat on the floor, starting with your waistline (as we define it, your waistline is the small of your back, your second lumbar vertebra). Where is your belly wall now? Is it falling back? If it is, your psoas is listening to you and has started to work. Only through balance can this movement happen. As you get up from this position and stand upright, what happens to your abdomen? What happens to your waistline? Can you find it? Now, can you voluntarily bring it back? If you're having trouble finding your waistline (at the back, not the front, of your body), try shifting your weight to your heels. As your psoas begins to answer your demand (it may if you shift your weight), you can become aware of your waistline, especially the *back* of your waistline.

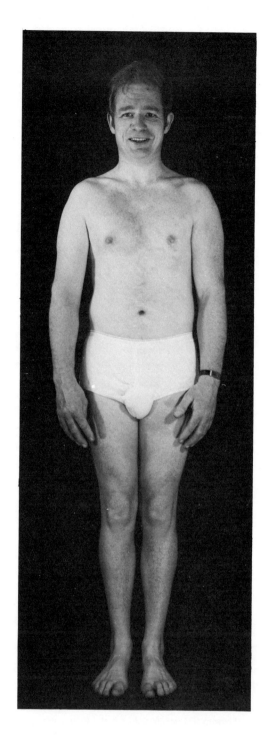

7-19 The psoas becomes more competent after processing through consistent reciprocal activity of psoas and recti in all body and leg movement. The groin area flattens and widens with movement. The picture is one of greater support: the trunk begins to fit over the legs; the torso loses its chronic flexion and allows the ideal horizontals to be seen.

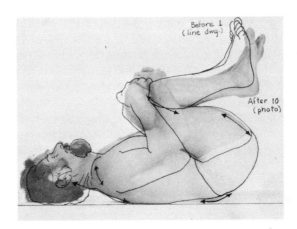

7-20 Arrows indicate areas of greater extension. The outline of a Before 1 photograph of Mr. J has been superimposed on an After 10 photograph, showing the change not only in the contour but also in the movement excursion after integration. Note that the photograph clearly shows better balance of body masses (especially apparent in the head and neck). Before processing, he seemed able to draw his knees closer to his chest, but this excessive flexion reflects poor psoas structure. As the psoas becomes better balanced, the excursion of the leg is lessened as body masses in general become better balanced.

There is also a more advanced test for psoas competence, but it is apt to confuse beginners. Lie on your back and extend your legs skyward. What happens to the belly wall (the recti abdominis) as you flex in this way? Probably it shortens, thickens, hardens, and mounds up. Any gymnast will tell you this is normal. He'll say, "This is the way it is; this is the way the recti behave. This is their function, this is normal." But we take exception to this statement. We say it is *average*, not normal; it is the random pattern. This mounding of the abdomen means that the psoas has been overwhelmed by the recti. When competent psoas-rectus reciprocity exists, you can raise your legs to a vertical position with no hardening of the recti. When you can do this, your psoas muscles have passed their Ph.D. examinations —they are competent for their complex job.

Competence in any field, muscular or otherwise, is ex-

7-21 In a balanced body, as the legs are drawn up, the waistline falls back. In other words, the coccyx and apex (lower end) of the sacrum turn under, the base (upper end) of the sacrum and lumbar spine fall back toward the ground. Both psoas and recti abdominis are falling back, as seen in the relaxation of the adjustment in the gluteal group to accommodate this position, although this is not so apparent in the photograph. When the body can accept this position, the entire spinal length and the muscles of the pelvis seem to decompress and become sturdier.

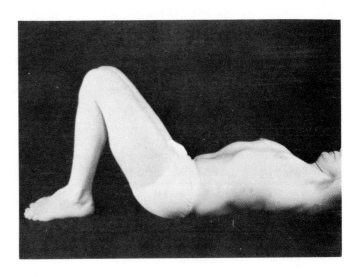

pressed in beauty and characterized by grace. Psoas quality manifests itself in stance and gait. Standing, which is the zero limit of balanced movement, makes demands on the psoas. In moving, walking or flexing, the abdominal surface (obliques as well as recti) adjusts with the easy, resilient sliding that characterizes free muscles. In movement, walking or flexing, we reiterate, the belly wall does not billow forward or slump forward—it falls back. This elicits a sophisticated grace of movement that, in a dancer, is a delight; in the average workaday citizen, it is a benchmark of personal excellence that gives him unending satisfaction as well as physical ease. He becomes aware of himself as an integrated man—he and his body are one.

Sadly enough, the psoas is too often unable to play a suitable part. In the random individual, it tends to be structurally retired, glued to the pelvic brim. It does not participate in the gait of the average person. Athletic training emphasizes repetitious movement of outer muscles at the expense of the inner (intrinsic); the psoas, more central to the body than the rectus abdominis, succumbs more rapidly to inappropriate exercise. In walking, skiing, dancing—any motor activity of the legs—the average man will flex by shortening the rectus femoris. Abdication of the psoas in favor of either the rectus femoris or the rectus abdominis is undesirable. The structure as well as the function of the psoas is unique; no other myofascial element can substitute satisfactorily. Some strands originate in the trunk itself at the lateral margin of the twelfth dorsal vertebra. By the time the muscle attaches at the lesser trochanter of the femur (thigh), it has reinforced the lumbar spine, traversed the pelvis, and crossed the pubes. In this way, the psoas unifies torso with thigh. Sturdy, balanced walking (in which the leg is flexed through activation of the psoas, not of the rectus femoris) thus involves the entire body at its core level. In such walking, each step is initiated at the twelfth dorsal vertebra, not in the legs; the legs move subsequently. Let us be clear about this: *the legs do not originate movement in the walk of a balanced body; the legs support and follow. Movement is initiated in the trunk and transmitted to the legs through the medium of the psoas.*

A random walk not only puts strain on crooked legs, it also pulls the diaphragm into the act. Tough fascial structures of the diaphragm, in supporting the ribcage, require their own "horizontals." To maintain these, the body block (that is, the thorax) must be able to act independently of lower-lying structures. This requires competent adjustment at the lumbodorsal junction and underscores the importance of the psoas-rhomboid balance, which makes this possible (see Chapter 13).

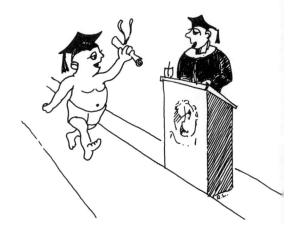

7-22

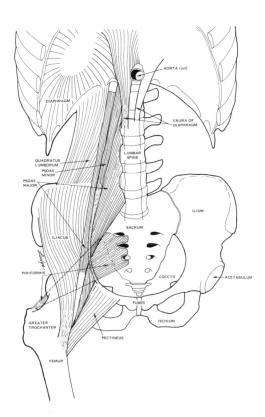

7-23 Anterior view: Notice the proximity of psoas and diaphragm. Obviously any weakness or problem in either will affect the other.

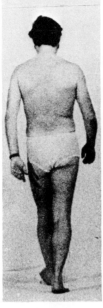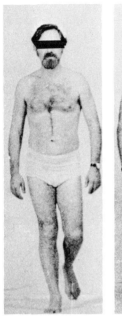

7-24 In a random body, the psoas is often inadequate. In these photographs of Mr. J walking, the wooden stiffness of his body between waistline and midthigh (the length of the psoas) is especially clear from the back. Instead of initiating leg movement with his psoas, he picks up his feet by shortening his rectus femoris. He is apt to walk with his shoulders as well as his knees.

Ribs, individually and collectively, have a large part in determining the respiratory pattern through their structural location and through reflex stimulation. Tying the diaphragm to the movement of lower-lying structures by an incompetent lumbodorsal junction interferes with rib function and therefore with respiration. The diaphragm attaches to lumbar vertebrae (1L, 2L, 3L), and thus lies adjacent to psoas fibers. During a lifetime, stresses of many sorts occur, and psoas and diaphragm, like myofascial neighbors throughout the body, may thicken and glue together, destroying their individual freedom of movement. Any such consolidation of fibers interferes with the normal pattern of breathing or of walking. This is sad, for respiration and the muscular interplays of balanced walking are, by design, a perfect and complete exercise.

Normal, balanced walking calls for a progression of the knee joint straight forward and straight back. After all, you intend to move the body-as-a-whole straight forward. Is it logical that your knee should describe the arc of a circle? Only the kind of flexion that features an active psoas allows this straight-forward, straight-back motion (assuming knee and ankle joints are straight). Interference of any sort with the independence of the psoas—whether from diaphragm, rectus abdominis, or rectus femoris—destroys the pattern.

Average, random walking is a very different movement (Fig. 7-24). It expresses the average poor posture and gives leg muscles a job for which they are not designed. This is the origin of so much of the trouble housed in the legs of middle-aged and elderly people. When the activity of the rectus abdominis or the rectus femoris overwhelms a dormant psoas, the adjustment in the rotators of the gluteal region is also much changed. In the random pattern, the individual "picks up" his knee (by activation of rectus femoris). The knee describes a rotational, circular motion that is exacerbated by badly shortened hamstrings.

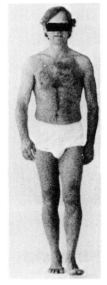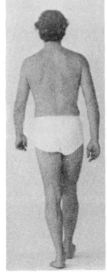

7-25 After Integration, when his psoas is activated in every movement, Mr. J's walk has changed. No longer does he walk by swinging his rotated femur around its head. The femur moves straight forward; the adjustment occurs around its head. In picking up his knee, he initiates action with the psoas. This brings his "waistline" (upper lumbar spine) back. There is a joyful lift to his body.

That the aberrated pattern is so widespread is understandable. It has been· inculcated from early childhood: "Pick up your feet," say Mama, Papa, and Uncle Ned. Johnny obediently responds by shortening his rectus femoris and iliotibial tract—that is to say, he picks up his feet. Neighboring hamstrings participate. By the time Johnny is an older walking individual, he is trapped in an inefficient gait that successfully bypasses the psoas and prevents its participation. Every step he takes involves activity in a great many muscles that should not be in action. In the baby, extrinsic* muscles comprise the bulk of the myofascia and seemingly are easier for the infant to reach. In any individual at any age, extrinsics are more readily accessible to consciousness than the intrinsics. Therefore, it is entirely understandable that the child will meet demands from adults by way of this pattern, which is more available to him even though it is more wasteful of energy. He thus expends an energy store that might better be used for more creative purposes, but at this age he can afford the waste.

In the random gait, the femur rotates in the hip joint, which is held rigid. In the more appropriate muscular economy, the pelvis is free to rotate around the femur. The normal pattern (involving the psoas), activates the lumbar and sacral plexi; an aberrant gait bypasses this. This is the inevitable result when lifting the knee is the primary movement in walking. When our little Johnny "picks up" his foot (and knee), consciously or not he must hold the pelvis rigid as he lifts the weight of his leg. And the result of this? The man who has a vested personal interest in gym work will show you with pride his capacious abdominal wall and bulging thighs. He will invite your admiration by punching it to test its hardness. "You see," he says, "you are

---

*Standard medical nomenclature defines *intrinsic* as *situated entirely within or pertaining exclusively to a part*. Thus, the intrinsic muscles of the tongue are those entirely within the structure of the tongue (uperior, inferior, transverse, and vertical linguinalis). We have used intrinsic and its correlate, extrinsic, to denote, respectively, muscular elements that are invested in the deepest fascial layers of the body (intrinsics), and their paired antagonists (or cooperators), the extrinsics, which are more superficial, occupy greater volume, and are more directly and obviously subject to the plastic changes of the integrative technique.

We have found it both convenient and logical to use this nomenclature in describing what is a functional rather than a descriptive parameter. Relatively little organized work has been done mapping the unexplored territory of fascial anatomy. Time and research in the future will certainly define these terms more clearly as scientific attention in the biological field focuses on the dynamic rather than the static aspects of humans.

wrong about bay windows. This one is pure muscle, not fat." Yes, it is pure muscle. Too much pure, rigid recti abdominis, obliques, and transversi. He does not have the leaven that could give him grace and the ability to accommodate to the demand of moving and living. Instead, his bay window exists as a mass of unyielding and too, too solid flesh. This is just as true of the ballet dancer. She will show you with pride her hard, muscular, overdeveloped thighs, the product of much concentrated effort. And most dancers will ruefully acknowledge the price they pay for all this overdeveloped rectus femoris—the price of restricted walking, early arthritis, "dancer's hip," etc.

What could change this picture is an adequate, functioning, competent psoas. When the psoas participates, walking is a peerless body organizer. Walking is primarily a locomotor function; secondarily, if psoas and rhomboids are included in the movement, its alternating flexion and extension contribute to basic physiologic processes. The freely moving psoas and rhomboids, supported by a mobile lumbar spine and adequate lumbodorsal junction, spell health in the pelvic plexi.

I sometimes wonder about overdeveloped athletes. Adequate plexi at lumbar and sacral levels express themselves in normal elimination. But in the man with a bay window, the hazard posed by his weak lumbar spine (and related plexi) is ever-present. Someday he will come to know about it consciously: he will develop symptoms. For that physical, muscular hardness, his pride and joy, is a shoring up against an underlying structural inadequacy, his anterior lumbar spine. It is as though his body, through this hardening, is attempting to reinforce its weakness by splinting itself. For a while this may be effective, but not forever.

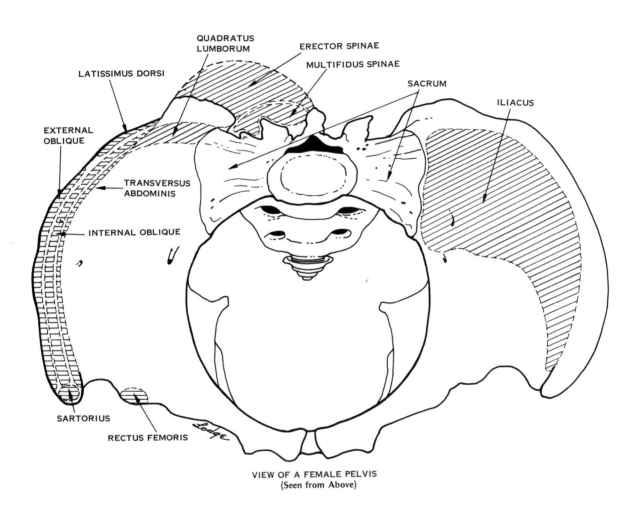

QUADRATUS
LUMBORUM

ERECTOR SPINAE

MULTIFIDUS SPINAE

LATISSIMUS DORSI

SACRUM

ILIACUS

EXTERNAL
OBLIQUE

TRANSVERSUS
ABDOMINIS

INTERNAL OBLIQUE

SARTORIUS

RECTUS FEMORIS

VIEW OF A FEMALE PELVIS
(Seen from Above)

8-1 View of a female pelvis, seen from above.

8
The Pelvis Has Many Facets

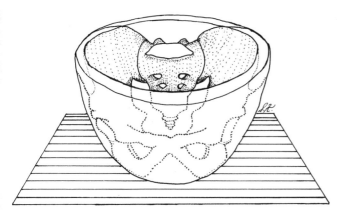

8-2 The pelvis is a bony basin.

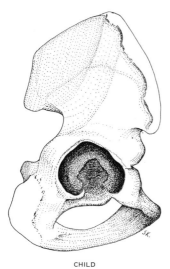

CHILD

Lateral View

8-3 Components of the pelvis. While the function of the bony pelvis can be summarized as that of a bony basin, it should be remembered that the development is from several smaller bones. Lateral views show the fashion in which these bones coalesce to form the pelvis and how the relative size of the individual segments alter and shift to form the pelvis from child to adult.

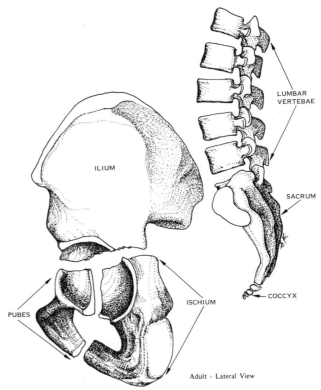

LUMBAR VERTEBAE

ILIUM

SACRUM

PUBES

ISCHIUM

COCCYX

Adult - Lateral View

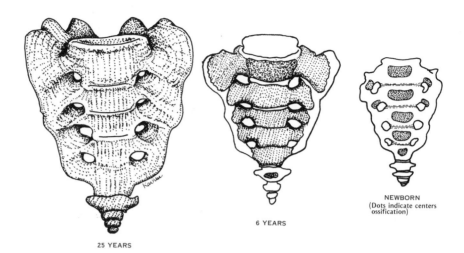

25 YEARS

6 YEARS

NEWBORN
(Dots indicate centers
ossification)

The simplified overview of the body and its keystone, the pelvis, must now be superseded. The newer model we describe has a greater depth and is a more finely tuned mechanism. Eventually a body must be recognized as an outer structure balancing an inner, an extrinsic structure balancing an intrinsic. This picture requires detailed understanding of what lies deeper, a realization of how deep ligamentous, tendinous, and other deep fascial structures balance softer outer tissue.

Even at this greater depth, the pelvis is still, as the anatomists have said, primarily a bony basin. But the pelvis is more complex and is constructed of several parts, several separate bones. Finally, the incomplete basin formed by these individual bones is closed and completed by the sacrum. The pelvis, like the sacrum, is a consolidation. In the young child, the three parts are still separate, united only by ligamentous bonds. Later, in adolescence, they fuse to make the adult pelvis. They are called, respectively, the ilium (os iliae), the pubic bone (os pubis), and the ischium (os ischii).

Adult bones are formed through the fusion of segments originally laid down as cartilage in the embryo, later developing to more mature bone in the young child and adolescent. The sacrum is such a unit. In the adult, to all appearances it constitutes a single bone, triangular in shape. This apparently single unit is a base for the spine. It is formed by fusion during early childhood of five separate segments. If the pelvis is to be seen as a single, closed bony basin, the sacrum must be included as part of it. Manifestly, this bone is not only part of the pelvic basin, it is also an important constituent of the vertebral column. Thus pelvis and spine together form one basic central structure. It is clear that strains from either end will peak at the level of

8-4 Anterior view: The Sacrum. Like the pelvis, it develops through the fusion of segments. The similarity of sacral segments to vertebral units is clear. Note also how the coccyx is proportionately shorter as the individual matures.

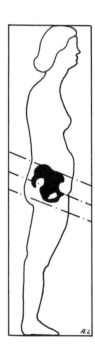

8-5 Here is the aberrated pelvis of a random body. Tipping of the pelvis is not limited to any one body type. Compare this with the following illustration in terms of stance, the way thigh and leg transmit weight, and the pattern in which the neck balances lower-lying aberrations. (This is Ms. F, pictured previously in Chapters Six and Seven).

124

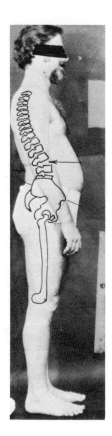

greatest structural weakness, usually the lower lumbar spine (at the fourth or fifth lumbar vertebra), just above the sacrum. Stress of any sort directed into a part may become manifest as serious pain and functional incapacity. Such is the usual history of the ubiquitous lower-back syndrome. Stress here is a functional complaint advertising a structural weakness.

If stress is to be relieved, it is important that no myofascial component contributing to pelvic balance be overlooked. In addition to the abductors and adductors of the thigh already considered, other muscle groups also participate in pelvic movement—hamstrings, the gluteal group (maximus, medius, and minimus), and the so-called rotators underlying the gluteus maximus. Together, they are a bridge between the ischial structure of the pelvis (sacrum and hipbone) and the thigh. Hamstrings, in that they attach below the knee, weave the leg itself into a web connecting lower extremities and spine. All these myofascial elements determine pelvic position; in so doing they unrelentingly create or limit pelvic freedom.

8-6 Forward tipping of pelvis and sacrum place heavy strain on the entire vertebral column. In the body pictured here, the strain is transmitted to the lumbar area. As in any lordosis, some individual vertebrae are wedged apart, some crowded together. Compensations will show as rotations in individual veterbrae.

As the individual grows older and is subjected to various strains, too much stress may be transmitted to the sacroiliac articulation by way of the ilia or lumbar vertebrae. This may be more or less severe — a chronic dull ache or the screaming intensity of acute displacement. But all lower back pain is a sensory report of this type of structural strain.

ROTATORS

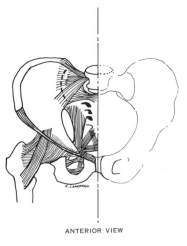

ANTERIOR VIEW

8-7

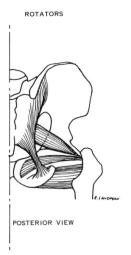

POSTERIOR VIEW

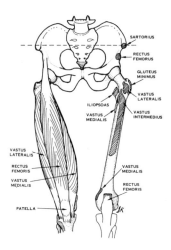

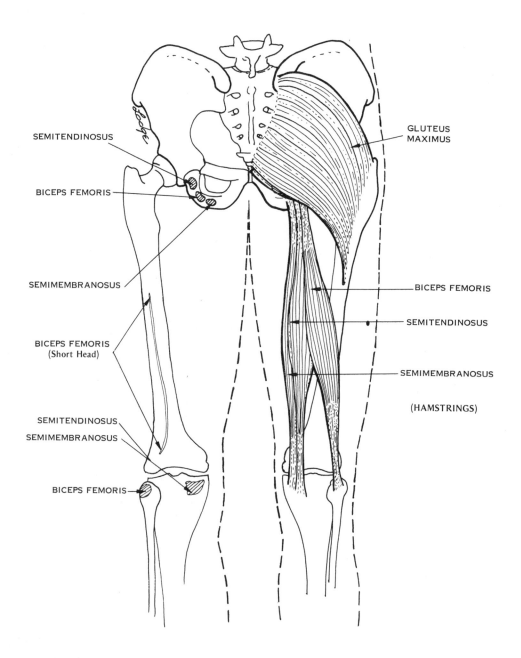

SEMITENDINOSUS

BICEPS FEMORIS

SEMIMEMBRANOSUS

BICEPS FEMORIS
(Short Head)

SEMITENDINOSUS
SEMIMEMBRANOSUS

BICEPS FEMORIS

GLUTEUS
MAXIMUS

BICEPS FEMORIS

SEMITENDINOSUS

SEMIMEMBRANOSUS

(HAMSTRINGS)

8-8 Posterior view: The hamstrings and gluteus maximus. The hamstrings are among the most powerful muscles of the body. They traverse the back of the thigh, joining the pelvis (ischial tuberosity) to the leg below the knee. They shorten and thicken as a result of overemphasis on leg exercise. Some degenerative diseases, particularly arthritis, modify their chemistry. It is clear that these three hamstrings, in such close proximity to one another, may become "glued" together, losing independent movement by shortening. When this happens, the contour of the back of the leg at midthigh bulges.

When these muscles shorten from any cause, freedom in both knee and hip joint is lost and the lower limb becomes stiff and sometimes painful in movement. Hamstrings are overlaid by the gluteus maximus, which reinforces and protects them. Only the attachments of the hamstrings are shown at left, emphasizing the mechanism by which they act. In this posterior view of the gluteus maximus and hamstrings, the areas of attachment are shown on the left leg.

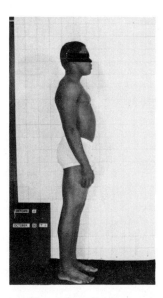

8-9 Shortened hamstrings are easy to spot; bulging contours on the back of Mr. P's thigh betray them. According to the ideas of standard physical education, such bulging contours indicate strength. According to Structural Integration, they are manifestations of imbalance and restricted movement — the beginning of weakness, not strength.

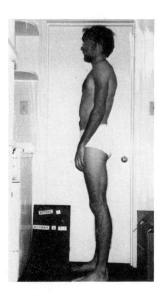

8-10 The bulging contour from the back of this thigh indicates that this young man, although structurally very different from Mr. P is also suffering from shortened hamstrings. Note how the knee and lower leg are pulled backward to accommodate these, and how the area between knee and pelvis is rotated asymmetrically. This indicates that the hamstring distortion is greater in one leg than in the other.

The function of bone, any bone, is to serve as a sophisticated, curved, thrusting bar, holding softer myofascial tissue apart. The position of the pelvic bones makes possible subtle, effectively directed tendinous and ligamentous pulls. Nowhere else in the body is this function to be seen as clearly as in the surfaces of the "hipbones," the ilia. The overwhelming importance of the pelvis, which is stressed throughout this work, becomes clear once its potential for determining balance by directing thrust and muscular pull is appreciated. The three-dimensional realities of the word *balance* become more evident. The Tantric assumption that the pelvis is the seat of the soul becomes more plausible. Be that as it may, it is certain that no soul can be really comfortably seated in a three-dimensional world without the appropriate contribution of the pelvis.

Chapter 7 has examined many of the elastic (or, too often, inelastic) attachments of both ilia and pubes. Up to this point, however, we have given no consideration to the very important group of muscles originating on the ischium. In English, these are called the hamstrings; in German, they are the *Gesässmuskel* and attach to the *Sitzbeine*. Recognizing that these words mean, respectively, "sitting muscle" and "sitting bone" gives a new understanding of comfortable sitting and its dependence on hamstrings.

Specifically, the term hamstrings applies to three important muscles (semimembranosus, semitendinosus, and biceps femoris) that bind the pelvis (at the ischial tuberosity) to the leg (below the knee). The adductor magnus also functions as a hamstring. Their tendons are visible as tough, inflexible, round bands along the sides of the knee joint. Hamstrings are especially prominent in athletically inclined men (Fig. 8-9). In these athletes, they tend to look and feel like steel cables and have almost as little resilience.

At the level of the hip, the hamstrings are covered by a big, fan-shaped muscular pad (gluteus maximus), which cushions us against a tough world. Those who think nature has been too generous in their endowment of cushion complain loudly. But their dissatisfaction lacks the bitterness of people less affluent in this respect; poorly cushioned ischia, when seated on a chair or bleacher seat, feel like raw, unprotected bones. Like all muscles, the gluteus maximus depends for its shape and position on the fascia of adjacent structures, even sometimes of structures very far afield. When, for example, the ankle is reorganized in Structural Integration, the gluteus may often be seen reorienting itself. Or if the gluteus is too tightly bound, it thrusts the femoral head, even the leg itself, out of line, transmitting strain to all lower structures. Applying energy—directional pressure and appropriate movement—at the contracted fascial

127

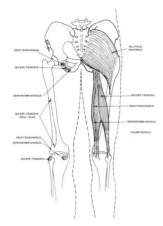

8-11

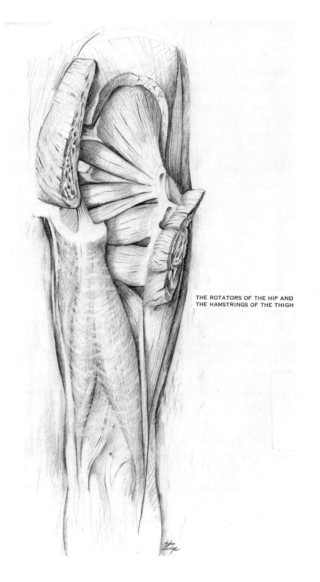

THE ROTATORS OF THE HIP AND
THE HAMSTRINGS OF THE THIGH

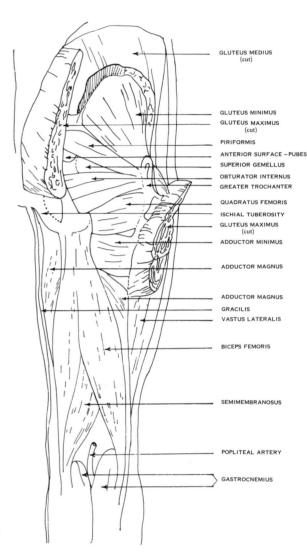

GLUTEUS MEDIUS
(cut)

GLUTEUS MINIMUS

GLUTEUS MAXIMUS
(cut)

PIRIFORMIS

ANTERIOR SURFACE – PUBES

SUPERIOR GEMELLUS

OBTURATOR INTERNUS

GREATER TROCHANTER

QUADRATUS FEMORIS

ISCHIAL TUBEROSITY

GLUTEUS MAXIMUS
(cut)

ADDUCTOR MINIMUS

ADDUCTOR MAGNUS

ADDUCTOR MAGNUS

GRACILIS

VASTUS LATERALIS

BICEPS FEMORIS

SEMIMEMBRANOSUS

POPLITEAL ARTERY

GASTROCNEMIUS

8-12 Posterior views: These schemata of the hamstrings and rotators emphasize the mechanism of "gluing." Individual muscles are encased in fascia, and groups of muscles are encased again in containing and restricting myofascial sheaths. Given the tendency of fascial sheaths to glue together when they are in trouble, the knots and thickenings that can be palpated below the skin become understandable.

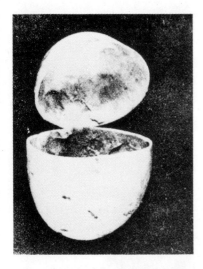

8-13 **This photograph shows the egg - shaped deposit of hardened exudate formed around a point at which air and oil have been injected into fascial tissue. This pouch, from a rat, shows both inner and outer surfaces and great regularity of thickness if its wall. In any adult body, hardened areas of this sort can be felt in palpation. Fascial tissue responds to stress or other tissue insult in various ways, "gluing" being one of the most frequent. (From Selye, THE STRESS OF LIFE, Fig 3; After H. Selye, courtesy of the** *Journal of the American Medical Association.)*

attachment on the femur can return the gluteal group to greater flexibility and more effective function. Then the overendowed in terms of hips find themselves happy to be more "contained"; the formerly underprivileged note with delight that their "sitting bones" are now feeling protected from the unrelenting world.

The hamstrings, which underlie the gluteals, arise from the ischial tuberosity of the pelvis. These myofascial units are particularly prone to chronic shortening. Their vulnerability, especially in arthritics, creates problems. They are powerful flexors of the knee, perhaps the most powerful flexors in the body. The gymnastics and calisthenics used in our culture for strengthening the legs and/or abdomen contribute to shortening, thickening, and "gluing" the fascial wrappings of these hamstrings one on the other (or even on the adductor that is their closest neighbor, the adductor magnus). Sometimes just by looking at a body, constrictions resulting from the gluing process can be clearly seen.

"Gluing" is an interesting phenomenon. In practically all bodies, in one muscle or another, small lumps or thickened, nonresilient bands can be felt deep in the tissue. The lumps may be as small as small peas or as large as walnuts; the bands may be one or even two inches in length. They apparently form when the fascial envelope of one muscle attaches itself to a neighboring fascial surface. How this happens is unclear; perhaps the "glue" is a dried exudate secreted in healing a muscle trauma; possibly it results from imperfect healing when a virus has attacked a muscle or tendon. Hans Selye's book *The Stress of Life* shows pictures of sacs about the size of walnuts resulting from artificially introducing air into fascial sheaths (Fig. 8-13). Some similarly injurious process no doubt gives rise to the lumpy knottings we have noted.

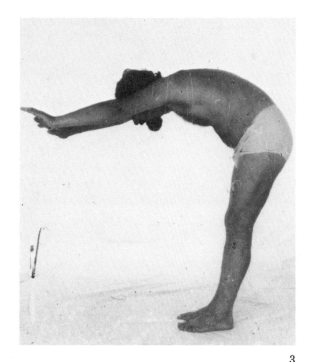

3

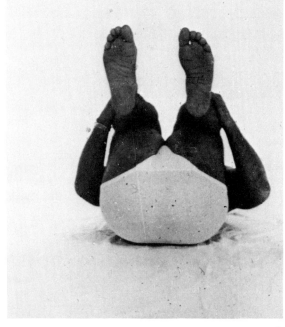

2

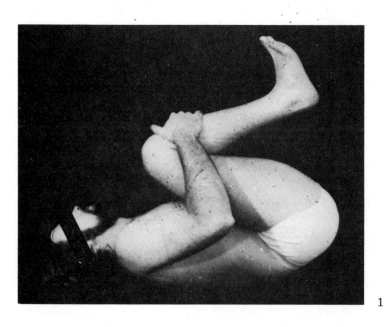

1

8-14 When hamstrings are too short and inelastic, flexion becomes difficult. As a body flexes at the groin, it should give a picture of widening across the sacral and buttock area; any other picture promises trouble. In 1, not only are the knees unable to meet the chest, but the short neck becomes shorter and pulls into the shoulders. Pictures 2 and 6 emphasize how the knees pull apart to accommodate the short hamstrings. In 3, the compensation shows chiefly in the knees and lower legs. Numbers 4 and 5 also show how, in bending, the legs accommodate to shortened hamstrings; in both, the hamstrings have distorted the knees and seriously imbalanced leg support;

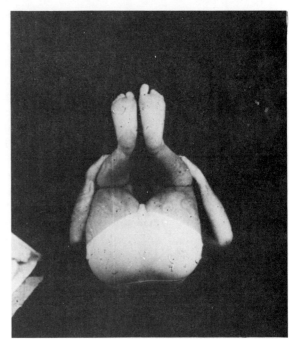

6

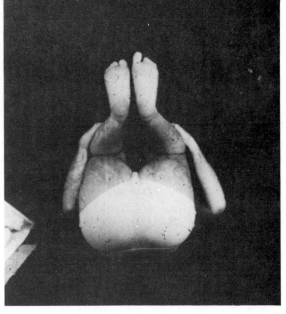

5

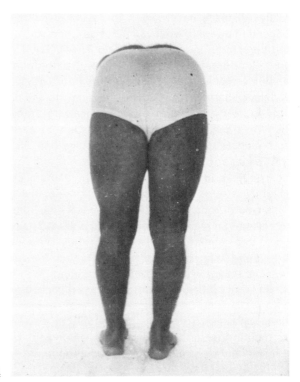

4

Shortened hamstrings bring many penalties. Their chronic thickening causes discomfort in sitting; there is always too thick a pad between leg and chair. The tendency of people to cross their legs is a way of relieving this kind of strain. In standing as well as in sitting, they unbalance the knees, which then are never comfortable; the joint feels too short and too compressed. The hamstrings arise on the ischial tuberosity and insert below the knee. When they are short, the joint is compressed or, worse, rotated. The individual who is unable to touch his toes or the floor in flexing is probably suffering from shortened hamstrings (Fig. 8-15). More significant than the problem at the knee is the sense of compression in the pelvis from the increasing ischial tug when chronically thick hamstrings are unable spontaneously to lengthen. In this case, when the body flexes, the buttocks (glutei) rotate instead of widening, further compressing the ischial structure. As a body flexes at the groin, it should give a picture of widening across the sacral and buttock area; any other picture promises trouble.

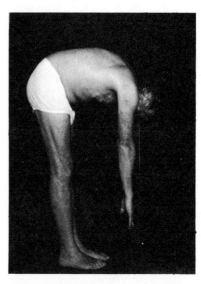

8-15 This kind of flexion emphasizes shortcomings of the hamstring group.

Do you want to test your own hamstring function? It's simple: Lie on your back. Flex your knees upward as far as they'll go, keeping them together. Do they touch, or even approach, your chest? Good; you're better than average. How does your lower back feel as you flex your knees? Does it widen, or does it seem to pull together? Don't settle for the irresponsible shrug and "I can't feel a thing." You can, really. All that's necessary is to devote a few minutes to becoming aware of what you perceive when you stop pushing perception away from consciousness. Try it; you may well be surprised. Perhaps you feel that the part of your anatomy that you just sit on is unimportant. Whether it widens or narrows as you flex is a minor detail concerning only yourself and your tailor. Cosmetically this may be true. But functionally the behavior of the lowest part of your spine and its attachments is unbelievably significant to you.

The second common picture of pelvic disorganization appears in the sacrum itself. The sacrum can rotate (slightly) around its own vertical axis (a sagittal rotation). This type of rotation can be determined by palpation. One lateral margin of the sacrum seems too deep. The other may seem to be a mere superficial bony ridge. These sacra may be slightly painful to the touch; in this pain, they record the tension under which they are struggling. Well-balanced sacra seem covered and protected by a fairly thick, resilient, myofascial pad. Sacra under strain lose this elastic pad; their pad seems stringy and inadequate; it may even seem as though the surface of the bone lies immediately under the skin and lacks elastic protection altogether.

People who have these types of problems are apt to be

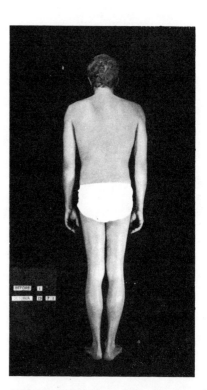

8-16 Most distortions of the sacrum consist in a forward displacement of the bone itself. A posterior displacement is also possible, as shown in this picture.

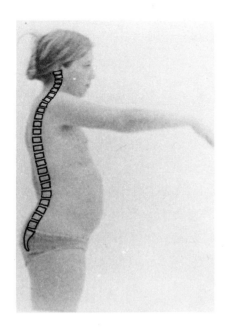

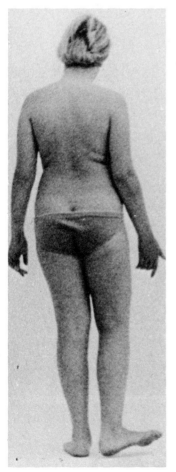

complaining of pain from time to time, and this is under-standable. Any such displacements give rise to primary tensions throughout the lower half of the body. The upper body, lacking balanced support, generally shows tension as well, even though it may be secondary and seem unrelated.

Very often, the sagittal rotation of the sacrum allows the sacrum as a whole to move anteriorly. This happens more often to women, but it also occurs in men. In reference to the resulting lack of support, the body attempts to reinforce the lower area, and the result is the wide-hipped figure of Fig. 8-17.

The sacrum, like all bony members of the spinal-pelvic complex, is balanced by the myofascial webbing of post- and prevertebral muscles and ligaments. The weight of the upper body tends to force the upper part of the sacrum (its so-called base) forward. Its apex and the upper coccyx may or may not compensate by rotating backward. Very strong ligaments bind the sacrum in place; their function is to resist these rotational tendencies. An interosseous sacroiliac ligament unites ilium and sacrum. This is reinforced by the sacrotuberous ligaments. In myofascial health, this pair weaves a joint of great strength that holds the sacrum fast against lateral rotation. The sacrospinous and sacrotuberous ligaments resist the tendency of the base of the sacrum to rotate forward. The anterior surface of the sacrum is lined by the piriformis, a member of the rotator group. Therefore, through the piriformis muscle, deviation of the sacrum is transmitted as strain to the rotators of the thigh. A sacrum that is too deep, either unilaterally or bilaterally, causes as well as reflects inadequate support from the related rotators. Imbalanced rotators transmit disparate support; one or both femurs (together with the legs) will then be aberrated. Sagittal rotation of the sacrum can be and usually is passed along to the neighboring coccyx, for the coccyx depends on the sacrum and its ligaments for even, balanced suspension. The pelvic floor in turn reflects support from the coccyx.

8-17 So-called soft bodies usually reflect lack of support from the sacrum. The sacrum as a whole may have moved anteriorly, or it may have tipped so that the upper part is anterior with respect to the lower part. In this girl, the base of the sacrum has been displaced forward.

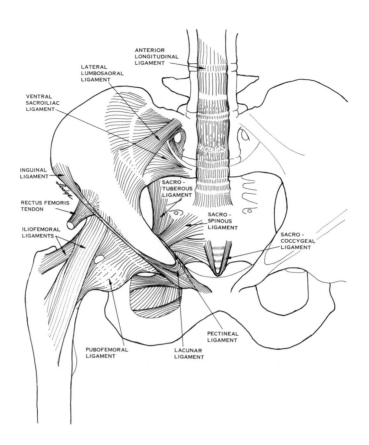

ANTERIOR LONGITUDINAL LIGAMENT

LATERAL LUMBOSAORAL LIGAMENT

VENTRAL SACROILIAC LIGAMENT

INGUINAL LIGAMENT

RECTUS FEMORIS TENDON

ILIOFEMORAL LIGAMENTS

SACRO-TUBEROUS LIGAMENT

SACRO-SPINOUS LIGAMENT

SACRO-COCCYGEAL LIGAMENT

PUBOFEMORAL LIGAMENT

LACUNAR LIGAMENT

PECTINEAL LIGAMENT

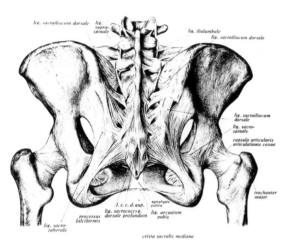

8-18 Anterior view at left; posterior view at right: The functional reality of the pelvis is not in the bony basin but in the tough, myofascial web of ligaments that connect the bones, prevertebral as well as postvertebral; These ligaments, in offering attachment for muscles, determine structural balance in the legs as well as throughout the body. (Posterior view from Sobotta, ATLAS OF HUMAN ANATOMY , Vol. 1, Fig. 259)

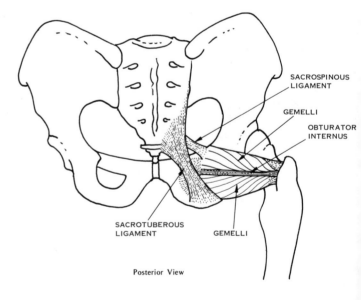

SACROSPINOUS LIGAMENT

GEMELLI

OBTURATOR INTERNUS

SACROTUBEROUS LIGAMENT

GEMELLI

Posterior View

8-19

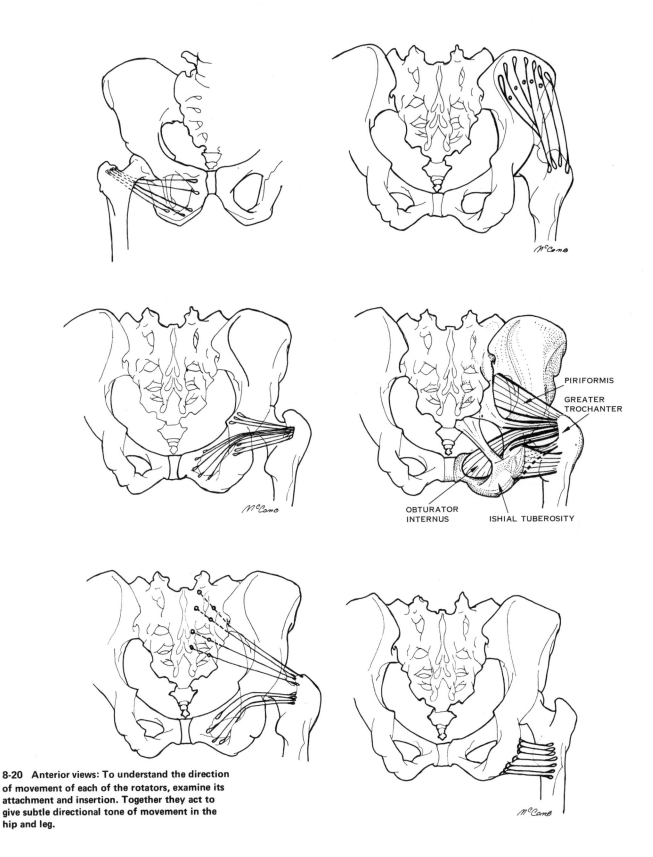

PIRIFORMIS

GREATER TROCHANTER

OBTURATOR INTERNUS

ISHIAL TUBEROSITY

8-20 Anterior views: To understand the direction of movement of each of the rotators, examine its attachment and insertion. Together they act to give subtle directional tone of movement in the hip and leg.

Several years ago, Dr. Arnold H. Kegel, an inspired gynecologist, observed that the health and positioning of a small, seemingly insignificant muscle of the pelvic floor (the pubococcygeus) appeared to be directly concerned with the over-all well-being of his patients. His work has been abstracted in *Reader's Digest* and is reported simply and comprehensibly in a book titled *The Key to Feminine Response in Marriage.** The importance of this relatively thin sheet of muscle is more readily apparent in the female body, although it has a significant function in males as well. Originally it was called the levator ani—the "muscle that raises the anus." This name called attention to one of its very important and more obvious roles—contributing to the placement and function of the anal sphincter. More recently, anatomic nomenclature has been revised so that muscles are now tagged with names designating their origin and insertion. Under the modern system, this muscle is called the pubococcygeus.

The importance of a pelvic floor containing and supporting pelvic organs and abdominal contents is self-evident. The pubococcygeus forms the most important component of this floor. Its significance and function, particularly its importance to women, are described with succinct clarity in the presentation of *The Key to Feminine Response in Marriage.* The diagrams from this source transmit one idea, convey one message (Figs. 8-21 through 8-24). But it is implied rather than spelled out. As we would say it, the muscles—the pubococcygeus and its neighbors—must be balanced in tone and balanced in direction if optimum functioning is to be attained.

The physiological activities influenced through the muscular hammock of the pelvic floor involve a wide, seemingly unrelated range, as Deutsch's book makes very clear. Satisfaction in the personal, physical, and emotional sexual relation and undoubtedly also the closely related physiological situations of fertility and childbirth are involved. Especially in the female, urinary continence and satisfactory bladder control and function at any age seem to reflect the tone and well-being of the pubococcygeus. Although the relation is less apparent in the male, it seems that this significant set of muscles may contribute to the contractions of orgasm. Therefore, in both sexes it is vital to sexual satisfaction.

The pioneering contributions of Dr. Kegel have been outstanding. They have vastly extended modern realization of how physical mechanisms and emotional expression interlock. His research in urogenital disturbances has been of inestimable value to countless women, especially those

*Ronald M. Deutsch (New York: Random House, 1968).

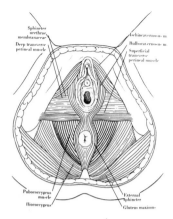

8-21 View from above: The three lower muscle diaphragms of the pelvic floor. (From Deutsch, THE KEY TO FEMININE RESPONSE IN MARRIAGE, Fig 6)

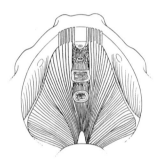

8-22 View from above: The pubococcygeus muscle after removal of the more superficial muscles. Note how the fibers surround the urinary passage, vagina, and rectum, interlacing with other muscle fibers of these organs. (From Deutsch, THE KEY TO FEMININE RESPONSE IN MARRIAGE, Fig. 7)

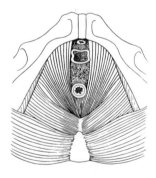

8-23 The pubococcygeus muscle seen from above. (From Deutsch, THE KEY TO FEMININE RESPONSE IN MARRIAGE, Fig. 8)

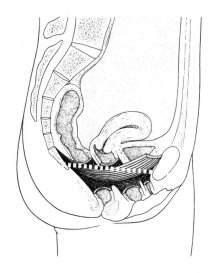

8-24a A lateral view: The pubococcygeus muscle with good tone and proper position. (From Deutsch, THE KEY TO FEMININE RESPONSE IN MARRIAGE, Fig.9)

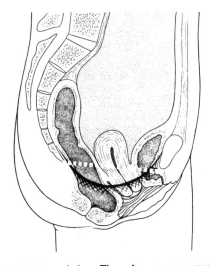

8-24b Lateral view: The pubococcygeus muscle with poor tone and position. Note the sagging of structures due to weak support. (From Deutsch, THE KEY TO FEMININE RESPONSE IN MAR— RIAGE, Fig. 10)

beset by complications following childbirth. Dr. Kegel has offered a system of voluntary exercises for strengthening these muscles. The figures quoted by Deutsch from the files of the American Institute of Family Relations bear witness to the efficacy of Kegel's method. They report that 65 per cent of the thousand cases of so-called "frigidity" recorded in their files have been helped.

But what of the other 35 per cent? Do they all have "deep-rooted emotional problems"? Is there no physical and relatively simple way of initiating change in such people? The premises of our book suggest that effective function in the pubococcygeus is directly determined by structural balance. This is another way of saying that substantially equal tension and span is called for in the fibers of the basic muscle (the pubococcygeus) and its immediate neighbors (iliococcygeus and ischiococcygeus). It is our postulate that the tone and fiber direction of these (as of all) muscles depends on the position in space of the bones to which they attach. As we have implied earlier, muscles and bones are spatially interdependent. Our results indicate that the position of bones is determined by the span and direction of the attaching soft tissue. The soft tissue must change before the bones can permanently shift. (In spite of this conviction, in these discussions we bow to the consensus and describe soft tissue in terms of the more apparent location of bones. This contradiction is a matter of convenience, not conviction.)

The pubococcygeus inserts into the coccyx, at best a vulnerable area. Fused from three to five small bony segments, the coccyx is united to the sacrum only by the relatively delicate sacrococcygeal disc. Otherwise unsupported and at the base of the spine, the coccyx becomes a target for physical impacts of all kinds. Every time a youngster falls out of a tree, or off a horse, or on the ice and lands on his derrière, it is his coccyx that receives the blow. When the coccyx is forced out of line, the span of the pubococcygeus is unbalanced. The entire floor of the pelvis suffers. When you palpate a coccyx, your finger often reports aberrated structures.

The question follows, What must happen to the pubococcygeus when the coccyx to which it attaches loses its appropriate space and/or tilt? Inevitably, hyper- or hypotoned fibers then invade the tissue. More than most muscles, this delicate sheet requires smooth spanning and homogeneous tone. (The same problem arises if the bony pubic symphysis has been aberrated. The symphysis, however, by placement is less vulnerable.) Are these structural facts the answer for the other 35 per cent, the ones not helped by Kegel exercises?

Pictures in standard anatomy books show conventional positions for the bony basin of the pelvis. However, the structure as "seen" by your fingers as you palpate a standing subject may be quite different. Your finger may have to search deeply to contact the pubic symphysis. You realize suddenly that the pelvis involved must be in "this" position; no other is possible. The observed individual must follow this general pattern. In other words, the pubic symphysis is too low. This pelvis is tipped; the abdominal contents seem to be spilling (Fig. 8-25).

All too often, such a pelvis has resulted from physical trauma—a bad fall, a difficult birth, an automobile accident. If its genesis has been in this kind of trauma, it is highly probable that the pelvis also is not symmetrical to the mid-vertical line (the so-called mid-sagittal plane), the plane that in imagination divides the left side from the right. In this event, how do the two halves of the pubococcygeus relate to each other? Will they balance? Can they balance? No, of course not. Furthermore, if the aberrative imbalance is sufficient, exercise will serve only to further shorten and tighten the side that is already hypertoned, exacerbating the imbalance. It would be interesting to investigate statistically how many recalcitrant pubococcygeus muscles suspected of being "deep-rooted emotional problems" are in fact manifestations of muscular and skeletal imbalance.

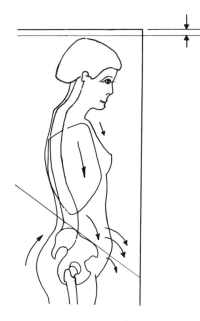

Fortunately, we have a logical remedy available. Our proposed solution refers to our basic premise: balance the whole man, or the whole woman, in the gravitational field. First of all, the pelvic basin must be made to conform as nearly as possible to the horizontal. In the course of accomplishing this, the displaced coccyx will be more appropriately positioned and the too low or too deep pubic symphysis raised. What effect this will have in terms of Dr. Kegel's measurements can only be determined by a well-planned scientific investigation.

In Fig. 8-25, it is strikingly apparent that pelvic contents must be displaced forward and downward. Not merely are the basin and its contents tipped as a whole, but within the basin the contents will and must sag. This is what determines the chemistry that we see and feel and call tone. Good "tone" can only occur, as we have said, when structures, particularly supporting myofascial structures, are balanced in space. Tone is the name given the outward manifestations of homeostatic chemical balance of the body. It applies to the balance of the individual as a whole as well as to the chemical well-being of particular areas or organs. According to the thesis of this book, the body needs a uniform tone level. If deep-lying structures manifest aberrant, deteriorating chemistry, a deviation of tone (and

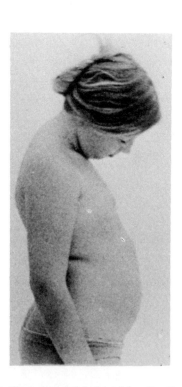

8-25 When the pelvis is tipped, locating the pubes by palpation may be difficult. In the light of the schema, this is understandable.

138

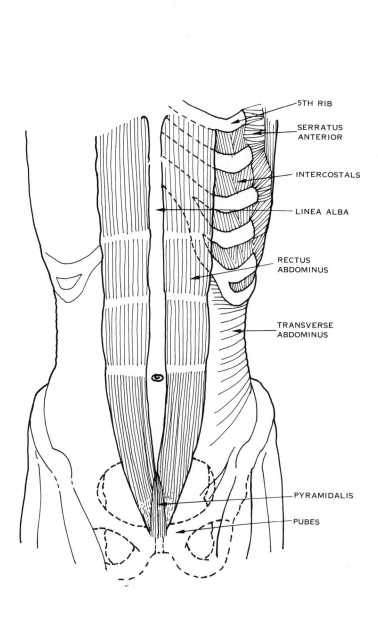

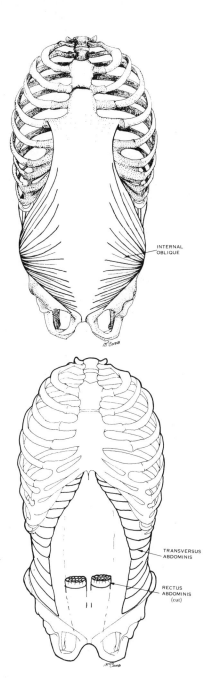

8-26 Anterior views: The abdomen is encased in tough myofascial walls consisting of three levels of muscles. The most superficial is the rectus abdominis already described. Underlying and more lateral to this are two layers of obliquely directed muscles, the external and internal obliques. Their lower attachment is at the iliac crest, their upper along the costal arch of the ribcage. They overlie a more simply structured muscle, the transversus abdominis, whose fibers more nearly approximate the horizontal. All three layers are readily accessible to change.

Alterations in both ribs and pelvis are quickly reflected into these abdominal muscles. Displacement of their bony attachments is rapidly compensated by a changing span. This is what underlies the many and varied abdominal contours to be seen in people. While it is true that fluid containing droplets of fat, etc., can and does collect between these musclar layers, the popular notion of the gross, pendulous abdomen as "fat" is erroneous. Basic to this distorted abdomen is a failure in direction, in tone, and in span of these important muscles.

therefore chemistry) will also be apparent in the overlying superficial layers of the body. Aberrations in tone, while they may peak at certain areas, cannot be isolated.

Thus if deep muscles and tendons tip the pelvis, overlying and/or supporting muscles must also deteriorate. The tone of such muscles as the obliques, the recti abdominis, the gluteal and rotator groups—all attaching to the pelvic bone—furnish an index to the general health and well-being of pelvic and abdominal organs. Poor tone in these superficial muscles necessarily means poor tone in the pelvis itself. The ligaments that support uterus and ovaries in the female, the important reproductive structures of the male (especially the prostate), the bladder and lower intestinal tracts in both sexes will all lack appropriate support, and their tone and function will suffer. A sagging potbelly and gluteals are not merely cosmetic offenses. They relate to the heavy, dragging gait of the individual. At a deeper, nonvisual level, they tell of sagging organs, reproductive and eliminative, a retroverted or anteflexed uterus, beleaguered prostate, and ptosed colon.

The pelvis is the key to man's well-being, as wise men have taught from time immemorial. But it is not the pelvis per se which is the key to beneficence. It is the relation of the human being, through the pelvis, to the gravitational field of the earth. Perhaps the ancients' fabled seat of the soul referred not to a structural entity but to a relationship—the relationship of the pelvis to the gravitational field.

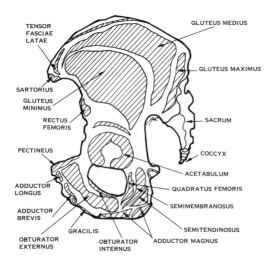

8-27

TENSOR FASCIAE LATAE
GLUTEUS MEDIUS
GLUTEUS MAXIMUS
SARTORIUS
GLUTEUS MINIMUS
RECTUS FEMORIS
SACRUM
PECTINEUS
COCCYX
ACETABULUM
ADDUCTOR LONGUS
QUADRATUS FEMORIS
ADDUCTOR BREVIS
SEMIMEMBRANOSUS
GRACILIS
SEMITENDINOSUS
OBTURATOR EXTERNUS
OBTURATOR INTERNUS
ADDUCTOR MAGNUS

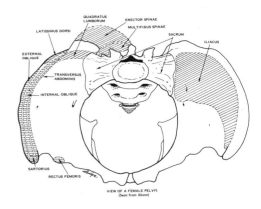

QUADRATUS LUMBORUM
ERECTOR SPINAE
LATISSIMUS DORSI
MULTIFIDUS SPINAE
SACRUM
ILIACUS
EXTERNAL OBLIQUE
TRANSVERSUS ABDOMINIS
INTERNAL OBLIQUE
SARTORIUS
RECTUS FEMORIS

VIEW OF A FEMALE PELVIS
(Seen from Above)

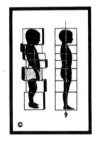

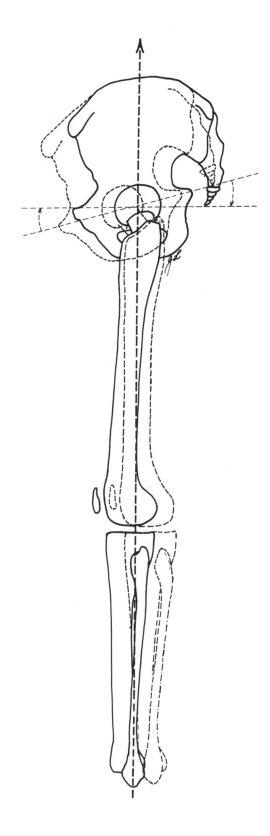

9-1

9
The Joint That Determines Symmetry

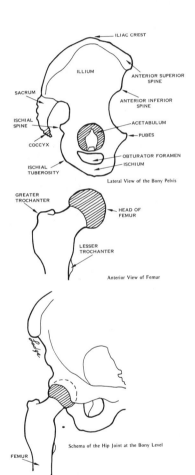

9-2 Lateral views: The position of the femoral head is the second factor influencing freedom at the hip joint. Depending on aberrated pulls by muscles of the thigh (especially the rotators) and distortions within the lower leg, ankle, and/or foot, the femur may be rotated in the hip joint. The distorted pulls must be released where they originate before the joint can move freely and in pattern.

We have placed a great deal of emphasis on an analysis of the pelvis and its individual attachments and separate parts. At this point, our goal is to look at the elements of the pelvis with respect to how they synthesize into a functional moving structure. Central to this must be the workings of the hip joint. This is the meeting place of pelvis and leg; this is the joint that determines symmetry.

Balance and/or integration implies symmetry—of the individual pelvic bones and in the relation of pelvis to gravitational field. In terms of flesh and bone, this means that in the standing position, the bony basin must be horizontal. The two high points, the most prominent points (anterior superior spines) on the crest of the ilium, must be on a horizontal line. This is obvious, you say? Are yours? Are the bony projections that mark the anterior superior spines of the ilium to be found in a horizontal line in your body? Or is one hip higher than the other, bigger than the other, broader than the other, farther from the midline than the other?

If the anterior superior spines are level, the ischial tuberosities will also be level. When you sit on a hard seat, do you feel your weight transmitted evenly to both ischii? Or does one bone take much more weight? These are functional and structural indices of the degree of balance in the pelvis. If you fail to pass these tests, you may assume that your pelvis is rotated as well as tipped. Any deviation from the horizontal by the ischial tuberosities always involves a rotation. There are many patterns in which pelves may be rotated. In the flesh-and-blood man, rotations are never simple, never in one plane only.

It would seem logical in terms of structure that the anterior superior iliac spines in a horizontal pelvis lie in a

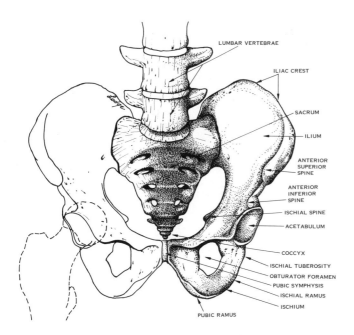

Labels in figure:
LUMBAR VERTEBRAE
ILIAC CREST
SACRUM
ILIUM
ANTERIOR SUPERIOR SPINE
ANTERIOR INFERIOR SPINE
ISCHIAL SPINE
ACETABULUM
COCCYX
ISCHIAL TUBEROSITY
OBTURATOR FORAMEN
PUBIC SYMPHYSIS
ISCHIAL RAMUS
ISCHIUM
PUBIC RAMUS

9-3 Anterior view: The integrity of the joint depends on the position of the hipbone (ilium) and the position of the femur. The plane of the ilium is defined by the relation of the anterior superior spines to the pubes (they should be in a vertical plane) and the realtion of the tip of the coccyx to the pubes (they should be in a horizontal plane). If these conditions are met, then the head of the femur can fit into the acetabulum in a fashion that allows free rotation.

plane vertical to the pubic symphysis. In living bodies, vertical planes are harder to determine than horizontals. Therefore, in one's own body, this is harder to determine than a horizontal plane defining the anterior superior spines. Since living bodies are usually random, living pelves by definition are usually not horizontal, so this vertical plane is rarely seen.

If this horizontal-vertical construction of the pelvis is the appropriate one, the ideal, then what factors have determined that even in a broad sample of the population this configuration is so rarely found? The answer is simple enough, but needs endless reiteration. Bones are where they are because of the position of the related myofascial structures.

Any accident, any illness that leaves a chronic scarring in soft tissue interferes with equipose. Inelastic scar tissue in one or several related fascial sheets makes matched movement by antagonists impossible. When movement is demanded of one of such a glued pair, both answer; if, as is often the case, the two are agonist and antagonist, both try to respond to the stimulus. As a result, movement is inhibited. Deterioration of movement is progressive; consistent inhibition of a movement is followed by local atrophy to a greater or lesser degree. Eventually the muscle can no longer be stimulated, and movement is taken over by neighboring groups. When this happens, coordinated movement in the area (and in the whole body) is no longer possible.

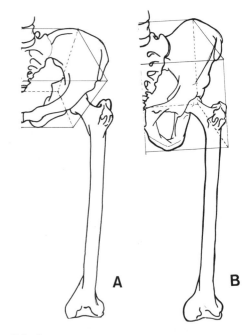

9-4 Anterior views: The imaginary cubes overlaid here call attention to the difference in weight organization in a rotated versus a horizontal pelvis. Pelvis A is horizontally tipped rather than laterally rotated, but even this simple distortion shows the difference in the way weight is transmitted through the femoral head. Consider, too, the difference in strain at the lumbar vertebrae.

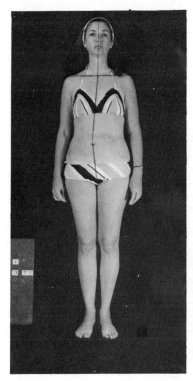
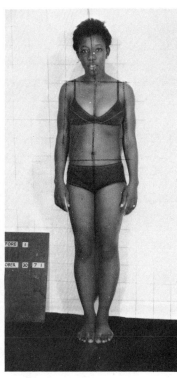

9-5 In these two photographs, the complicated pelvic rotations (involving sagittal, horizontal, and coronal planes) are pointed up by the construction lines. Lines such as these drawn over any photograph make your analysis of rotations easier.

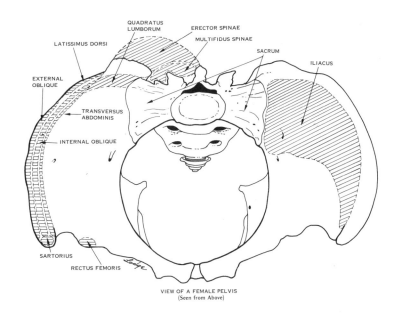

QUADRATUS LUMBORUM
ERECTOR SPINAE
MULTIFIDUS SPINAE
LATISSIMUS DORSI
SACRUM
ILIACUS
EXTERNAL OBLIQUE
TRANSVERSUS ABDOMINIS
INTERNAL OBLIQUE
SARTORIUS
RECTUS FEMORIS

VIEW OF A FEMALE PELVIS
(Seen from Above)

9-6 View from above: The close crowding of muscles attaching at the crest of the ilium is apparent in this drawing. Most of the muscles finding attachment on the crest are structures that bind the upper half (trunk) to the pelvis (the sartorius, iliacus, and rector femoris are exceptions).

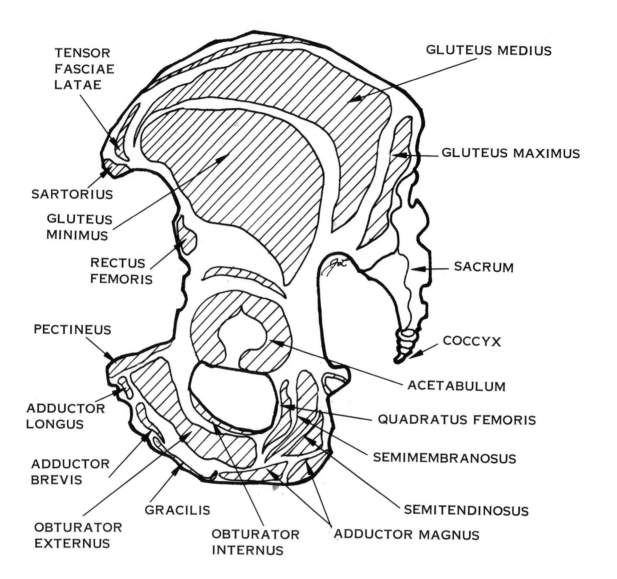

TENSOR FASCIAE LATAE

GLUTEUS MEDIUS

GLUTEUS MAXIMUS

SARTORIUS

GLUTEUS MINIMUS

RECTUS FEMORIS

SACRUM

PECTINEUS

COCCYX

ACETABULUM

ADDUCTOR LONGUS

QUADRATUS FEMORIS

SEMIMEMBRANOSUS

ADDUCTOR BREVIS

GRACILIS

SEMITENDINOSUS

OBTURATOR EXTERNUS

OBTURATOR INTERNUS

ADDUCTOR MAGNUS

9-7 Lateral view: The well-rounded, sturdy, lateral contour of the hip encloses a variety of muscles serving a variety of functions. Rectus femoris, sartorius, tensor fascia lata, iliopsoas, adductors, and hamstrings bind the leg to the body, as does the gluteal group. Others (including the superior half of the iliopsoas) extend upward, uniting upper and lower halves of the body.

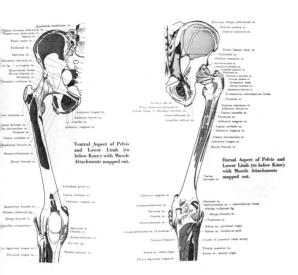

Ventral Aspect of Pelvis and Lower Limb (to below Knee) with Muscle Attachments mapped out.

Dorsal Aspect of Pelvis and Lower Limb (to below Knee) with Muscle Attachments mapped out.

9-8 For more serious students, these beautiful schemata by Hepier show both distal and proximal areas of attachment of the muscles joining leg and pelvis. (From Sobotta, ATLAS OF HUMAN ANATOMY, Vol1, Figs. 311 and 312)

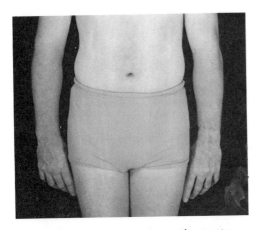

9-9 A hip well-nourished is a sturdy structure.

With this typical progression in mind, let us look at the intricate fashion in which its attached muscles determine the position of the bony pelvis. Figs. 9-6, 9-7, and 9-8 give some idea of the closeness of muscular tissue. Even on the limited surface of the crest of the ilium, myofascial attachments form a close, crowded pattern, as shown. When even one member of such an intricate complex fails, what happens is unpredictable, but any failure has far-reaching consequences.

A well-nourished hip is a solid, sturdy structure, well-clothed with flesh. Its adequate chemistry and appropriate physiology allow the joint to move freely under its well-supported superstructure. Competent structure and function create their own contour; it looks like this (Fig. 9-9). Here muscles are really free to move; the fascial sheath of one slides over the surface of its neighbor. This flow of movement and energy spells security. Our pictures deliver their own message. They emphasize that legs must not only support the pelvis as the man stands, they must, as he moves, create a dynamic balance, emphasizing the role of the ball-and-socket joint.

The design of this joint clearly suggests that the lower limb should be able to take a great number of positions vis-à-vis the pelvis. Its position at any given movement will be determined by adjustments of antagonists appropriately separated in space by bone. Ideally these adjustments respond to voluntary control and direction by the person himself; chronic restriction, inelastic fibers, or degenerative attachment to neighboring elements limits the range. It is commonplace to find an individual whose femur habitually comes to rest in some deviant rotation. He is unaware—unable to be aware—of this deviance; still less can he control it.

Any person should be able voluntarily to rotate his leg in the hip socket both laterally and medially. But watch people! Is the movement of leg to hip too free, therefore toneless? Or is the leg fixed; has it a limited range in its rotation? Can the man voluntarily change the rotation, or is he unable to reach it? Any of these constitutes aberration.

Joint limitation, wherever found, generally results from some accident that has stretched one muscle or muscle group beyond its limit of elasticity. Without outside help, the muscle cannot return. Without the addition of outside energy, it becomes permanently fixed. Failing this, delinquency must then be compensated by structures elsewhere in the body. On any joint, this describes the progressive limitation too often oversimplified as "aging." Shoulder as well as hip joints are highly susceptible to traumatic accident. But in the hip, poor adjustment carries

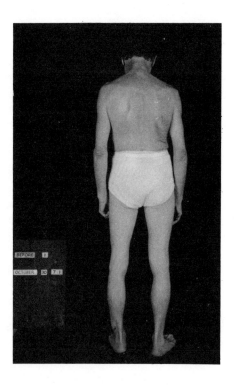

9-10 In order to support a pelvis, legs must underpin it. In the case of Mr. H, legs not only do not efficiently support the pelvis, they cannot be seen as underpinning it either. Recognizing how badly this pelvis is rotated, we can understand this failure.

more serious physiological hazard in that compensations here aberrate the pelvic floor and interfere with pelvic physiology.

Theoretically, an infinite number of adjustments is possible at a ball-and-socket joint. In fact, however, only a limited spectrum of structural configurations meets the ideal requirements of horizontal planes at ischia and ilia. Bodies are not perfect; the precise symmetrical planes of theory are not actualized in nature. Differences in habitual muscular use (right- or left-handedness) as well as visceral structure (liver complex on right side compared to heart and stomach on left) preclude literal symmetry. Nevertheless, to ensure reasonable physiological health, weight-bearing must approach a practical balance.

Does appropriate integration of the pelvic structure actually require that its landmarks (anterior superior iliac spines, pubes, coccyx, and ischial tuberosities) all define horizontal planes in a standing position? If so, reorganization or readjustment must very apparently center about the insertion of the head of the femur (as part of the leg) into the acetabulum (as part of the pelvic bone). Three joints determine movement in the leg—hip, knee, and ankle. Clearly this number of moving surfaces has potential for a great variety of maladjustment and disorganization, and trouble below will reflect upward to the junction of the femoral head and acetabulum.

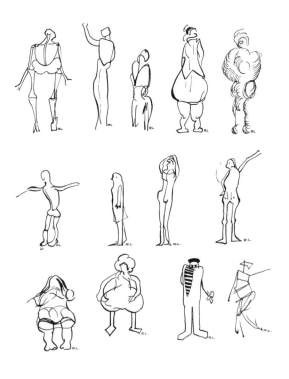

9-11

148

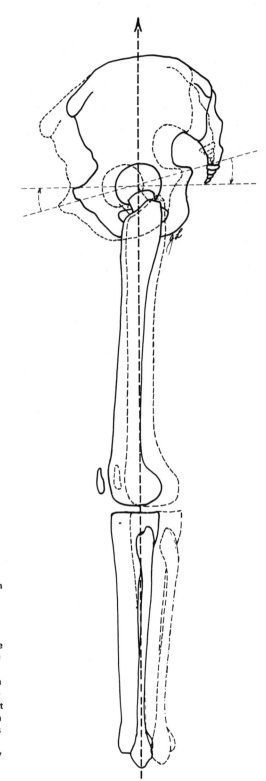

9-12 Lateral view: Limitation at the hip joint in
any body may be the result of direct impact
(an accident, a bad fall) on the joint itself.
(There can be other causes, as discussed previously.) The primary gravity requirement is that
the sole of the foot adjust to the ground. If the
foot is aberrated, tibia and fibula (at the ankle)
may have to compensate to allow this adjustment. Then the other end of the tibia and fubula
will have to reorganize, changing weight transmission through the knee. The femur must adjust
at both knee and acetabulum, which may in turn
tip the ilia. In its solid lines, this schema shows
the position of a horizontal pelvis. The broken
lines indicate an aberrant position the pelvis may
have taken to accommodate strains from the
underpinning legs.

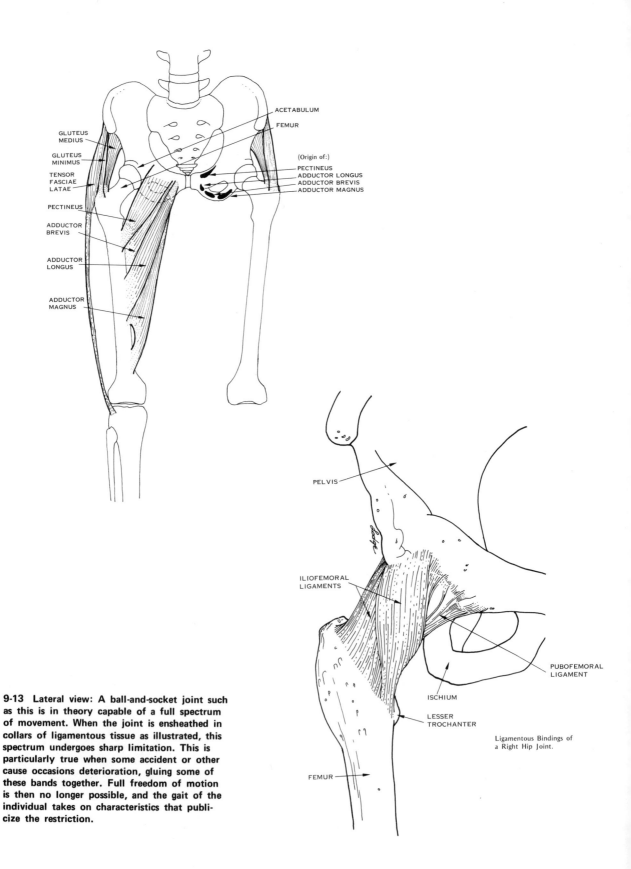

GLUTEUS MEDIUS

GLUTEUS MINIMUS

TENSOR FASCIAE LATAE

PECTINEUS

ADDUCTOR BREVIS

ADDUCTOR LONGUS

ADDUCTOR MAGNUS

ACETABULUM

FEMUR

(Origin of:)

PECTINEUS
ADDUCTOR LONGUS
ADDUCTOR BREVIS
ADDUCTOR MAGNUS

9-13 Lateral view: A ball-and-socket joint such as this is in theory capable of a full spectrum of movement. When the joint is ensheathed in collars of ligamentous tissue as illustrated, this spectrum undergoes sharp limitation. This is particularly true when some accident or other cause occasions deterioration, gluing some of these bands together. Full freedom of motion is then no longer possible, and the gait of the individual takes on characteristics that publicize the restriction.

PELVIS

ILIOFEMORAL LIGAMENTS

PUBOFEMORAL LIGAMENT

ISCHIUM

LESSER TROCHANTER

FEMUR

Ligamentous Bindings of a Right Hip Joint.

150

If you are thinking about body efficiency and its creation, it is important to realize that both superficial and deep organization are necessary for free movement. In other words, balance must exist between the deep ligaments, the bones pictured in Fig. 9-13, and the structures nearer the superficial contour. Elasticity—that is, capacity for adjustment of basic ligamentous structures—depends on freedom for movement of overlying muscles and their spatial relationship to their deeper relatives. As always, in biological situations, this is a circular situation.

The deep ligamentous structure of joints mirrors the state of more superficial members. The chemistry and physics of both levels are determined by the way the joint moves within the force field of gravity. Consistent stress interference with joint movement in this field is the first milestone on the road to chronic compensation and deterioration. Persistent stress at the hip interferes not only with ease but with precise support from the thigh. To the extent that the thigh is unable to deal with the overlying weight, the latter must be supported and moved by structures higher in the body. Thus it can often be seen that much of the body weight is literally being hoisted by the shoulders and/or rib cage. Obviously this is a completely inefficient pattern and the source of constant stress to its owner.

The unending random patterns highlighted on any beach or boardwalk emphasize that pelvic balance at the hip joint is the key to all movement in the individual (Fig. 9-14).

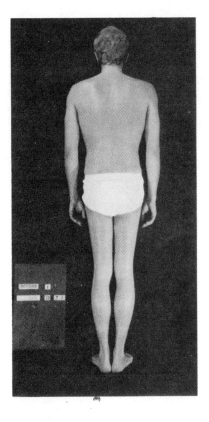

9-14 To the casual observer, this man seems to present a fine figure — broad of shoulder, narrow of hip, etc. His complaint: always feeling as if he were confined in a strait-jacket. It sounds unwarranted, the complaint of a hypochondriac. The sophisticated eye looks more deeply and sees the fierce tension in the legs that makes them so slender. Shortened calf muscles pull the foot to the side to accommodate shortened tendons. The slender thighs tell the same story; the hamstrings particularly cannot accommodate to the adductors. The tension has compressed the hip joint. It has no freedom, and a rotation of the pelvis has tried to adjust to this. The man's walk is so restricted that he tries to carry his weight from his shoulders. When we have really understood these various problems, we appreciate his complaint and the restrictions under which he is laboring.

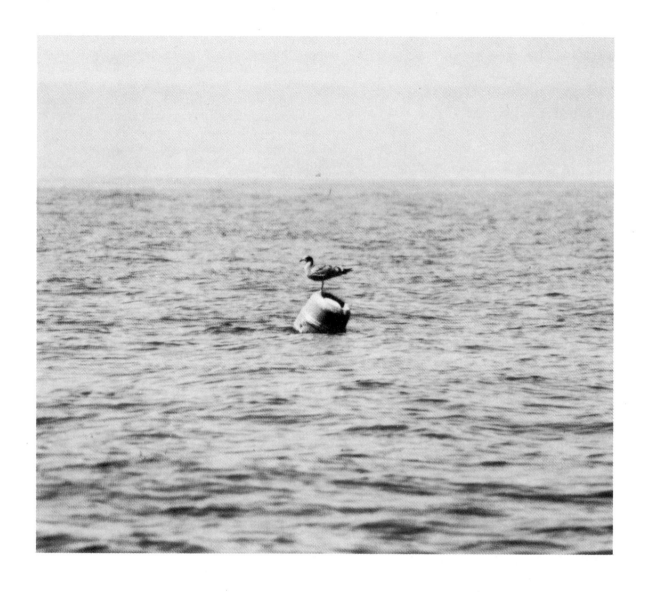

10-1 <u>Movement</u> is a term whose limits are hard to define. This also applies to the word <u>stillness</u>. We think of the gull on a buoy as still, but his need for continual adjustment to the moving water keeps his muscles in an unceasing inter-play of movement. In humans, no matter how still a man may be, he is always adjusting to his respiratory needs, his circulatory needs, his perceptual needs (The saccadic movements of the eye are so slight that they have only recent-ly been recognized.) In an organic world, there is no such thing as complete lack of movement.

10
Function Is
Movement

Anatomy studies a projection of the static body, but function in the living body requires more than static recognition. Function is movement; movement is life. Movement is the index of life, its outstanding expression. While it is alive, no human or animal body is ever completely still. We see a gull sitting on a buoy; we exclaim over its stillness. Close inspection shows that the bird is not still; he balances and rebalances continuously in an interplay with the rippling water. A human, too, is constantly readjusting by moving himself in one way or another. For example, take respiration. Contrary to the general idea, normal respiration in a balanced body involves movement not merely in the thorax, but from the sacrum all the way up to the cranium. In normal inspiration, the spine lengthens from one end to the other; in expiration, it shortens.

Physical personality is reflected in psychological personality. So, too, physical movement colors psychological behavior. Through movement, humans sense the driving force of change. Movement is the physical acceptance of change; awareness of this tends to be below the individual's conscious awareness. For the therapist of the psyche as well as for the therapist dealing with the physical man, the goal is appropriate movement. The psychotherapist senses immobility in the dimension of time rather than of space. The individual bogged down, unmoving in time, unable to escape from his infantile or adolescent assumptions or traumata, manifests this physically as well as psychologically. His lack of movement, his general or localized rigidity, are unequivocal in their statement. Movement induced in the physical body (as all dance therapists know) will loosen psychological chains. The job of the psychotherapist thus becomes easier.

In the human body (as in any segmented biological structure), movement is determined by joints. Therefore, appreciation of anatomical joint structure offers to the

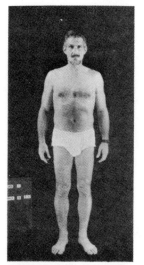

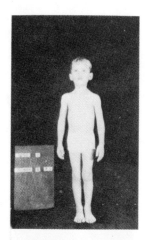

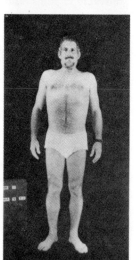

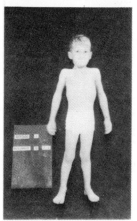

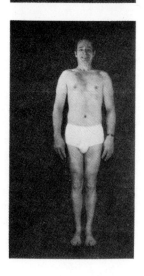

10-2 These three people are responding to a request for deep inhalation. In the father-son pair, the photographs were taken before they had experienced the organizing of Structural Integration; the movement seen in these two random bodies is an expansion of the chest by lengthening the anterior chest wall. Mr. R, on the other hand, has had a considerable amount of processing; in his integrated body, inhalation lengthens the spine as well. In a random body, the spine does not lengthen in respiration. In these two particular random bodies of father and son, it is apparent that the shortened, immobile spinal structure is forced forward (rather than lengthened) by the inhalation movement of the chest wall. Thus each breath involves far more work than is necessary in the more balanced body. Although the boy does not have the same aberrations as his father, his style of movement strikingly mimics the adult's, demonstrating the way movement is transmitted from generation to generation (like father, like son).

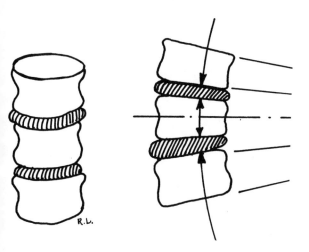

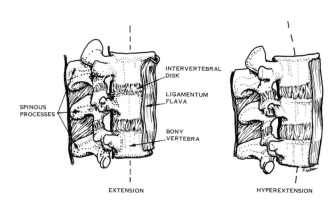

SPINOUS
PROCESSES

INTERVERTEBRAL
DISK

LIGAMENTUM
FLAVA

BONY
VERTEBRA

EXTENSION

HYPEREXTENSION

10-3 Lateral views: Of the various joint patterns, the cartilaginous is the most powerful, the most widely distributed. All vertebral joints are cartilaginous. Body movement is possible only through the adjustment of joints. Thanks to its segmented jointing, the spine flexes and extends. Yet chronic flexing, as in old age, causes permanent anterior compression and thinning of the discs.

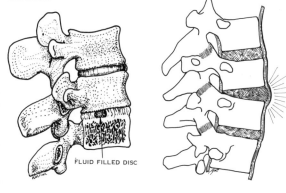

FLUID FILLED DISC

10-4 Lateral views: Discs are not solid cushions of cartilage. Rather, they are fluid-filled sacs (left), and so they have a greater potential for movement. Local tensions within individual fibrous bands of cartilage determine the "home" position of each bony vertebra. This position of "rest" should be one of balanced extension. At any local level, however, chronic compression of an anterior ligament expresses itself in chronic flexion; compression of posterior ligaments expresses itself as chronic hyperextension. If the disc structure is aberrant or the chemistry poor, the strain of movement may spread the fibers of the ligament. This weakened spot permits the fluid to seep through. The result, the so-called herniated disc (right), may cause much distress and, after healing, chronic restriction of spinal movement.

therapist one key to understanding normal process and putting it to work for healing. Segmental junctions make gross body movement (gesture) possible. In addition, joints permit the finer adjustments that appear as integrated physiological and psychological behavior patterns within the body. Free interplay within joints is therefore both an index to health and the road that must be followed to get there. This is another circular situation, another gradient scale.

A joint is usually defined as the interface of two bony surfaces. Anatomists describe several basically different joint patterns, each with its optimal type of movement.

Most important and widely distributed of these are the cartilaginous joints, which bind and integrate (for example, the segments of the spine); synovial joints, which permit the far-reaching and diverse motor activities at hip and shoulder, knee and elbow; and syndesmoses, which bind bones like the tibia and fibula.

Spinous segments (Figs. 10-3 and 10-4), which are the most important of the cartilaginous joints, are involved in weight transmission. So are many of the synovial joints. Logically, certain structural similarities may be expected. In addition to being merely a juxtaposition of two bony interfaces, such joints must include a cushion of some sort (usually fibrocartilage) to allow alternating contraction and spread during movement. In the spine, these are called discs. The cushion should be sturdy enough to protect the bony surface from irritation; naturally, it must be tough (not easily subject to damage) and highly elastic. Spinal joints illustrate all these qualities. Cushion and bony segments are tightly bound together by very tough ligamentous bands. For greater strength, the bands are short; although tough, they are nevertheless elastic. They must be, in order that relatively free flexion, extension, or rotation can take place.

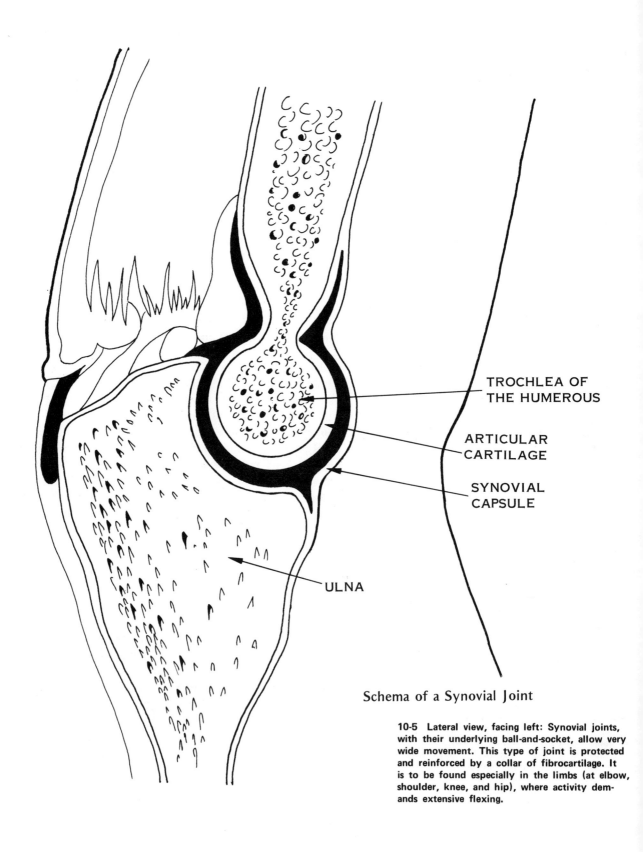

TROCHLEA OF
THE HUMEROUS

ARTICULAR
CARTILAGE

SYNOVIAL
CAPSULE

ULNA

Schema of a Synovial Joint

10-5 Lateral view, facing left: Synovial joints,
with their underlying ball-and-socket, allow very
wide movement. This type of joint is protected
and reinforced by a collar of fibrocartilage. It
is to be found especially in the limbs (at elbow,
shoulder, knee, and hip), where activity demands extensive flexing.

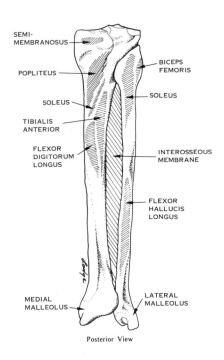

SEMI-
MEMBRANOSUS

POPLITEUS

SOLEUS

TIBIALIS
ANTERIOR

FLEXOR
DIGITORUM
LONGUS

BICEPS
FEMORIS

SOLEUS

INTEROSSEOUS
MEMBRANE

FLEXOR
HALLUCIS
LONGUS

MEDIAL
MALLEOLUS

LATERAL
MALLEOLUS

Posterior View

10-6 Anterior view: Syndesmosis is the name applied to a joint where two bones, closely related in function, are held together by an interosseous ligament. The lower leg (shown here) and the forearm are typical of this joint.

Constituents of all moving joints show certain similarities. In accordance with the physiological function to be served, the cushion may be thick or thin, tough or fragile, elastic or rigid. In spinal joints, cushioning depends especially on that part of the disc that is fluid. This in turn allows free movement of the smoothly plated articular surfaces within the encapsulating sleeve of collagenous tissue. Adjacent vertebrae are further joined by a tough cartilaginous band or ligament. This blueprint—articular surfaces, cushion, sleeve, and ligaments—is an over-all picture of many joints in addition to the cartilaginous spinal joints; for example, the synovial joint at hip, knee, shoulder (Fig. 10-5), and wrist.

Some joints are designed for very little motion. Even in these, limited spatial change can be brought about by improving the tone of the interosseous membrane or the innermost ligaments. Such a joint is called a syndesmosis, a structure in which bones that are spatially a short distance apart are held together by interosseous ligaments (Fig. 10-6). The functional union of tibia and fibula, of radius and ulna, are examples. Finally, there is a limited number of joints in which physiological requirement for movement further decreases; as it approaches or actually reaches zero, the union is known as a suture. Such interfaces join the bones of the skull (Fig. 10-7). But even here a thin, fibrous sutural ligament cushions the junction of the bones. In later life (middle age), this junction may ossify.

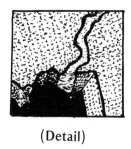

(Detail)

10-7 Even the joints called sutures, which by design are capable of only minimal movement, consist of a union of two bones joined by a cartilaginous pad.

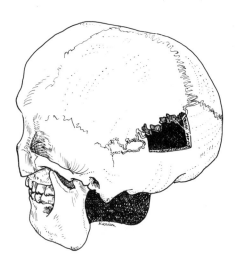

All too often, a joint is vaguely thought of as the immediate neighborhood of articulating surfaces of two bones. Considered as a structural-functional unit, a joint is much more than this. In the context of movement, a joint is the interplay of muscles and ligaments overlying the bony junction or attaching to it. Circumduction at the hip joint, for example, summates activity of simultaneous abduction-adduction, flexion-extension, and rotation. Each of these functions needs to be examined in turn; the summation of these individual contributions expresses the movement (Fig. 10-8).

Muscles and ligaments making up any synovial joint leave clues to their basic function in their pattern of distribution around the bone. In the primary function of the leg that is walking (a progression forward), anatomical provision must be made for flexion and extension of the leg and foot. In an unmoving body part, tissue energy expenditure should approach zero—the part should be at complete rest. In real life, of course, this rarely happens. To approach zero, a rather precise equilibrium is necessary between antagonists controlling the joint. Chronic shortening in any one fiber of a flexor means that to prevent unwanted movement its antagonist (the extensor) must maintain a constant counterbalancing tension·or contraction in a similar degree. In other words, the extensor must expend energy continuously. In this case, energy equilibrium in the body part (and therefore in the body in general) comes to what looks like rest at a point something above the zero point. It thus never truly rests. In the evocative words of the old-fashioned manipulators, the body "leaks" energy. The "leak" manifests itself in various symptoms—a sense of weariness, or of weakness in a part, or even chronic dull pain.

In analyzing movement, muscles about any joint separate into significant functional categories—abduction-adduction, flexion-extension, rotation, circumduction. In walking, pelvis, thigh, and leg cooperate in the total movement, and all these categories may be called upon. In general, straight-forward walking should not stimulate rotators of the thigh. These should remain balanced, at "rest."

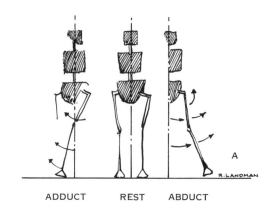

ADDUCT   REST   ABDUCT

Anterior View

EXTEND   REST   FLEX

Lateral View

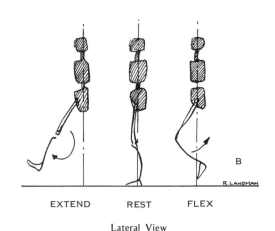

INVERT   REST   EVERT

Anterior View

10-8 The term flexion applies to a movement that draws the more distal part nearer to the center, decreasing the angle at the hinge. Extension reverses this, increasing the angle. Rotation moves a bone around its longtitudinal axis in a plane at right angles to the axis; abduction moves a part away from the midline; adduction moves it toward the midline; circumduction is a summation of all these.

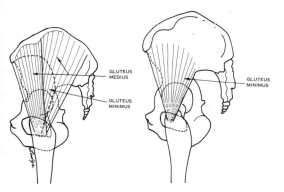

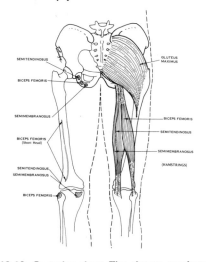

10-9 Lateral view of gluteal rotators. The gluteus minimus and medius abduct and medially rotate the hip joint.

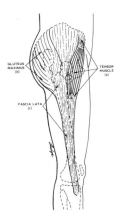

10-10 Posterior view: The gluteus maximus extends and laterally rotates the thigh on the hip. Hamstrings, close neighbors of the gluteal group, are powerful extensors of the hip joint, acting in antagonistic relation to the flexors on the front of the thigh (iliopsoas, sartorius, pectineus, and rectus femoris).

Abduction—pulling the thigh away from the midline—is one of the most powerful movements of the lower limb. It is a primary function of three muscles that attach to the pelvis near the anterior superior spine of the ilium. Of these, gluteus medius and minimus insert near the greater trochanter of the femur (Fig. 10-9). The third and most powerful of the three, the iliotibial band together with its tensor, runs along the femur (Fig. 10-11). This band spans the femur without attaching to it, inserting just below the knee into the lateral condyle of the tibia. The length of this (or any) muscle indicates its potential strength and the distance through which it can move the related parts. In spite of their potential, these three primary abductors form only a small part of the volume of the thigh. It should be noted that they are quite superficial muscles. (Muscles powerful in their action and able to move body parts through long distances are situated near the surface of the body.) The strength of the leg in abduction derives from the powerful, tough fascia lata (iliotibial band). In the young male, the natural toughness of this fascia is exaggerated by our present fashions in sports training.

Adductors (muscles that draw toward the midline) form a slightly larger group in terms of volume of the thigh. For the most part, they originate from the pubic area and the ischiopubic rami. Only one, the adductor magnus, arises from the ischial tuberosity, thus adjoining the hamstrings. In many ways, it thereby shares the weakness of the hamstring group. These muscles form an interesting spatial pattern, a simple fanlike design that should, in theory, allow abductors and adductors to balance. Sadly enough, they seldom do. For some reason, perhaps our cultural pattern of foot eversion, adductors seem to suffer more than other groups. One or several individual muscles become atrophied, stringy, persistently painful to the touch. Then, as usual, neighboring structures try to compensate. If the deterioration is unilateral, the pelvis begins to rotate, distorting its position around its horizontal axis and sagittal plane.

10-11 Lateral view: The so-called iliotibial band joins the ilium (pelvic bone) to the tibia of the leg. This very powerful fascial band contracts and relaxes by the action of the relatively small muscle at its proximal end, the tensor fascia lata, abducting the thigh.

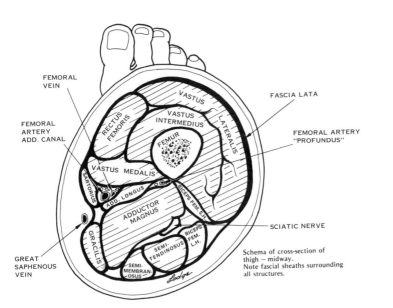

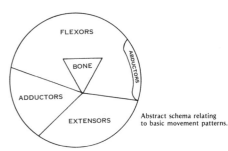

Abstract schema relating
to basic movement patterns.

Schema of cross-section of
thigh — midway.
Note fascial sheaths surrounding
all structures.

10-12 View from above: A cross section of the upper thigh suggests the volume relations of antagonistic groups. It also emphasizes the off-centered position of the bone of the thigh (femur).

Flexors:

sartorius
pectineus
rectus femoris
adductor longus
adductor brevis
adductor magnus
   (anterior head)
tensor fascia lata

Extensors:

gluteus maximus
semitendinosus
semimembranosus
biceps femoris
adductor magnus (posterior head)

Abductors:

gluteus medius
gluteus minimus
tensor fascia lata
sartorius
piriformis

Adductors:

adductor magnus
adductor longus
adductor brevis
gracilis
pectineus
quadratus femoris
obturator extermus

Muscles can perform several of these different functions, depending on the movement demanded.

Centerfold

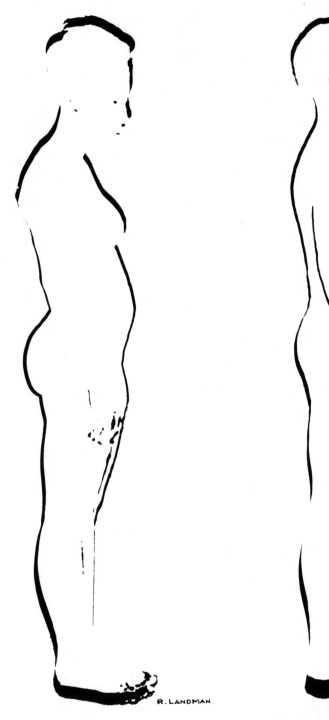

R. LANDMAN

R. LANDMAN

CF-1,2 It is hard to believe that this vital, well-organized young black woman is the same as the dreary, depressed figure on the left. Ten hours of processing over a period of five weeks have accomplished this.

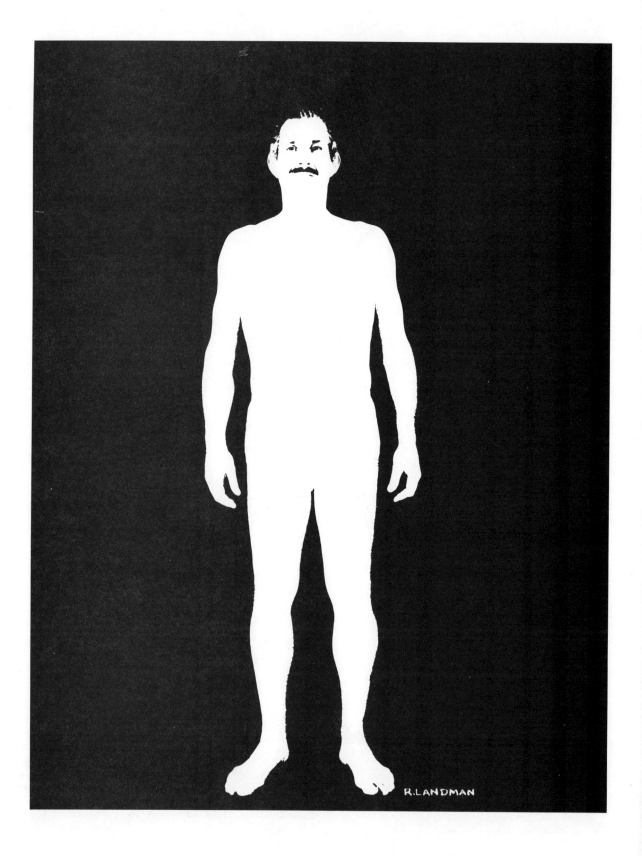

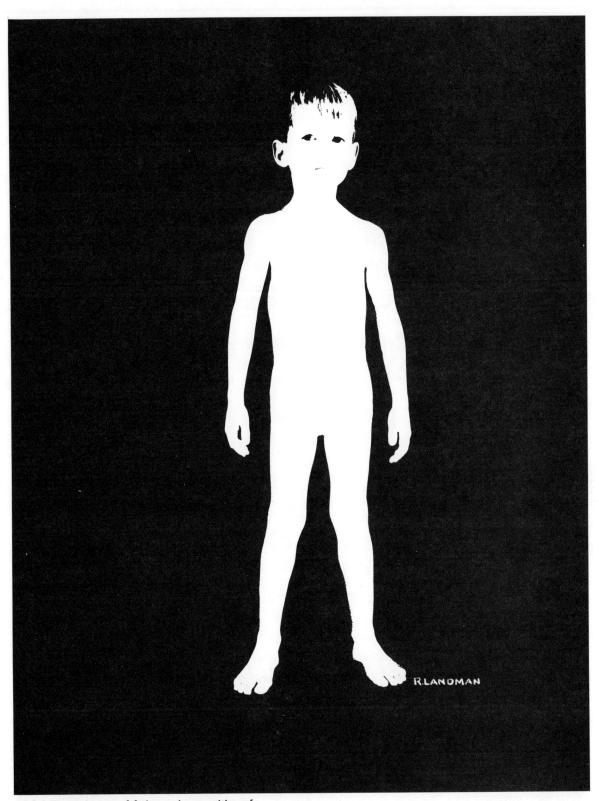

CF-3,4 These pictures of father and son, neither of them processed, demonstrate the similarities to be found in families. Some of this is certainly the result of genetic endowment; but probably more has to do with the environmental and cultural factors fostered within family groups. "Like father, like son."

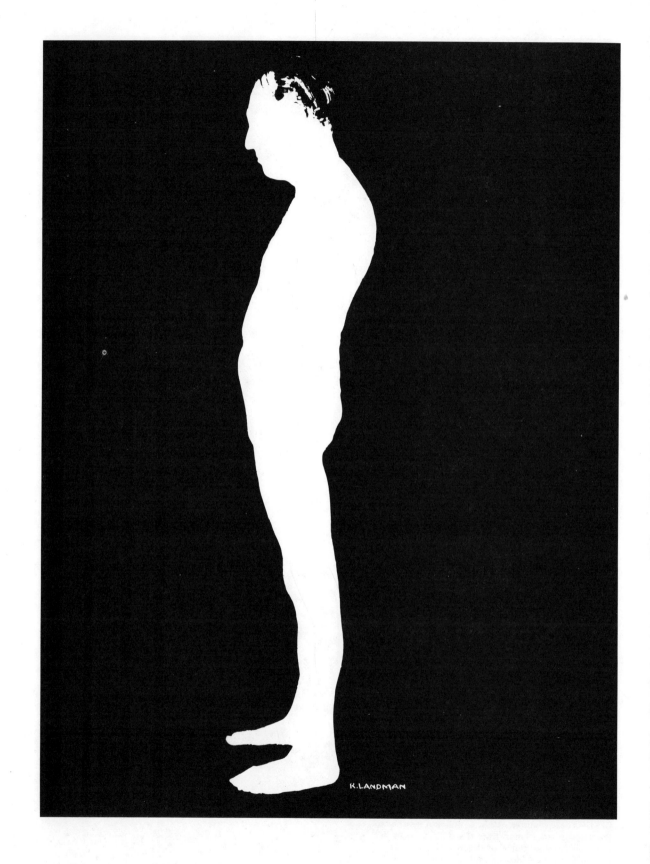

K.LANDMAN

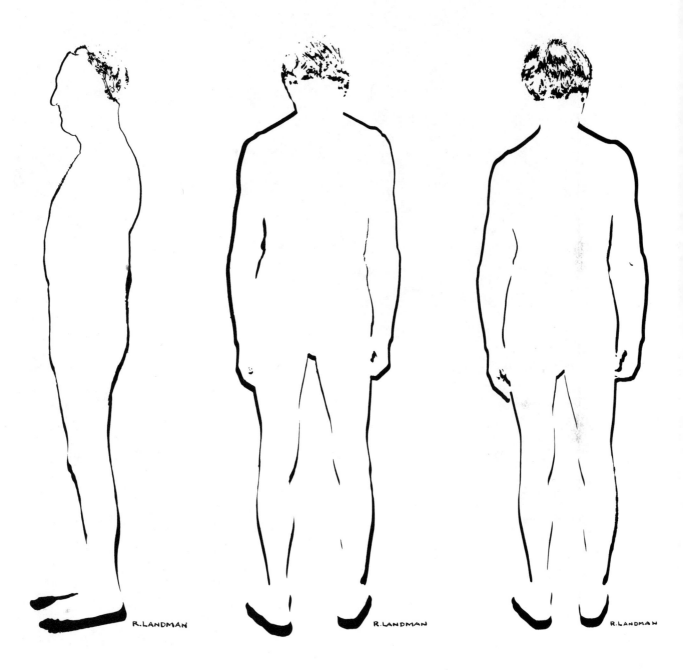

R.LANDMAN

R.LANDMAN

R.LANDMAN

CF-5,6,7,8 These solarizations, made from photographs of Mr. H, document his change over a
five-week period.

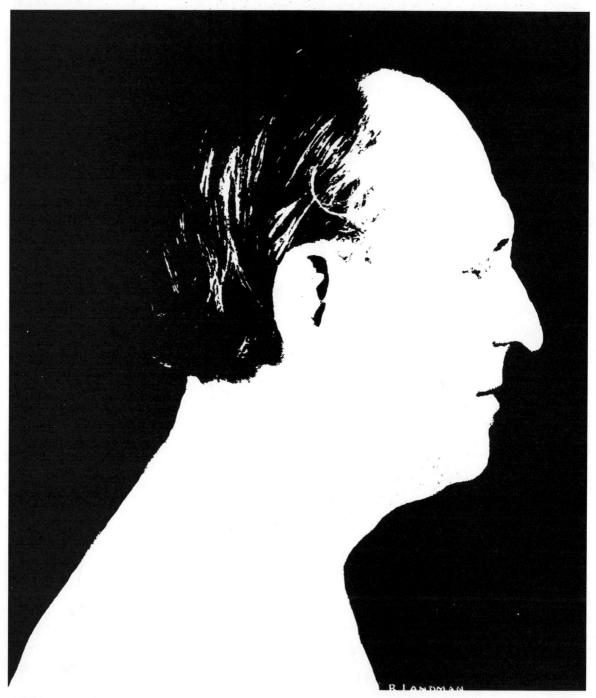

CF-9,10 These record the visible changes in head and neck conformation of Mr. H in one significant hour of Structural Integration — the seventh. At this point in the processing, the entire hour is devoted to organizing head and neck. In the case of Mr. H, the success of this hour's work is clear. The change in facial expression evoked in personality expression.

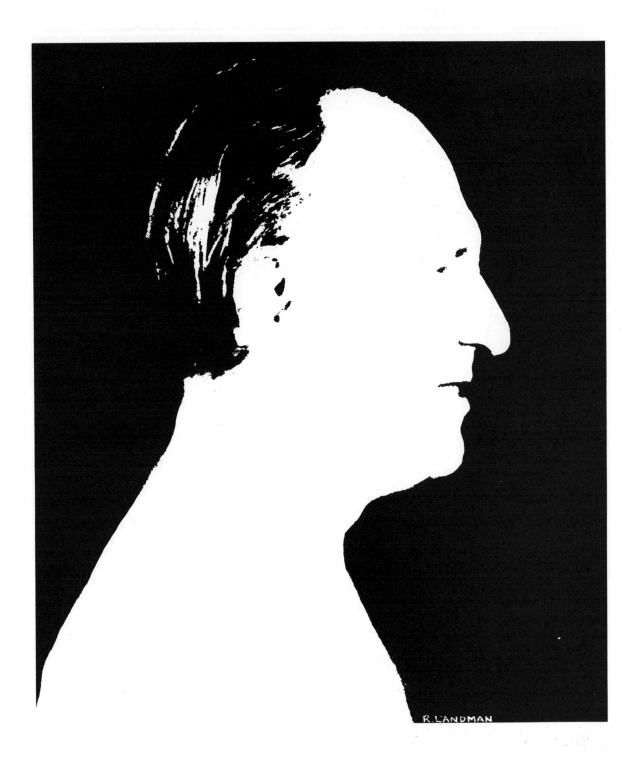

R.L'ANDMAN

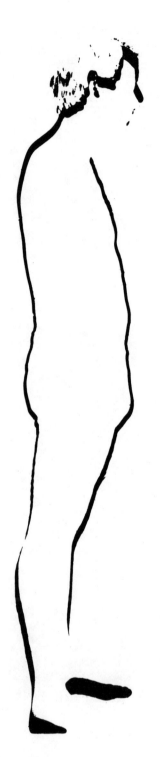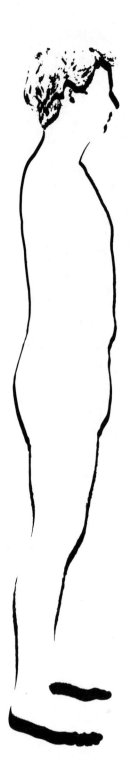

CF-11, 12, 13, 14 These two pairs of photographs
record the changes in each of these two men occurring as a result of one hour of processing.

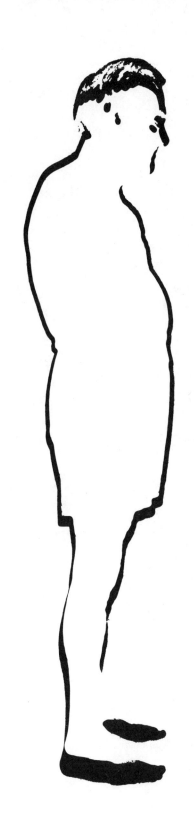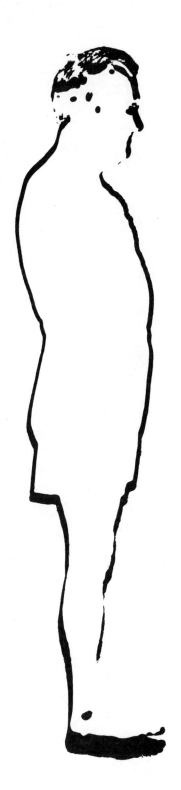

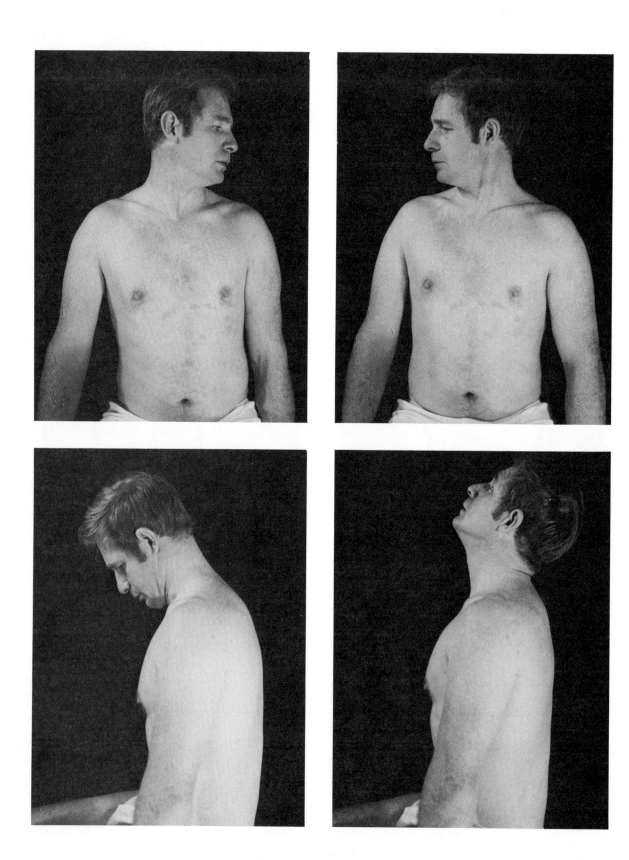

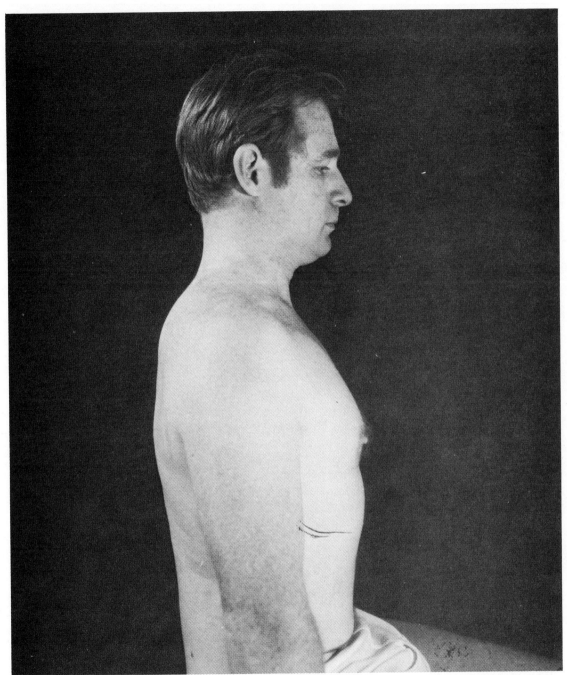

CF-15, 16, 17, 18, 19 The five photographs shown here depict neck movement as it manifests in an integrated body. Mr. R, a practioner of Structural Integration, has been the subject of many hours of processing in the course of his training. As a result, his spine shows sturdy resilience. This contrasts with the hypermobile body and posterior lumbar spine he showed as a child, and is evidence of the value of Structural Integration to young people. Note the way his head rotates on deep lying muscles, with little or no disturbance of the superficial shoulder and neck muscles. The way the cervical spine extends upward and lifts as he tips his head backward, and the position of his ear over his shoulder; both are signatures of a more adequate cervical spine. The verticality of the sternocleidomastoid muscle as the neck rotates is an indication of developing balance in cervical muscles.

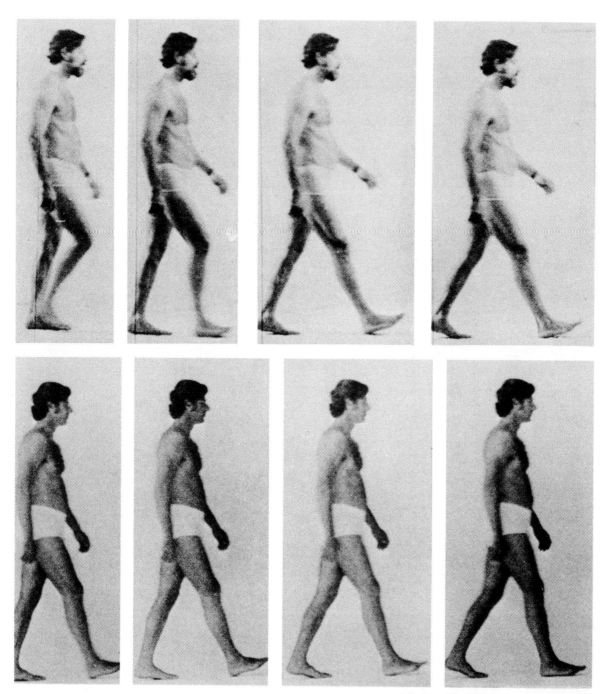

CF- 20 — 38 This final set of photographs records
the movement of Mr. J during his two training
classes as a practitioner — a period covering eighteen
months. They are self-explanatory. Fortunately for
the record, Mr. J shaved his very becoming beard
during the period, and there can be no mistaking
even at a superficial glance which are the "before-
processing" pictures, and which are the "after."
It is instructive to realize that the basic structural

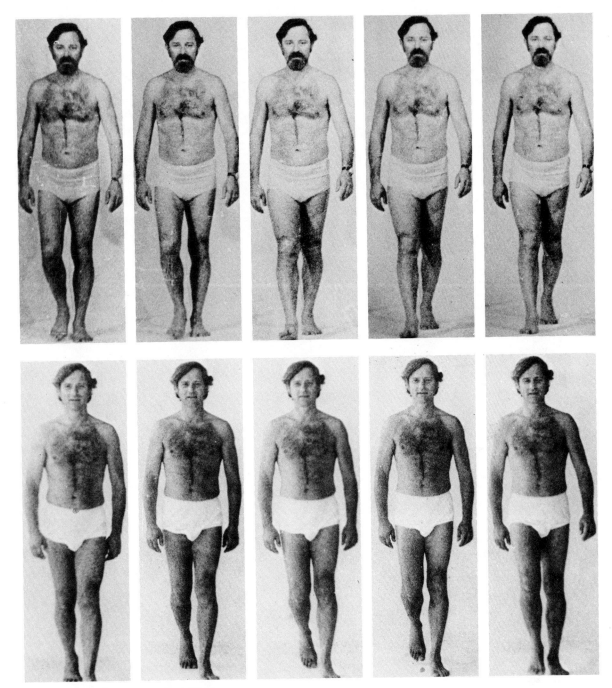

problem in this body is the very anterior lumbar
spine area. As this assumed a more normal position, his entire movement pattern changed. This
is evident in the knees accepting a straight-forward
direction, in the neck slowly becoming longer and
further back, and in the freeing of arms and elbows,
thus transferring responsibility for arm movement
from arm muscles to the broader, sturdier muscles
of the trunk.

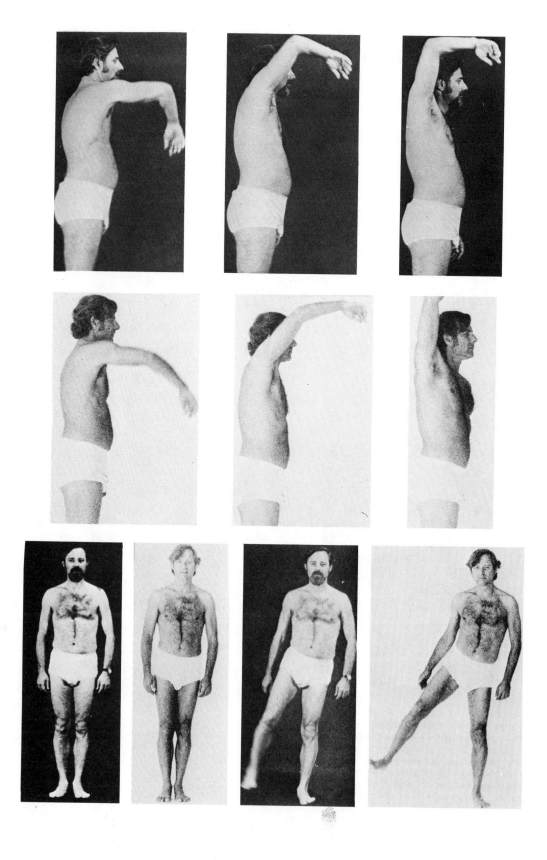

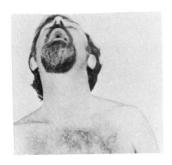
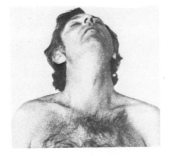
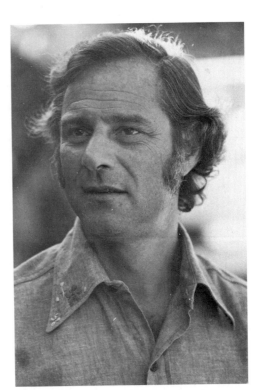
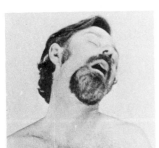
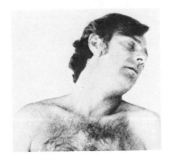
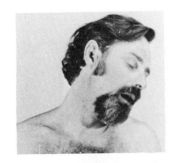
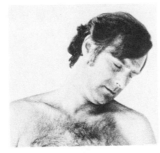
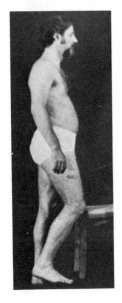
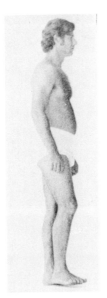
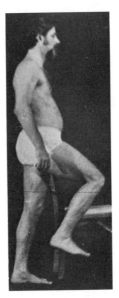
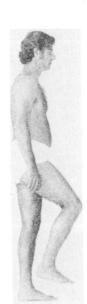

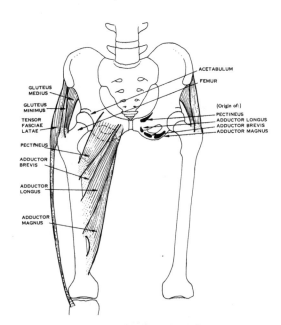

Functional differentiation between flexors and extensors is often quite difficult. The muscle that acts as flexor in one situation frequently plays the role of extensor in a different movement. Even in one movement, it will sometimes act as flexor at a nearer joint and extensor at a more distant segment. This is particularly true of large, complex muscles like the quadriceps femoris. In this powerful complex, four parts (*quadriceps*) almost encircle the femur. Of these, one head (rectus femoris) is the most powerful flexor of the thigh. In a single contraction of the quadriceps femoris, one head (rectus femoris) flexes the thigh, while simultaneously three sister muscles (vastus lateralis, vastus medialis, and vastus intermedius) act as extensors of the leg. (Fig 10-14ab). (Technically, the word *leg* refers to the lower limb below the knee; *thigh* refers to the upper segment.)

10-13 Anterior view: This schema of the adductor group indicates clearly how the adductors balance the gluteus medius and minimus. By holding the femur in an appropriate position, the glutei establish the spacing of the adductors (this is, of course, an oversimplification: rotators and abductors also participate).

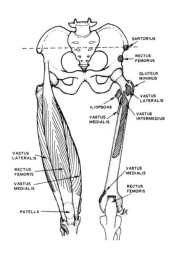

10-14 Extensors and flexors must cross the joint to move it. Quadriceps cross the knee, extending the leg below the knee (vasti lateralis, medius and intermedius, and rectus femoris). The rectus femoris attaches on the pelvic bone; thus it is a flexor of the thigh as well as an extensor of the leg below the knee. The gluteus maximus and the hamstring group: (biceps femoris, semitendinosus, and semimembranosus) cross the hip joint; they are extensors of the thigh, antagonists of the quadriceps.

Muscles act by shortening. In a balanced body, movement involves shortening one muscle or group (agonist) as the antagonist lengthens. To flex the thigh, for example, the rectus femoris (and other muscles on the front of the thigh) must shorten; on the back of the thigh, the hamstrings will lengthen. In random bodies, the tendency is for all these muscles to contract (flex); the result is inhibited, therefore unbalanced and uncoordinated movement.

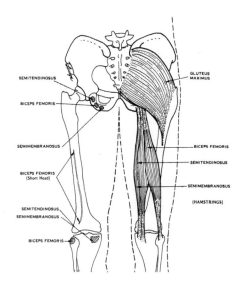

In theory, abduction-adduction and flexion-extension are simple actions, each creating movement in planes 180 degrees apart. In point of fact, very few muscles of the lower limb are free to act unidirectionally. Most have fibers that shorten in moving, and thus rotate the thigh. Normally the muscle should move as a whole. This shortening of individual fibers is *not* a normal pattern, but the result of accidental changes. Any consistent exercise, any repetitious posture or movement, if it shortens fibers, will tend to change the home position of the femoral head. Repeated often enough, the modified posture becomes chronic (unconscious). When the overlying gluteal structure cannot fit snugly, the hips seem too wide, and the problem is emphasized in the individual's slightly rolling gait (Fig. 10-16 ab).

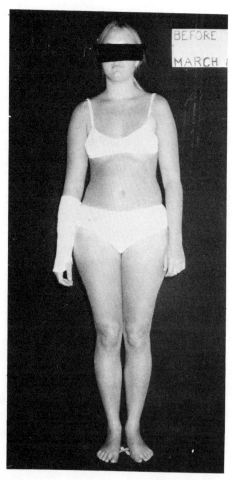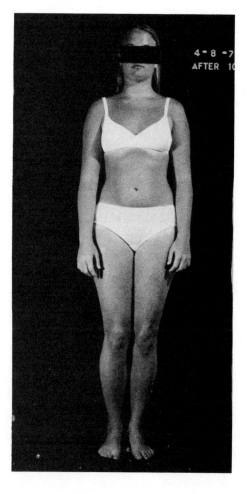

10-15 When the overlying gluteal structure cannot fit snugly, the hips seem too wide.

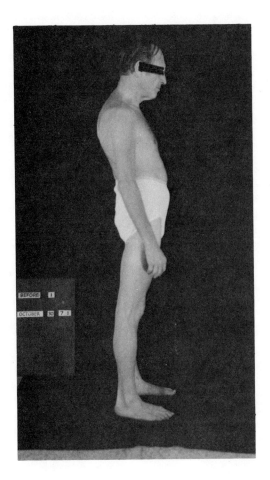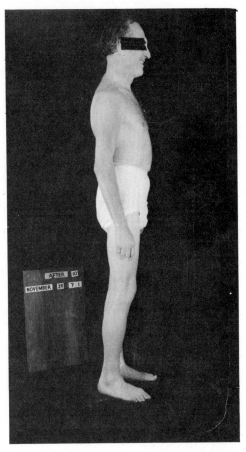

10-16 The man on the left is approaching seventy and looks aged — tired, disheartened, ill. Even visual examination, however, suggests that there is something that can be done to improve the situation. Reorganization at the hip joint will, in turn, support the upper body. The picture of the same man, on the right after ten hours of processing, confirms this interpretation.

But let there be no mistake. If help is to be had through Structural Integration, it is not possible to start locally at the hip joint. To induce appropriate change in the hip, it is necessary to start with the feet and ankles and to progress through a sequence that at moments may seem far from the weak point of the hip. Nevertheless, this is the approach and the sequence necessary to effect the change recorded here.

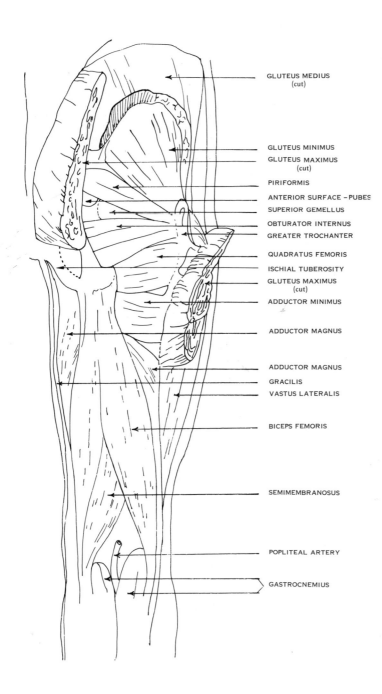

GLUTEUS MEDIUS
(cut)

GLUTEUS MINIMUS
GLUTEUS MAXIMUS
(cut)

PIRIFORMIS

ANTERIOR SURFACE – PUBES
SUPERIOR GEMELLUS
OBTURATOR INTERNUS
GREATER TROCHANTER

QUADRATUS FEMORIS
ISCHIAL TUBEROSITY
GLUTEUS MAXIMUS
(cut)
ADDUCTOR MINIMUS

ADDUCTOR MAGNUS

ADDUCTOR MAGNUS
GRACILIS
VASTUS LATERALIS

BICEPS FEMORIS

SEMIMEMBRANOSUS

POPLITEAL ARTERY

GASTROCNEMIUS

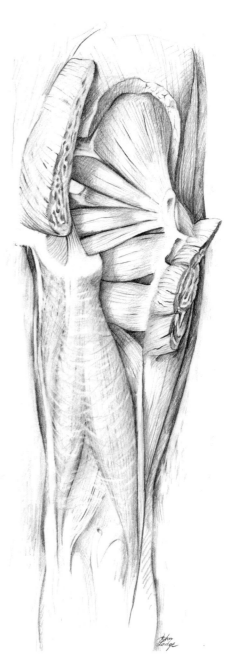

THE ROTATORS OF THE HIP AND
THE HAMSTRINGS OF THE THIGH

**10-17   Posterior views: Pencil sketch of all
rotators and key diagram.**

166

The simple rotation just described is apt to operate on a superficial level. But there is a group of muscles, the rotators, lying at a deeper level and performing a more complex function. Their general direction is roughly horizontal. They lie deep enough within the body to modify directly the plane of movement of the bony pelvic basin. They can and do transmit tension to individual bones of the pelvis (sacrum, ischium, etc.). Their attachment near the trochanter passes tension along, and thus the thigh is also involved. The profound effect of these muscles on gravitational balance is matched only by the psoas. Five individual muscles constitute these primary rotators. From above downward, they are piriformis, superior gemelli, obturator internus, inferior gemelli, obturator externus, and quadratus femoris. Clearly, all bind the trunk to the lower limbs (Figs. 10-17 and 10-18).

Two of the rotators (obturator internus and piriformis) share certain similarities with the psoas. All three of these arise within the trunk and attach to a peripheral unit, the thigh. These sophisticated diagonal pulls make more precise adjustment of the pelvis possible. But it is also this diagonal directional pull that makes all three potentially so powerful in aberrating gravitational balance. The obturator internus lines the medial wall of the ischium, traverses the lesser sciatic foramen, and inserts into the trochanter; in so doing, it stabilizes the ischial tuberosity. The piriformis lines the inner surface of three segments of the sacrum and, passing through the greater sciatic notch, connects all these structures with its point of insertion on the greater

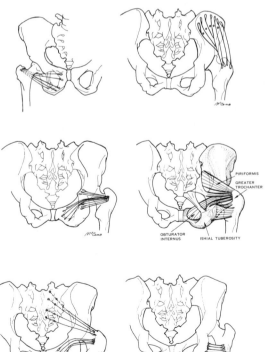

PIRIFORMIS

GREATER TROCHANTER

OBTURATOR INTERNUS   ISHIAL TUBEROSITY

10-18 Anterior views: These schemata show the individual attachments and insertions of each of the rotators. Fibers from any of these may interweave inappropriately in the random body. For example, when the sacroiliac junction is in lesion, fibers of the piriformis become involved in the confused cartilaginous disorder. Similarly, fibers of the pelvic floor may become entangled with the adjacent iliacus. Balance between gemelli and obturators is a major factor in the vertical and horizontal axes of the pelvis. When the vertical is interfered with, the span of the adductors becomes distorted (as evidenced, for example, in the position and movement of the knee).

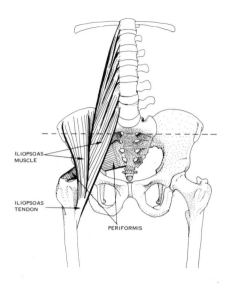

ILIOPSOAS
MUSCLE

ILIOPSOAS
TENDON

PERIFORMIS

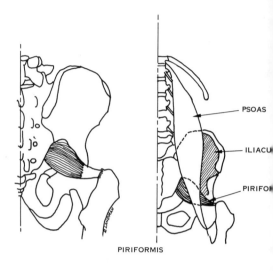

PSOAS

ILIACU

PIRIFO

PIRIFORMIS

trochanter (Fig. 10-19).

The psoas, arising on the anterior surfaces of the lumbar vertebrae (a higher level), crosses the pelvic brim near the pubes and inserts into the lesser trochanter. The piriformis and obturator internus, originating from a lower level (not the surface of the lumbars but the more inferior sacrum and pelvic wall), emerge through the greater sciatic notch and lesser sciatic foramen, respectively. In this fashion, these three muscles offer the variety of cross-directional pulls balancing pelvis on femur. (The term *foramen* applies to apertures through which muscles, nerves, or blood vessels pass; in many instances, they are formed by the tough ligaments joining adjacent bony structures, though occasionally they are actually apertures remaining after bone originally segmented has formed a stable junction.)

The group of rotators is covered by the more superficial gluteus maximus, which acts as a rotator of the thigh as the individual voluntarily rotates his leg outward. If the thigh is chronically rotated laterally, the gluteus maximus on the same side will be shortened. It may also safely be inferred that the quality of the underlying rotators will leave much to be desired. A similar inference may be made about the man who complains that he has never had anything to sit on. The quality and tone of his rotators have deteriorated, probably over much of his life. It is easy and seems logical to conclude that such a situation is irreparable—the muscles are lacking, nothing can be done. This is far from the truth. Appropriate balancing of gravitational units (which often includes shifting the position of the bony sacrum) allows lacking muscles to be reactivated and rebuilt. No structural situation in the living man is totally irreparable.

10-19 Anterior views: Prevertebral muscles establish and maintain the sturdy verticality of the spinal structure; their contribution to spinal well-being cannot be overestimated. In health, the anterior cushion of the prevertebral muscles prevents undue anterior displacement of the spine; by this support, they relieve the burden of the postvertebral extensors. In this sense, the well-being, resilience, and adaptability of all prevertebral myofascia is of great importance to economy of the body as a whole. The piriformis is an important component of the prevertebral group, as are the psoas and its sister muscle, the iliacus (which offer major support to the spine at the lumbar level). Deterioration in these prevertebral muscles is the beginning of major weakness in the spine.

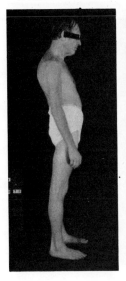
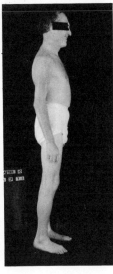

10-20 These photographs of Mr. H record and summarize the collapse of the overlying body. This happens when the piriformis fails to give adequate support to the sacrum, which then moves anterior. The compensating distortion within the spine, the failure of the rotators of the thigh to maintain support from thigh and leg, and the overshortened hamstrings that prevent balanced gait all are integral parts of the failure of the sacrum.

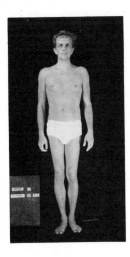

10-21 In this front view of Mr. W, his ineffectual leg structure is secondary to the problems visible at his groin. Even to the eye, the iliopsoas tendon lacks resilience and the legs are crowded into the torso. As a result, the ilia are drawn too closely together. Necessarily, the rotators of the thigh are also involved in the problem.

Thanks to the piriformis, relations between sacrum and rotators are reciprocal. If the rotators lack tone, the unsupported sacrum will be too far anterior. Any maladjustment of the sacrum is an indication of a lack of sturdy interplay in the rotators. The piriformis—the primary connecting link —arises from the inner surface of the sacrum. But many sacra, like the ones in Fig. 10-20, are terminals to very distorted spines. Where normal symmetry between lumbar vertebrae has been lost through some accident, the sacrum and attached piriformis may be subjected to abnormal unbalanced pulls. Sister rotators necessarily will be seriously distorted as well. Similarly, any accident that results in chronic rotation of the thigh will subject sacrum and overlying spine to pulls they may not be able to withstand. Both sacrum and spine then take refuge in compensatory distortion.

Reciprocal balance between lumbar spine and sacrum is of major importance. Lower-back problems indicate a deterioration of the normal internal balance between lumbar spine and pelvis. The very significant piriformis determines anterior-posterior placement of the sacrum and thus forms the foundation for the equally important compound iliopsoas. Whereas the piriformis establishes balance between sacrum and ilium, the psoas acts at the next higher level, at the lumbar spine. Both psoas and piriformis arise prevertebrally, within the trunk; both insert into the femur (thighbone). In arising on the anterior surface of lumbar and sacral vertebrae, they form a supportive web, coaxing these back toward the dorsal surface and helping them support the thoracic structure of the body. (The contribution of the iliacus is much the same. It forms a web on the inner surface of the ilium.)

The psoas is part of a greater complex, the iliopsoas. The iliacus, the other half of this complex, lines the inner wall of the bony ilium. About two-thirds of the bulk of this fan-shaped muscle arise from its inner surface; the lower part is free to adjust to the requirements of the tendon it shares with the psoas. Disorder in the psoas at any level transmits to the iliacus and thereby to the bony ilium. When the common tendon is under tension or deteriorated, the wings of the bony basin (the ilia) seem to draw closer together. It is often quite apparent visually that in a given individual the anterior superior spines of the ilia seem too close (Fig. 10-21). It is fascinating to watch these landmarks return toward a functionally more adequate distance as the tendon of the iliopsoas lengthens and becomes more elastic.

The piriformis attaches to the lateral aspect of the femur (greater trochanter); the iliopsoas attaches to the medial (lesser trochanter). By its attachment, the psoas is a direct

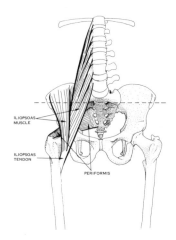
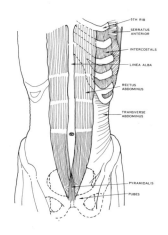
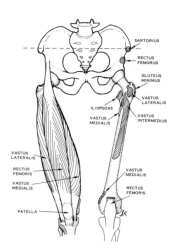

connection between the anterior surface of the intervertebral discs, the margins of the lumbar vertebrae, and the femur. The piriformis similarly connects the anterior surface of the sacrum to the femur. The iliacus lines the ilium; through a common tendon with the psoas, it shares its linkage to the femur. Piriformis, psoas, and iliacus form a continuous, steadying prevertebral web, which not only connects the spine with the femur but, when balanced, maintains appropriate distance between vertebral units. The iliopsoas tendon crosses the pelvic brim lateral to an adductor (the pectineus) and inserts into the lesser trochanter. In thus inserting on the medial side of the femur (the rotators insert more laterally), the psoas major can function as a medial and internal rotator of the thigh, balancing external rotators. Because of this essentially structural balance, any interference with movement, circulation, or metabolism in either group will affect the physiology of the other. It is of such tenuous threads that the intricate patterns of compensation are woven. The strands that make up these compensations, however confused, can be disentangled.

Together with the iliacus, the psoas should act as the major flexor of the thigh on the pelvis in all leg movement, especially walking. This would ensure the metabolic health of the embedded lumbar plexus. But, as we have seen before, flexion is too often quite inappropriately taken over by the rectus femoris. After this happens, the psoas, no longer in active use, usually deteriorates and no longer participates in any flexion. In this sequence, the recti femoris then perform the flexion. Recti, rather than the psoas, come to balance the glutei and supplement the recti abdominis. The psoas is bypassed; lumbar function suffers.

10-22 Anterior views: In balanced walking, the common tendon of the psoas and iliacus must lengthen as the rectus abdominis shortens. In this way, the pelvis rotates around an imaginary axis joining the heads of the femur. Psoas and rectus abdominis act as a pair to maintain horizontal balance. These schemata emphasize the fashion in which muscles from above and below can change the plane of the pelvis.

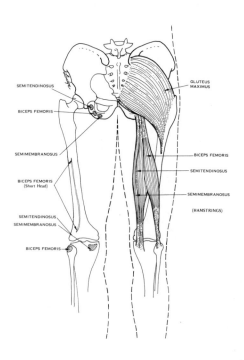

10-23

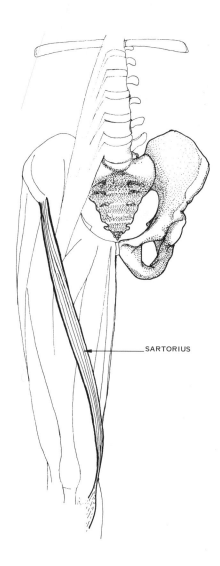

One other group of powerful thigh muscles, the hamstrings, further determines the spatial position of the pelvis. This complex consists of the biceps femoris, semimembranosus, and semitendinosus. Arising from a relatively small area on the pelvic bone at the ischial tuberosity, they rapidly become bulky and constitute about one-fifth of the total volume of the thigh. All attach below the knee. Through much of their length, they run close together; about two-thirds of the way down the leg they part company. The tendon of the biceps inserts into the head of the fibula on the lateral side of the leg. The other two hamstrings attach to the tibia, on the inner (medial) side. Thanks to these spacings, they extend the thigh and straighten the knee. At the same time, by shortening tendons to the tibia and fibula, they can flex the lower leg at the knee. These are among the most powerful of all the body muscles. Anything interfering with their equilibrium seriously disturbs the entire gravity pattern. If the hamstrings of both legs shorten consistently and permanently, the bony basin of the pelvis tips backward. If the shortening is unilateral, the pelvis rotates. No other single myofascial structure can compensate shortened hamstrings adequately. Only specifically lengthening the hamstrings themselves can bring the pelvic basin back to the horizontal.

One other powerful superficial thigh muscle participates in the complex that determines pelvic location and movement: the sartorius (Fig. 10-24). From the anterior superior spine of the pelvis, this longest muscle of the body runs diagonally across the thigh, inserting in a complicated interweaving pattern on the medial side below the knee (tibia). In shortening, it flexes both thigh and leg. Like the other flexors (rectus femoris, iliopsoas) and four of the adductors (pectineus and adductors longus, brevis, and magnus), it performs in an agonist-antagonist role with the three hamstrings. A chronically short sartorius can seriously restrict the ventral half of the thigh. Such a shortening forces a compensating thickening of the rectus femoris in that the origins of both muscles are very close together. Since the sartorius attaches at the medial aspect of the knee, this can cause not only contraction but also rotation at the knee joint. Both anterior superior and anterior inferior spines of the ilium are dragged forward and downward, thereby disorganizing all muscles attaching to the pelvic bone. Repeated or habitual sitting "tailor fashion," with legs crossed, or some yoga sitting patterns such as the Lotus can shorten the sartorius on one side more than on the other. This persistent pull on one anterior superior spine will rotate the entire pelvis.

It must be remembered that the word *rotation*, like the

SARTORIUS

10-24 After crossing the front of the thigh obliquely, the ribbonlike sartorius becomes a small tendon that spreads out into an aponeurosis. This curves around the insertion of the gracillis. If these two muscles, through inactivity, become glued together, the familiar mound at the inner side of the knee develops, and knee movement is pulled off its straight-forward-and-back track.

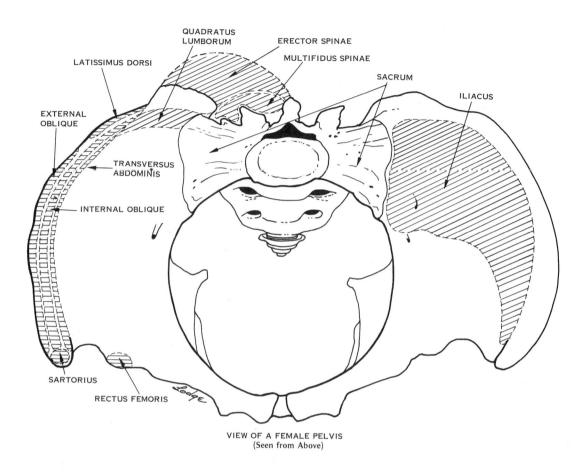

QUADRATUS
LUMBORUM

ERECTOR SPINAE

MULTIFIDUS SPINAE

LATISSIMUS DORSI

SACRUM

ILIACUS

EXTERNAL
OBLIQUE

TRANSVERSUS
ABDOMINIS

INTERNAL OBLIQUE

SARTORIUS

RECTUS FEMORIS

VIEW OF A FEMALE PELVIS
(Seen from Above)

word *curvature,* really expresses nothing more frightening than the fact that one muscle (or set of muscles) is pulling more than its structural antagonist is able to balance. This is another situation that can be changed. Sometimes in curvatures such as spontaneous idiopathic scolioses, some individual elements resist complete balancing, or may even be lacking. In spite of this, a significant degree of structural organization, which makes the individual more comfortable and more effective, is always available.

This is the story of the living pelvis. It emphasizes not the static but the dynamic. The pelvis *is* the key to the well-being of the individual. But it is a dynamic key, a process key. Technically and anatomically, the pelvis is a bony basin. Vitally and physiologically, it is a relation of energies. Optimal performance of such a system occurs only at the narrow peak of balance. This is, of necessity, precise.

10-25

10-26 Again you are looking at the left hip-bone from the left side. Here the hip has rotated around a horizontal axis. In this way, the relation of all muscles to the horizontal plane (and to the vertical gravity line) has been changed. Note particularly that the changed position of the hamstrings with reference to the horizontal plane distorts the position of the sacrum by altering the strain on the sacrotuberous and sacrospinous ligaments. Conversely, a sacrum seriously aberrated spatially by an anterior or rotated fourth or fifth lumbar will exert a continuous asymmetric drag on these ligaments. In turn, balanced, resilient stretch of the hamstrings is no longer evoked.

As a consequence of these disorganizations, physiological functions deteriorate; lacking the stimulus of use, eventually they atrophy. In many bodies, palpation locates the attachments of the hamstrings as lumps of gristle, no longer capable of the give-and-take required of the normal muscle, the normal ligament. Such deteriorated hamstrings interfere with the degree of flexion demanded of the psoas in normal walking. As "normal," we define the gait resulting from the rotation of the pelvis about the femoral head. It is axiomatic that in the normal body the agonist flexor is balanced by the antagonist extensor, that a given degree of shortening in a flexor is compensated by the same degree of uninterrupted lengthening of the antagonist extensor.

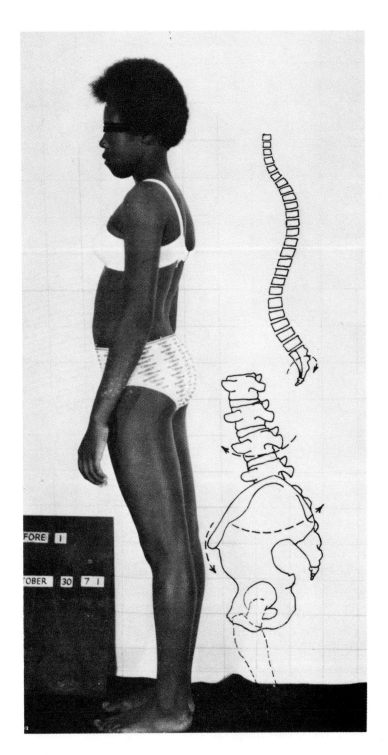

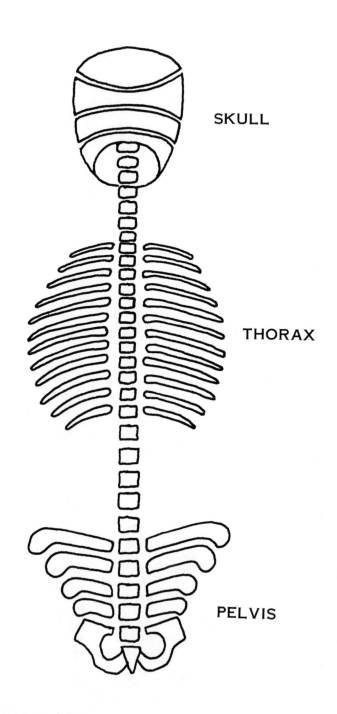

SKULL

THORAX

PELVIS

11-1 Schema of the human skeleton. (After Kahn, MAN IN STRUCTURE AND FUNCTION, Vol. 1, Fig. 62)

11
The Function of a
Normal Erect Spine
Is to Distribute Weight

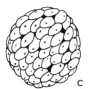

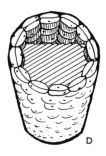

11-2 The fertilized ovum (A) proliferates (B). A sphere forms (C) and fluid collects. Finally, the sphere becomes hollow and cylindrical in shape — a blastula (D). This is the history of every human being within hours after fertilization (After Kahn, MAN IN STRUCTURE AND FUNCTION, Vol. 1, Fig.12).

The spine rests in the pelvis much as a person sits in a rocking chair. Although we consider the pelvis basic to the physical and emotional well-being of the individual, his optimal dynamic functioning requires structural integrity from the soles of his feet to the crown of his head. In relation to gravity, the spine is the connecting rod of the body, a segmented armature resting in the pelvis. Its two polar terminals, embodied in pelvis and head, make the spine a vital core that integrates the human with his gravity environment, poorly, well, or adequately, as the case may be.

Classically, the vertebral column (the spine) is regarded as a fundamental structural support. This has been considered its most important function. In a limited sense, this assumption is true; the spine does act as a pole or lattice about which to relate myofascial structures. It not only supports the muscular man, it also acts as scaffolding for his autonomic nervous system. In addition, it gives protective casing and support to the ontologically more recent system housed within the vertebrae, the central nervous system. The health of all important nervous tissue is closely tied to well-being in the spine.

The dual function of support and protection is emphasized in the embryological development of the spine. After fertilization, the one-celled egg rapidly proliferates into a many-celled, fluid-filled sphere (Fig. 11-2). The sphere flattens, forming separate layers; the upper, outer one is called ectoderm; the lower, entoderm. Later, the entoderm folds into a hollow tube running the length of the unit, giving form to an intestinal tract. The whole is rapidly enwrapped by a developing third layer, the mesoderm (Fig. 11-3). The elongated cylinder, the cells of the entoderm, has by now formed an intestinal tube. At the same time, the ectoderm grooves into a closed tube, later to be called the neural tube (Fig. 11-4). (Still later, this becomes the spinal canal, and will be encased in the spine.) All nervous components develop from this original ectodermal tissue. The spine, developing from the mesoderm, begins its intimate relationship of support and protection with the ectodermal nervous system when it closes around the neural tube. The rest of the ectoderm separates from the neural tube, proliferates, and finally enwraps the entire developing organism as skin.

The middle layer, the mesoderm, develops into the structures that are the primary concern of this book. From it evolve blood and bones, cartilage, fascia, and muscle. Early in this development, a line of thirty-three denser spots appear; these will differentiate into bony segments. The spots first develop into a cartilaginous casing; later, this becomes true bone and supplies protection to the central nervous tissue. Some of this general supportive and protective function of the mesoderm is supplied through growth in the ventral direction. Later in their development, we call these bony bands *ribs*. Lower in the body, they become the individual units of the pelvis. As ribs, the bony bands protect the vital units of heart, lungs, and upper viscera. As the bony basin of the pelvis, they guard and support the lower viscera.

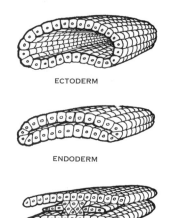

ECTODERM

ENDODERM

MESODERM

11-3 Meantime, a flat middle germ layer develops, called the mesoderm. From it differentiate the body systems with which we are primarily concerned — myofascia, cartilage, and bone. This layer folds upward, encasing the neural tube. This is the beginning of the protective armor later called the spinal column. It also extends downward enclosing parts of the intestinal tube in a casing of ribs and pelvic basin. (After Kahn, MAN IN STRUCTURE AND FUNCTION, Vol. 1, Fig. 13).

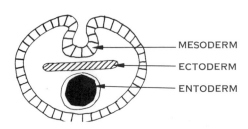

MESODERM

ECTODERM

ENTODERM

11-4 Within a day or so, the cylindrical blastula becomes a three-layered flat disc called a gastrula. The most interior of these layers is known as the internal germ layer (entoderm). It coils into a hollow tube, which later develops into an intestinal tract. The outer layer (ectoderm) completely encloses the two other layers. It develops as an outer integument, or protective skin. A dorsal surface becomes distinguishable, and along this surface, an additional small tubular structure appears. This is the neural tube; from its cells develop what will later be known as the nervous system. (After Kahn, MAN IN STRUCTURE AND FUNCTION Vol. 1, Fig. 15)

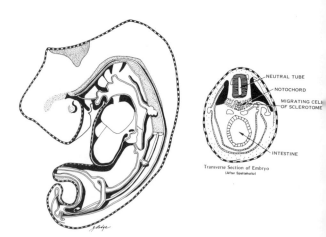

NEUTRAL TUBE

NOTOCHORD

MIGRATING CELL OF SCLEROTOME

INTESTINE

Transverse Section of Embryo
(After Spalteholtz)

11-5 At right, a transverse section of the early human embryo. As days progress into the very early weeks of embryonic life, a more complex and somewhat more solid individual appears (left). Many of the earlier structures are still recognizable, particularly the entoderm (now developing as an intestinal tract) and the ectodermal neural tube encased by the mesodermal vertebral structure (A after Spalteholz, ATLAS OF HUMAN ANATOMY, Fig. 309)

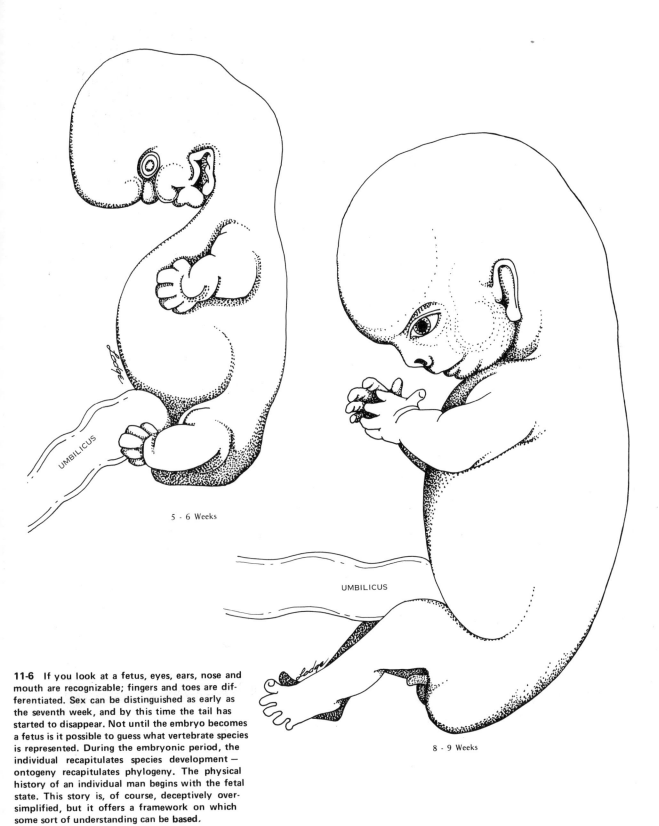

UMBILICUS

5 - 6 Weeks

UMBILICUS

8 - 9 Weeks

11-6 If you look at a fetus, eyes, ears, nose and mouth are recognizable; fingers and toes are differentiated. Sex can be distinguished as early as the seventh week, and by this time the tail has started to disappear. Not until the embryo becomes a fetus is it possible to guess what vertebrate species is represented. During the embryonic period, the individual recapitulates species development — ontogeny recapitulates phylogeny. The physical history of an individual man begins with the fetal state. This story is, of course, deceptively oversimplified, but it offers a framework on which some sort of understanding can be **based**.

Much of the tissue developing from the mesoderm is collagenous. (A more detailed discussion of this was given in Chapter Three.) The earliest and most primitive units of the mesoderm, the gelatinous stellate cells, rapidly undergo change. Through the development of interpenetrating fibers, the original jellylike mass evolves into fibrous connective tissue, varying in texture, compressibility, elasticity, etc. It has become collagen. Collagen fibers are able to plait or braid into extremely strong and very tough ligamentous units (Fig. 11-7). They lend support to basic nervous tissue. The brain and the central nervous system, for instance, are enwrapped in fascial sheets, first in the delicate arachnoid mater and pia mater, then in the tougher dura mater. All these very different layers derive from the collagenous fascia of the mesoderm.

At its early stage, connective tissue is avascular. During the second month of intrauterine life, minute blood vessels make their appearance, ensuring a source of nutrition. It is then that tiny ossific centers (chemically, calcareous deposits) begin to appear. More calcium is deposited and chemically unites with the collagenous matrix; this new material forms the early spongy bone of fetus and infant. This continuing process builds the bony framework of the body, the skeletal structure. Final fusion of the surfaces at which this bony growth takes place (epipheseal lines) occurs later (as early as in the fetus, as late as the late twenties). Cervical vertebrae, for example, may not fuse before the third year, although primary centers for each half have appeared during the seventh week of intrauterine life; secondary centers fuse later. Sacral segments, which make their first appearance about the twentieth week, are subject to complicated time schedules. Fusion, which may begin at the seventh to tenth year, will not reach final stabilization before age twenty-five.

It is important to realize that skeletal structure is in the process of fundamental change during more than half the life span of the average individual. The outward changes of the child and youth take place before our eyes. These rapid shifts are the physical expressions of the behavioral differences we call the generation gap. The average adult mistakenly tends to think of the young person, even the young child, as a miniature adult. This concept is not realistic—is even misleading. The average notion of bones and their growth, for example, is erroneous. Even in the adult, bones are not hard, tough, solid units, invariable and unchangeable. They are aggregates, a calcareous deposit within an organic collagenous matrix. During the entire life span of the individual, calcium is laid down within this matrix, and calcium may be picked up from it. The direction of travel of

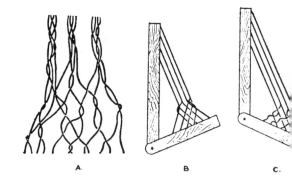

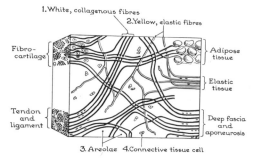

11-7 At left, A, collagen fibers of a tendon are plaited. B and C show how in different positions of a joint different fibers take the strain (After Mollier). At right, scheme to indicate that the four ingredients of areolar tissue (viz., collagenous fibers, elastic fibers, areolar spaces, and cells), when blended in different proportions, form other tissues (e.g., adipose, elastic, collagenous, ligamentous, and fibrocartilaginous) and that one may merge into another. (A and B from Basmajian, GRANT'S METHOD OF ANATOMY, Figs. 31 and 53)

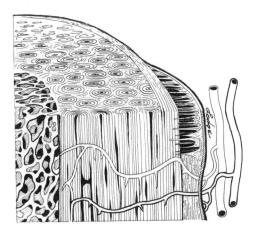

11-8

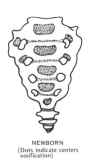

NEWBORN
(Dots indicate centers
ossification)

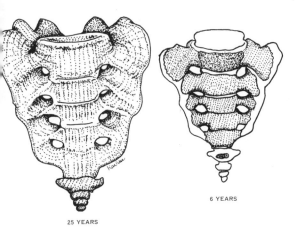

6 YEARS

25 YEARS

11-9

calcium will depend on the chemical homeostasis of surrounding tissue and body fluids. The miracle of it is that this complex interchange goes on in accordance with the laws of spatial patterning specific to man.

Realistic understanding of the process we call the body necessitates the rejection of a vast core of simplistic information. Assumptions about the separateness of bones, muscles, cartilaginous discs, ligaments, etc., are particularly misleading. Embryological development shouts this loud and clear. So does the actual anatomical structure of the adult. In the classic, static view, each is seen as a solid, separate element. In the living man, skeletal structures must be appreciated as integral parts of more complicated compound structures. Cartilaginous discs, for example, are not units separating bones; they are part of a bone-disc complex, bound together by ligamentous bands. Functionally, the whole acts unitarily. The implications of this unified, in-process design are most significant. In terms of the human body, they spell the possibility of change—change as long as life shall last. Change need not be negative deterioration (so-called aging); it may well be a positive evolving construction, a mechanism through which greater maturity (physical and psychological) may be achieved.

The body of any living organism is not a simple unit. Nor is it just an aggregation of separate elements (as much earlier we temporarily postulated, for simplicity's sake). The body has an intrinsic organic wholeness. In the matrix of the developing embryo, cartilage and bone are laid down together. While this unity has been separated and analyzed into its parts to further an ongoing understanding, still, the integration, the wholeness, resulting from unitary interplay is the basic fact. Through maturing and developing this premise, the techniques of Structural Integration have allowed us to create well-being, wholeness, health.

Contributing to this wholeness is the reciprocity of body chemistry with body physics, body metabolism with body structure. Foodstuffs find their way to tissues by way of fluids (e.g., blood and lymph). The freedom of flow here depends on structural integrity. The more freely fluids can flow or seep into and out of local areas, the greater the opportunity for positive change as needed to maintain spatial or genetic pattern. A soft, fluid-filled tissue such as the liver is subject to much more rapid change than muscle. Even bone itself is fed by small arteries, which penetrate to the marrow; therefore, even bone changes. This change can be amazingly rapid, especially in the young.

Realigning body structure thus implies realigning a flowing river of fluid-borne nutrients. Currents within the river flow at different rates. These chemical substances are not merely three-dimensional material particles floating in an aqueous medium. This is an oversimplified notion, another surface disguise. The underlying reality pattern is once again one of energy currents, energy interplays—energy transfers from less dense to more dense media and back again. As one substance or nutrient attaches to another in metabolic transfer, or as they detach in a catabolic phase, we call the exchange "chemical." With equal justification, we can see it as an energy phenomenon. Application of pressure (energy) through muscular expansions and contractions fosters these transfers. To get more economical flow, we must start at the macrolevels of muscular and fascial systems in order to influence the microlevels of cellular metabolism.

In our experience, the finest and most minute tissues of the body can be reached by way of the coarser layers; thus body structure can be integrated and ordered throughout. The start must be from the outside, the periphery. Loosening and stretching of superficial fascia permit liberation of underlying layers. Interaction between these freed intermediary muscles and tendons and deeper fascial layers allows the deepest-lying elements (the bones) to find their place and exercise the function appropriate to their structural design. The relocation of more peripheral soft tissue and appropriate organization of its mass directly affects chemical changes. The body that emerges through this balancing of structures is one of great resilience and lightness, the benchmark of effective metabolism.

In this kind of body, the vital myofascial tissue is the primary support—the more static bones are secondary (Fig. 11-10). As in our tent, where the tension created by the fabric and ropes of one side pulled up the other side, so in this body, agonist countering antagonist creates the span of balance. The function of the bone in this design is not primarily support; rather, it is the precise separation of myofascial tissue required to achieve span and balance. A spine barely more than semierect, merely a support for pendant muscles, acts as a dragging, weight-burdened, earthbound unit (Fig. 11-11). The lightness, the movement, the lift of the integrated body has nothing in common with it. The differences begin with the unit of the whole spine, not merely its individual bones.

Our forebears, limited by their lack of modern technology, regarded the spine as a collection of bony vertebrae stacked in a straight line. To complete this picture, a series of inserted cartilaginous discs cushioned the bony segments. A human spine, however, is much more highly developed and complex. Such oversimplification, while a useful primitive approximation, can be quite misleading. In a vertebrate

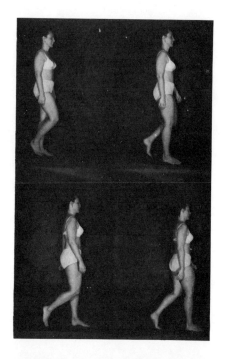

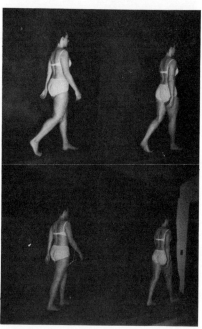

11-10 This woman (who has had a ten-hour Integrating series) shows how the body tends to lift itself upward in the gravity field. Her legs seem to walk under her lifted body, rather than her body being carried by her legs.

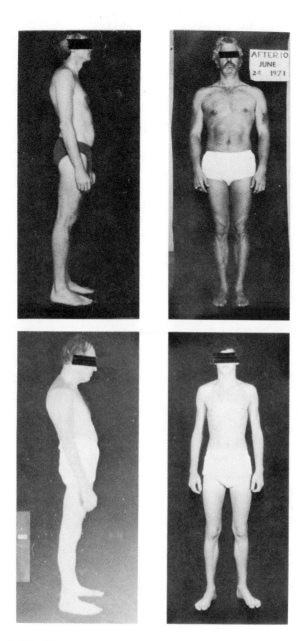

11-11 These bodies are at war with gravity, are earthbound, yet they show very different pictures. The "strong man" (top right) is very proud of his bulging, overdeveloped muscles. These are where and what they are in response to his requirement that his body be "held" erect against gravity. But there is no integration in this body, no interplay, no balance of intrinsic structure with extrinsic. His picture is one of continual effort to hold himself upright.

The others are classic examples of poor posture, of gravity versus man where gravity is winning. Only the bones contained within the skin prevent a collapse into formlessness.

species, struggling toward the erect, the spine has a central role in determining balanced, erect structure. Spine and pelvis may be seen as co-stars in this production. Therefore, a detailed layout of spinal structure and function is now in order.

Spine is a wider concept than the slightly less familiar term *vertebral column*. *Spine* refers to the column of thirty-three vertebrae that constitute the bony units of the body's core; it also includes the cartilaginous structures. The intervertebral discs seemingly hold the vertebrae apart; cartilaginous bands, ligaments, etc., span from bone to bone and serve to hold the elements together. Collectively, they comprise the spine; in the language of our grandfathers, they form the "backbone." An older generation used this term to designate not merely a physical structure but also a psychological attitude toward life. This was excellent observation on their part, for the individual's attitude toward his environment does mirror the sturdiness and adequacy of his spinal structure. A spine that consists of curves reversed with respect to the normal (a convex lumbar and concave dorsal, for example) is unable to pattern itself appropriately in space. The tone of the involved tissue cannot be normal. This poor tone is then often reflected in lack of psychological energy, of focused, purposeful drive. In attempting to understand man-as-a-whole, it is vital to appreciate his spinal structure—its tone, its conformity to or deviance from normal spatial position.

And the "normal"? What is it? The course of spinal growth and structure tells much about it. Spinal vertebrae, like many bones, are preformed in cartilage. There is no clean precision, no clear-cut separation between bone and cartilage. As the bone grows, cartilage persists at its ends and often knits imperceptibly into the tendons of the attaching muscles. In mid-life, at thirty to forty years of age, this type of cartilage may become calcified.

Wherever found, in whatever density, connective tissue has low fluid content. In general, it has few interpenetrating blood or lymph vessels; being without nerves, it is relatively insensitive. Three types of connective tissue can be distinguished as cartilage, all demonstrating basic collagen qualities. The shiny-white resilient material in which calcium salts are deposited to form bones and spinal vertebrae is called hyaline cartilage. A much thinner, more flexible cartilage (found in the external ear and the throat) is designated elastic cartilage. A tougher, more fibrous tissue is called fibrocartilage; this heavy-duty material makes up the intervertebral discs.

The ubiquitous "disc trouble" of the mid-twentieth century has made people aware that their spines, their "backs,"

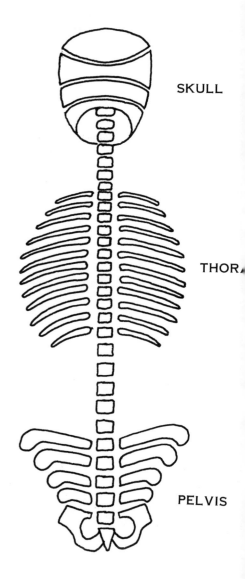

SKULL

THOR

PELVIS

11-12 This evocative schema suggests the vertical-horizontal pattern followed by the developing fetus. Ribs and pelvis emerge from units that develop at right angles to the spine. Horizontal pelvic segments later fuse into the bony basin. This diagram is, of course, suggestive rather than factual. (See Chapter Five for a more factual account of the development of the pelvis.) (After Kahn, MAN IN STRUCTURE AND FUNCTION, Vol. 1, Fig. 62)

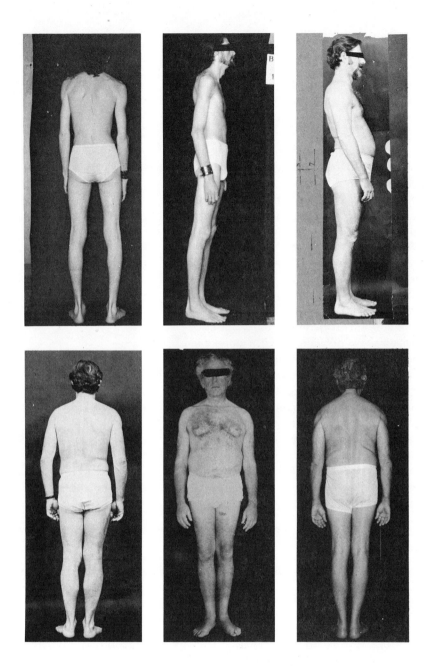

11-13 This series shows two basic spinal deviations. Mr. S is hypererect (this body type often is). His posture is the outward manifestation of an anterior dorsal and posterior lumbar spine. This reverses the average pattern; it is the deviation of an ectomorphic structure, and gives rise to an unusual pattern in the whole system. In this man, note the way in which the legs and shoulders have tried to compensate.

Classically, the spinal pattern of anterior lumbar and posterior dorsal has been called normal. It might better be called average. Messrs. J and L show such extensive exaggerations of this average structure that the spine is not able to lend adequate support to higher structures.

are constructed as much by elastic discs as by hard, bony vertebrae. The center of the spinal intervertebral disc, the so-called nucleus pulposus, is relatively soft, especially in early life. It is surrounded and protected by fibrous tissue, the annulus fibrosus. This tough fibrocartilage interweaves with the persisting hyaline cartilage edging the body of the bony vertebrae. Thus bony vertebrae and cartilaginous disc are structurally one unit. As the body ages, the softer center of the disc is replaced by fibrocartilage. The result is the lessened mobility called aging; chronology has little to do with it. Tissue age may be quite different from chronological age, and depends on the fluid content of the disc and on the elasticity of the ligaments that splint the vertebrae and discs together. Thus discs in a young person, having relatively high fluid content, can be subjected to heavier deformation strain and still recover. Experiments have shown that such individual discs can maintain properly distributed loads of 500-800 pounds without serious damage.

Discs constitute one-fourth to one-fifth of the spinal structure. Therefore, establishing or maintaining a good fluid balance in the discs is important in maintaining healthy spinal performance. By implication, this means ingesting an adequate amount of fluid daily (six to eight glassfuls). Exercise involving bending and straightening measures function in the discs and also acts as a pumping mechanism, bringing foodstuffs and oxygen to disc structures. Therefore bending can be a specific remedy for discs that are in chronic rather than acute trouble. Acute disc pain is a matter for medical care.

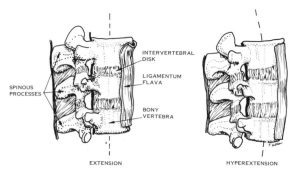

SPINOUS PROCESSES

INTERVERTEBRAL DISK

LIGAMENTUM FLAVA

BONY VERTEBRA

EXTENSION

HYPEREXTENSION

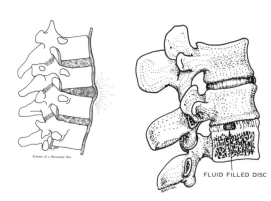

Schema of a Herniated Disc

FLUID FILLED DISC

11-14 Lateral views: Cartilaginous discs are not units separating bones; they are part of a bone-disc complex, bound together by ligamentous bands. They act as a single unit.

Biologically older humans are characterized by connective tissue with:

* Less fluid
* More fibrocartilage
* Sometimes accompanied by deposition of calcium.
* Increasing lack of mobility

Biologically younger individuals show connective tissue with:

* More fluid
* Collagen tissue with greater elasticity
* Mineral content probably lower, with less calcium
* Greater elasticity, faster recovery from injury, much greater mobility

All patterns show gradual desiccation after age thirty

11-15

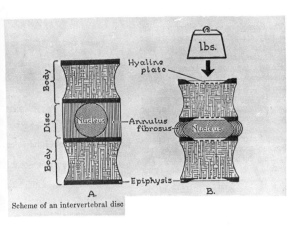

Scheme of an intervertebral disc

11-16 The universal disc troubles of the twentieth century all show the strain on spinal discs caused by imperfect downward-weight transmission. If the myofascial pre- and postvertebral webbing is competent, disc trouble is non-existent. Weight no longer drags downward through bony vertebrae, but is distributed through accessorial myofascial structures. Weight transmitted straight downward is a distorting force. (From Basmajian, GRANT'S METHOD OF ANATOMY, Fig. 26)

In this day and age, an increasing number of people say that they have disc trouble. This generalization covers diverse situations, many of which can be inferred from an understanding of the structure of discs. In a free, erect spine, the relation of disc and vertebral body may be schematized as in *A* in Fig. 11-16. However, pressure on the spine from above can modify this scheme toward that shown in *B*. In real life, especially in older bodies, the second pattern is the more usual one.

In a free, erect spine, the extensor system of the back supplies support and span to the vertebrae. Unfortunately, this support is vulnerable; all too often the extensors are hypertoned and may be felt as inelastic ropes along the spine. Any consistent interference with a freely adjusting extensor system in the dorsum (the back) can supply a pressure causing discs to bulge. Extensors bring the body to an erect position; deterioration prevents both appropriate body stretching and body straightening (Fig. 11-18). Adding further emergency effort to such an already unbalanced flexor-extensor relation is all that is necessary to produce the acute situation registered as pain. Continual bad posture or inelastic, chronically contracted lumbar fascia can easily supply the basic strain for the "slipped disc." Then, to produce the permanent bad back or the "sacroiliac," only a minor emergency is needed.

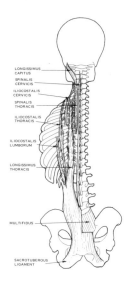

11-17 Posterior view: These are the erector spinae. It is obvious from their complexity how vulnerable they are. Deterioration in any member distributes imbalance throughout the extensors. Imagine, for example, what has happened to these erectors to produce the back of the young man pictured in the next illustration.

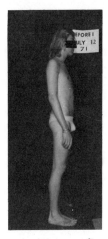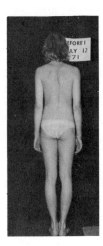

11-18 The shortening of the erector spinae group shows here in the bulges on both sides of the spine. This shortening helps force the bony spine forward. This young man shows the same basic reversal curves (anterior dorsal, posterior lumbar) as demonstrated in our ectomorph Mr. S, seen a few pages earlier. Mark how in this instance legs and shoulders compensate, although he is fifteen years younger than the other man, and therefore compensations have not had time to progress as far.

In youth, fibrocartilage has good resilience. A "slipping disc," released from distorting strain, can return to a position in which it will again integrate and coordinate with its neighbors. Later in life, as fibrocartilage desiccates, lessened resilience does not permit as easy readjustment to sudden traumatic shock or extreme muscular effort. If the chemistry of the fibrocartilage is poor, the disc may herniate (Fig. 11-19). Fibers of cartilage separate and allow the nucleus to seep through at the weakest point (usually the back of the disc, into the vertebral foramina and deep spinal structures). Such breakdown can be extremely painful; surgery is often required for repair. Fortunately, most "slipped discs" are not serious herniations; balancing the spinal muscles induces the disc to return to a more normal position, where spontaneous repair can occur. Chemistry is a determinant of the outcome; good chemistry in the local area fosters spontaneous repair.

Many chronic postural patterns contribute strain to spinal structure (Fig. 11-20). Persistently maintained flexed posture (the chronic flexion of age as well as the ubiquitous bad posture of youth) tends to thin the ventral aspect of discs; chronic lateroflexion will thin them on the flexed side. In youth, such unhappy structural developments may well remain unnoticed. In these earlier stages, little if any pain accompanies the deviation. Only as compensations to the situation spread to distant points of the body do symptoms develop. Finally, when pain makes the situation noticeable, some doctor demands an X-ray and the thinned disc becomes apparent. Its owner, terrified, decides he has "had it." His pessimism is entirely unjustified. Even after a certain degree of calcification starts to make the aberration permanent, muscular balancing and the ensuing more appropriate posture will elicit joint movement. The disc can then spontaneously reshape itself; restored structure restores function.

Discs are not only shock absorbers; they also offer a mechanism through which normal spinal movements of flexion and extension, lateral flexion, rotation, and combinations of these can occur. Discs determine the extent of spinal mobility; the thicker the bridging disc, the greater the movement possible. Thus greater movement is possible between lumbar vertebrae, with their thicker discs, than between the closer thoracic units.

Collagen is the basic constituent of all cartilaginous tissue of the spine, ligaments as well as discs. Ligaments guard joint integrity and alignment. Some, like the longitudinal spinal ligaments, run the entire length of the spine. Others, sheathing the sides of discs or connecting spinous processes, are short and interwoven, forming a strong web

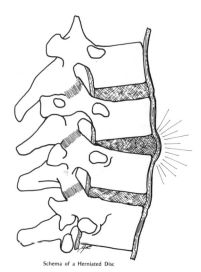

Schema of a Herniated Disc

11-19 Lateral view: A disc, a cartilaginous unit interpenetrated by fluid, is more vulnerable than a bony vertebra. Under strain, the cartilage "herniates" i.e. loses the pattern in which it can perform its spinal function. This is an anterior herniation; the posterior herniations are the ones that cause acute pain resulting from encroachment on the nerve. The victim says, " Yes, when I bent over to get something from the lower bureau drawer, I couldn't straighten up." Before the situation can be remedied, the disc must again become uniformly thick, thus removing localized pressure and inflamation.

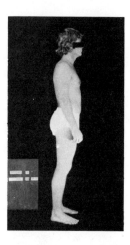

11-20 In a modern world, we do not expect to see a person carrying a bushel of coal or a basket of concrete on the head, thus creating bulging discs for himself. Nevertheless, it does occasionally happen. This very young man earned his living in the construction industry by carrying heavy burdens on his head. The response of his lumbar spine and the compensatory adjustment of his legs tell their own story.

186

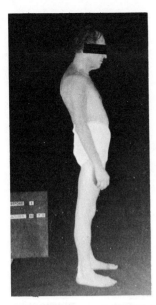

11-21 A man whose contour is like this is necessarily a man whose spinal structure is chronically under great stress. This inevitably reflects in poor physiological function at the level of greatest strain.

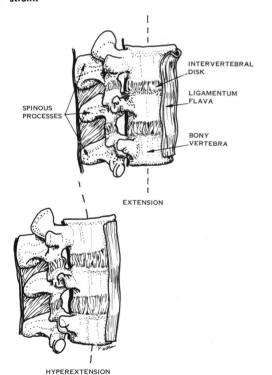

INTERVERTEBRAL DISK

LIGAMENTUM FLAVA

SPINOUS PROCESSES

BONY VERTEBRA

EXTENSION

HYPEREXTENSION

11-22 Lateral views: This is the type of adaptation which occurs in an early lumbar lordosis, stretching and thinning prevertebral ligaments and preparing for the chronic "bad lower back."

that limits the excursion of individual units. Ligament, disc, and bony vertebra together construct a whole that is different from (and greater than) the sum of its parts. The web truly integrates significant elements. In turn, chemical homeostasis in and around these tissues determines their sturdiness and the security of the spine (and thus of the individual).

In a body reaching toward equipoise, the spine distributes weight through balance rather than supports it. Here the myofascial structure becomes the key. The bony spine establishes and maintains span in myofascia. Within its limits, it can allow the balancing of soft-tissue counterparts. Thus one definition of a body in balance is a body in which the spine evokes myofascial equalizations. The average body seen on the streets or beaches is not in this class. True, its randomly distributed weight is more or less upheld by a spine; but, at best, the weight is unstable and becomes a heavy burden. We are again reminded of our ill-balanced tent, in which the center pole is off the vertical alignment, and the struggling owner must fight the weight of the falling canvas. In a tent, he sometimes wins and rights the structure. But in the complex reactions of a body, it is usually a losing fight. Gravity consistently wins.

In the ape-man (and in random bodies), the spine is placed like a slightly leaning, off-balance tent pole. It is used to support weight; under the conditions given, the weight must be supported off the center. (Once again, this is a game with an inevitable sequel: if the tent pole is off-center, its weight will drag it down; if it is upright, its weight will balance and keep it upright.) Thus the physiological function of a normal erect spine is to distribute weight. During the long evolution of the human body, from the semierect stance of the ape to the potentially light, erect balance possible in the structure of modern Homo sapiens, the spine has undergone many functional experiments. Obviously it is structurally more efficient to have the tent pole vertical, and man's evolution has moved in this direction. Most random bodies are still to be found at some point along the road from the ape-man to the truly erect human.

In understanding spinal function, there is still another outstanding confusion. We call the spine a column. We think of a column as underneath the structure it upholds. Thus the spine is obviously not a true column, since it is nearer the dorsal surface of the body. It is like a beam upended. In the four-footed animal, it acts as a relatively horizontal beam. In man, it shows as a beam becoming vertical and takes on the characteristics and necessities of such a support. This introduces problems that an erect central column would not pose. First and foremost, it means that even

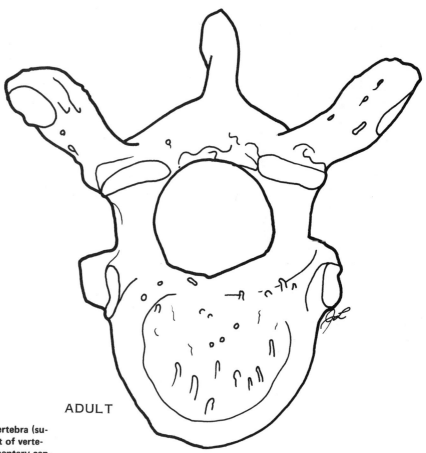

ADULT

11-23 Schema of the sixth thoracic vertebra (superior view). At birth, the development of vertebrae follows a standard pattern. Rudimentary centers of ossification laid down in the cartilage have become three bony units. At this point, they are united only by hyaline cartilage. During the latter half of the first postnatal year, the two halves of the neural arch fuse, forming the vertebral foramina in which the spinal cord lies. The bony walls of this canal form a protective armor for nervous tissue. As bone replaces cartilage, the spinous and transverse processes adapt to the requirements of the attached muscles.

The thoracic vertebra of a newborn indicates clearly how far development has to proceed before the vertebra of the adult is reached. Note the lack of well-developed bony processes able to contribute leverage to attached muscles. These processes will develop after puberty, in response to the directional demand of muscles. This means that the location and integrity of bone is, in a sense, a direct response to the functional demand of the moving muscles. In turn, this implies that through much, if not all, of life, structural integrity at any level (its direction and, within narrow limits, its pattern) can change over time in response to functional demand. At the present state of our knowledge, it would be highly arbitrary to assign a limit to this change, either with respect to structure or time.

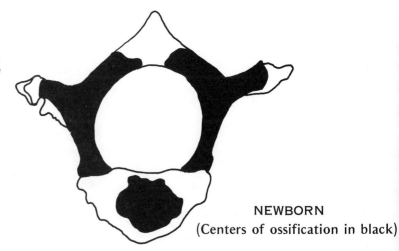

NEWBORN
(Centers of ossification in black)

though parts of the spine (bodies of the vertebrae) may function as weight-bearers, the off-center structure as a whole requires a tough set of adjustable guy wires to help maintain its upright position. The primary function of the powerful myofascial complex of the extensors of the back is to give such support, and to give it by suspension. When a segmented off-center beam is not fully upright, the tendency toward flexion inherent in the pattern renders this suspension mechanism inelastic and severely limits spinal mobility.

At birth, there are thirty-three bony (or, at this stage, cartilaginous) vertebrae. Later (at about age twenty), five vertebrae fuse to form a sacrum. Still later, the four very small terminal units unite; we call this last consolidation the coccyx. Thus in the fully adult spine, there are twenty-four true single bony segments, twelve of which bear ribs. Two composite units—the sacrum with coccyx, and the skull— form the two ends of the spine.

The developing tripartite spinal function of weight-bearing, protection, and scaffolding is displayed as the embryo unfolds. In this progression, the human spine as we know it seems still unfinished, still engaged in developmental experiments. In the earliest embryological period, three vertebral centers of activity develop simultaneously. One, the centrum (body), has characteristics that make weight support practical. Random individuals—off-centered and leaning beams—tend to make exclusive use of this pattern, which is easier for them; they depend on vertebral bodies to maintain posture. The centrum constitutes about half the volume of the vertebra. The neural arch, developing more slowly, gradually closes to form the vertebral foramina (vertebral canal). In so doing, it takes on its function as protective armor for that most important element, the central nervous system.

The spine's function as a scaffold or lattice supporting myofascial structures is a still later development, concomitant with functional demands for movement as the child grows. Spinous articular and transverse processes change as the spinal "beam" progresses from horizontal to vertical. This map, repeated in the embryological, fetal, and postnatal development of each individual, points unmistakably to the evolutionary possibility in all human bodies of a truly erect equipoise stance.

The vertebral scaffolding of spinous and transverse processes, ontologically the latest spinal development, supplies levers by which man-as-a-whole moves. These are the points of muscular attachment through which he can erect and elongate his body. These spinous and transverse pro-

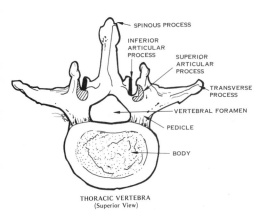

SPINOUS PROCESS
INFERIOR ARTICULAR PROCESS
SUPERIOR ARTICULAR PROCESS
TRANSVERSE PROCESS
VERTEBRAL FORAMEN
PEDICLE
BODY

THORACIC VERTEBRA
(Superior View)

11-24 Superior view of a typical vertebra, in this case lumbar. A body (centrum) is about half the volume of the vertebra; together with its epiphyses, it is basically designed for bearing weight. One spinous and two transverse processes offer projecting levers to which the web of extensor muscles attaches. Articular processes (four on each vertebra, two superior and two inferior) and their attaching muscles restrict random vertebral mobility, thereby protecting against the accident of forward displacement. To some extent, they direct intevertebral movement. They face in different directions at different levels of the spine, thereby very carefully monitoring movement of individual vertebrae. Failure within this mechanism allows the vertebra to slip, one of the causes of a "bad lower back."

189

cesses develop and change in response to the changing demands placed upon them as the child first crawls, then walks, and later takes on the precision movements of sports, etc. The hundreds of strong, tiny cartilaginous bands that interweave a spinal structure change position with the patterns of his activity and, as levers, exert their different pulls. In this light, a normal spine is an open-ended system; there is nothing final about it. This basic structure permits a very great variety of deep readjustments and reorganizations, though a program of consciously fostering development in this sense is rarely explored. (This would be a better focus for the physical-education programs to develop our young.)

Classical thinking has always recognized that there are four curves in the normal spine; two (sacral and thoracic) are concave ventrally; two (lumbar and cervical) are convex. In the embryo, the spine, accommodating to the confines of the enclosing uterus, is a single unbroken curve. By the time of birth, this curve has largely straightened, though some convexity persists in dorsal and sacral areas (Fig. 11-26). As a result, the design of dorsal intervertebral discs is thinner anteriorly. This dorsal convexity is called a primary curve. Such a design, however, does not permit the eyes of the individual to look straight out. The growing child, exploring his world, changes the position of his head to permit his eyes to look ahead. This sensory stimulation modifies the pattern, creating compensatory curves especially in cervical and lumbar areas. The change modifies the structure by (ventral) thickening of the intervertebral discs.

According to Wingate Todd, discs of the secondary lumbar curve constitute about 55 per cent of the total lumbar spine; thoracic (primary curve) discs are less than 30 per cent of the thoracic (or dorsal) vertebral length. In the thoracic region, the combination of disc and vertebra is held in place by the attached ribs. Consequently, since discs are plastic units, not only greater movement but change in form (relationship) is much more possible in the lumbar section, where the discs constitute a larger percentage of the structure. In this sense, the lumbar and cervical areas are secondary curves, relatively dependent on the less mobile dorsal curve. Clearly, if the spine as a whole is to be changed, the modification must occur through shifting the more plastic secondary areas.

If spinal structure were more uniform in the design of its individual parts, the diversity of movement and adjustment possible to modern man would be greatly reduced. A basic pattern of vertebra and disc exists throughout, but drastic modifications changing shape and potential movement function are to be found in individual areas. The neck, for

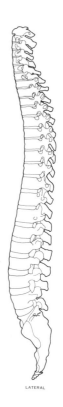

LATERAL

11-25 This schema presents a lateral view of a spine balanced according to the premises of this book. Here the spine reflects the lack of strain that follows appropriate stacking of body segments one above the other, thus allowing the myofascial structural components to accept responsibility for "lifting" weight rather than supporting it. It is important to realize that this is a goal toward which we are striving. We do not expect to attain to this degree of perfection, but significant progress is possible. All change in this direction adds up to greater well-being.

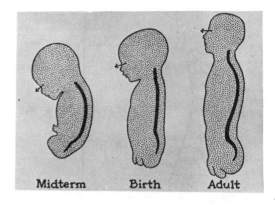

Midterm Birth Adult

11-26 (From Basmajian, GRANT'S METHOD OF ANATOMY, Fig. 22)

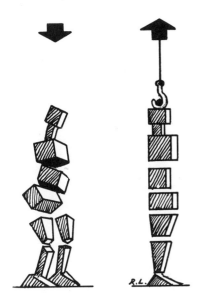

11-27 Meditation on our friend of the skyhook helps evoke the reality of balance. Even if a theoretical vertical line were to join the five significant point (ankle, knee, hip, shoulder, ear) of the body, unless the myofascial framework is able to balance the spinal structure, there can be no equipoise, no true lift, no vertical thrust.

11-28 Superior view: The topmost vertebra (first cervical) is called the atlas. It is unique among vertebrae in having no centrum (body). Fossilized reptilian remains seem to indicate that at one time in the history of vertebrates, the first cervical, like other vertebrae, had a centrum. Later (again as evidenced by fossil remains) this centrum apparently transferred from the atlas to its neighbor, the axis (second cervical). Here it develops as the odontoid process. A transverse ligament joins the two lateral halves of the atlas, thus forming a ringlike structure through which the dens of the axis can fit. This arrangement makes possible rotation of the atlas independently of its lower neighbors. The transverse processes of the atlas are very long; this length makes them efficient levers in the rotation of structures above and below. The capacious vertebral foramina of these two upper cervicals should be noted; it allows the head to turn without compression of the enclosed spinal cord.

example, is built around a core of seven vertebrae. In these seven, four basically different vertebral variations can be observed. The uppermost (atlas) is a flat, substantially diamond-shaped bone that fits over the second cervical vertebra (axis or epistropheus) as a ring fits over a finger. Thanks to this design, a man can rotate his head without involving his neck and shoulders. The fit is so precise that very slight modifications limit function and alter the rotational range of the head. Often, modification results from an apparently minor accident; it may even come from the swollen glands of the common cold, or, specifically, a sore throat.

At the mid-cervical level, the vertebrae become structurally lighter and simpler. The scaffolding to which muscles attach, especially the spinous processes, is better defined. The design here seems to emphasize the need for appropriate span in the postvertebral extensor muscles. Since the gravity adjustment is basically a flexor-extensor equilibrium, the relative position of the mid-lines of the spinous processes to which they attach is very important. The silhouette of a normal body clearly shows this equilibrium. The neck or cervical structure is centered with respect to both front and side contour. This contour underscores the design of the shoulder girdle as a yoke fitting over neck and upper dorsal spine, reminiscent of preautomation stereotypes of Dutch milkmaids fitted with wooden shoulder yokes.

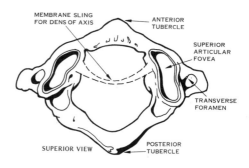

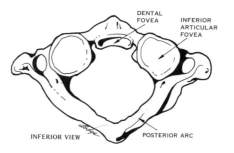

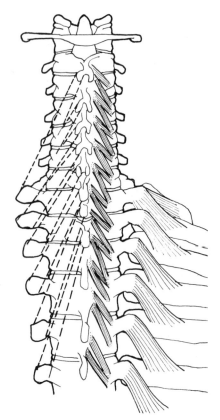

Schema of Rotatores, Multifidus (dotted lines),
and Levator Costae Brevis.

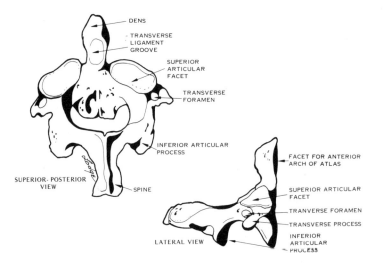

DENS

TRANSVERSE
LIGAMENT
GROOVE

SUPERIOR
ARTICULAR
FACET

TRANSVERSE
FORAMEN

INFERIOR ARTICULAR
PROCESS

SUPERIOR- POSTERIOR
VIEW

SPINE

FACET FOR ANTERIOR
ARCH OF ATLAS

SUPERIOR ARTICULAR
FACET

TRANVERSE FORAMEN

TRANSVERSE PROCESS

INFERIOR
ARTICULAR
PROCESS

LATERAL VIEW

11-29 The second cervical vertebra, the axis (epi-stropheus), forms the other half of the mechanism that makes efficient rotation of the head possible. The dens, an upward projection from the body of the vertebra, is, as its name suggests, a toothlike part that extends upward through an encircling ring formed by the bony anterior tubercle and the transverse ligaments of the atlas. The atlas turns around this pivot.

Heavy extensors of the spine (multifidus and semispinalis cervicis) terminate at this level. The spinous processes of the axis are usually bifid, thus allowing a greater surface for these attachments. In a normal (balanced) rotation, these extensors will lengthen when the head turns.

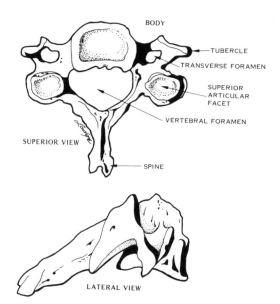

BODY

TUBERCLE

TRANSVERSE FORAMEN

SUPERIOR
ARTICULAR
FACET

VERTEBRAL FORAMEN

SUPERIOR VIEW

SPINE

LATERAL VIEW

11-30 Superior and lateral views: Mid-cervical units conform more clearly to the typical vertebral pattern: body, transverse processes, vertebral foramen, and spinous process. The spinous process here extends obliquely downward; in so doing, it creates a locking device that prevents a dangerous degree of hyperextension.

192

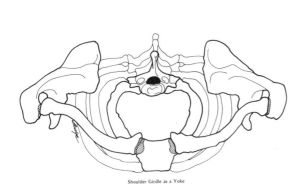

Shoulder Girdle as a Yoke

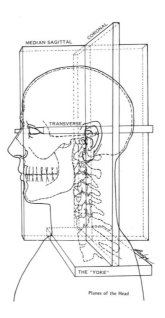

MEDIAN SAGITTAL
CORONAL
TRANSVERSE
THE "YOKE"

Planes of the Head

11-31 A balanced ribcage and shoulder girdle must be found under a head and neck balanced with reference to its three planes (medial, coronal, and sagittal). The shoulder girdle is the yoke. It follows that until ribcage and shoulder girdle can be balanced, head and neck cannot find the position of equipoise.

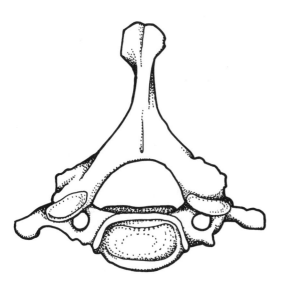

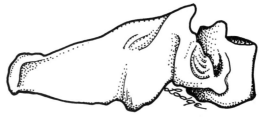

11-32 Superior and lateral views: The seventh cervical marks the transition between cervical and dorsal spine; in the average body, therefore, it is often a problem area. Such functional transition points in the spine are always vulnerable and often in trouble.

In order to fit the smaller core of the cervical structure into the larger overlying sleeve of shoulder girdle and rib-cage, a structural "gap" between cervical and dorsal sections of the spine must be bridged. Anatomically, this becomes the task of the vertebra prominens—the seventh cervical vertebra. Normally, the greater length of its spinous process provides transition between cervical and dorsal sections. When this vertebra is slightly displaced and overlaid by a fleshy pad of nonfunctioning tissue, it forms the nucleus of the common dowager's hump.

The bony core of the upper dorsal structure in a random body looks like this woman (Fig. 11-33). Here, it is clear that the lower cervical discs are consistently too wide, too deep, at the front; the spinous processes are forced closer at the back. Clothed in this flesh, the bones can only look like this. Clearly, such a neck can never evoke a smooth, effective line, outward signature of a competent underlying structure. This neck and the others pictured here (Fig. 11-34) can approach a gravity vertical only by changing the relation between cartilaginous disc and bony vertebra. The bony units must come closer together in front, farther apart in back, to call out organized horizontal lines. If a cervical shift is to be permanent, lower supporting spinal structures must also alter. Permanent change will include distant as well as adjacent regions, lumbar areas as well as dorsals. The complex interrelation of dorsal and lumbar spine, especially at the lumbodorsal junction, must be exploited for effective and permanent change, irrespective of where the original problem lies; all spinal areas function reciprocally.

The thoracic (dorsal) spine bridges between the light, shallow vertebrae of the neck and the square, massive segments of the lumbar spine. It consists of twelve vertebral segments, to each of which attach a pair of ribs. Like the cervical vertebrae, these differ in many details one from another, and this diversity makes body reorganization possible. For example, bodies of thoracic vertebrae vary progressively in contour. Of necessity, this must be so, for the shape of vertebral bodies will vary with function, in this case the amount of weight transmitted. Leverage requirements will alter the bony scaffolding (i.e., the transverse processes).

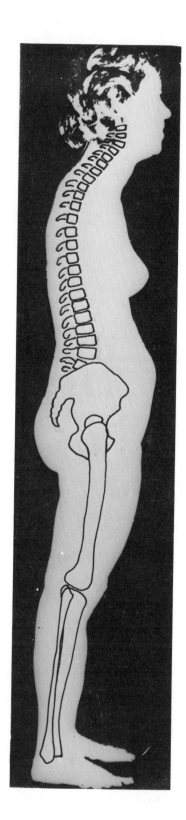

11-33 The so-called dowager's hump involves not merely an exaggerated curve at the cervicothoracic junction, but distortion of the relation between individual cervical and thoracic vertebrae. As in so many compensations, the body "splints" the underlying distortion with a padding of flesh.

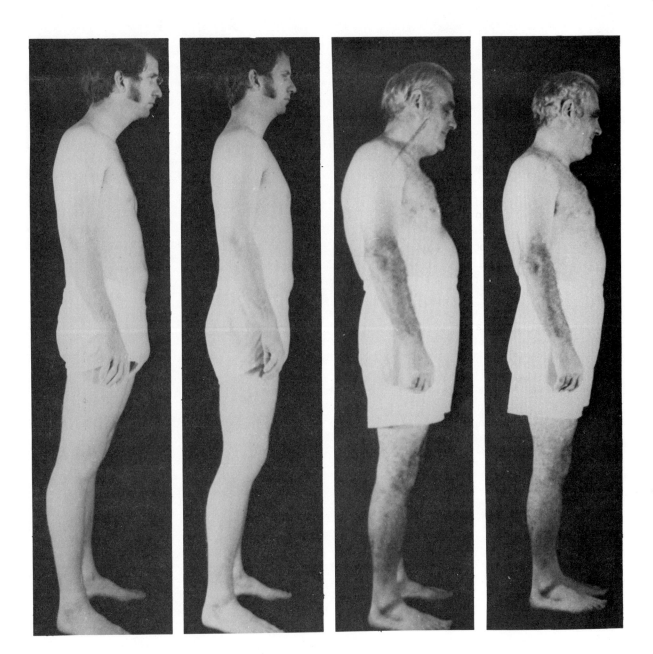

11-34 Many dowager's humps are points at which mechanical tensions from lower-lying distortions accumulate. These pictures illustrate the effect on the neck of relieving distortions of the lower spine, legs, and thighs during the first hour of Structural Integration. (Note that these pictures were taken before and after the first hour of Structural Integration.)

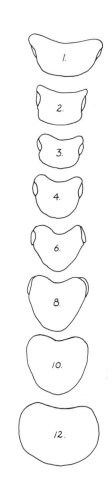

11-35 Superior views: The tendency to think of vertebrae as a group masks the facts. Vertebrae are adapted to their specific job very precisely. This schema suggests the variation in shape of bodies of the thoracic vertebrae. Note the progression through the dorsals from the relatively slight structure of T3 to the massive bulk of T12. All spinal junctions have points of special significance; T1 serves as a transition between the light cervical structure, which bears little weight, and the spinal dorsal. In that the first rib is attached to T1, it initiates a new spinal function: rib-bearing.

11-36 Lumbar vertebrae are massive compared with those higher in the spine. They can be recognized by their spinous processes, which no longer slope downward. Instead, the bulky processes, with ample space for the attachment of heavy muscles, are very nearly horizontal. The third lumbar vertebra is illustrated.

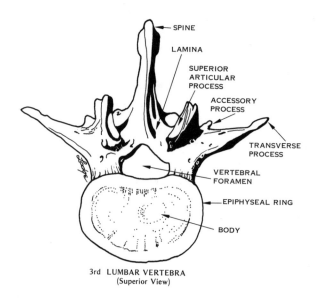

3rd LUMBAR VERTEBRA
(Superior View)

196

Both dorsal and lumbar vertebral spinous processes vary in slope. This tends to unify the spinal curve, emphasizing its character of supplying muscular support and span. This evidence points to the development and adjustment of the total spinal unit. Spinous processes of individual vertebrae determine the kind of movement possible in local areas; they also limit its range. For example, the steep inclination of the spinous processes in the dorsal area minimizes hyperextension (backward bending); in this way, the thoracic spine, especially the segments that innervate the heart, is protected from damage by excessive local movement. Intrauterine life limited the spine at birth to an unbroken, ventrally concave element. This fundamental tendency toward concavity persists throughout life. It is maintained by a lesser ventral depth of the vertebral bodies.

The amplitude of spinal movement or separation is limited not only by the spinous processes but by the character and volume of the discs. In the lumbar spine, where discs form about 55 per cent of the structure (as compared to 30 per cent in the dorsal), their elasticity encourages not only flexion and extension, but also extensive rotation. A competent lumbar spine is essential for fine control of generalized movement, but the same qualities that lend it mobility contribute to making it vulnerable.

As we progress down the spine, not only the discs but also the bodies (corpora) of the vertebrae change fundamentally in size and shape. Gradual at first, the shift becomes abrupt at the dorsolumbar junction. Here, the lighter dorsal spine, whose major function is rib-bearing, shifts into the heavier lumbar structure, whose major task is clearly weight-bearing. In the heavy units, the spinous and transverse processes no longer slope; they are substantially horizontal. Emphasis on the scaffolding function of the lumbars is unmistakable in both pre- and postvertebral muscles. The external postvertebral (transversus and quadratus lumborum) and the internal prevertebral components (psoas major and minor), together with the lumbar fascia, form a tough network. The spinous processes support this web, which in turn holds the spine in place. Weakness in any part permits a shift in the relations of the lumbar vertebrae. Thus, the very commonplace lumbar lordosis invariably reflects an incompetent, displaced, weak psoas group. A different lumbar pattern, a posterior spine, occurs when the tough postvertebral lumbodorsal fascia contracts to bonelike rigidity. This pattern is just as incompetent to support a vertical upper spine and torso, and the burden then necessarily shifts to muscle structures not designed for the task. Compensation, this universal response, is the message broadcast—it is often called rigidity.

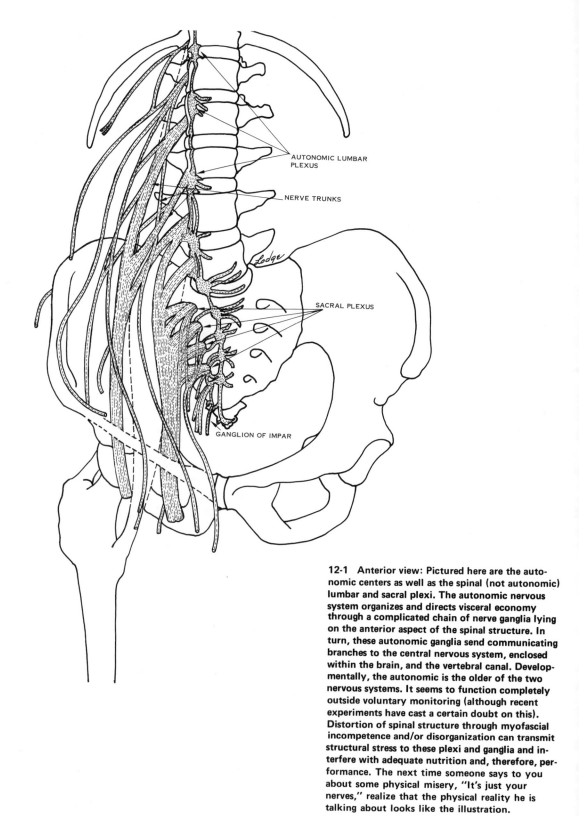

AUTONOMIC LUMBAR
PLEXUS

NERVE TRUNKS

Lodge

SACRAL PLEXUS

GANGLION OF IMPAR

12-1 Anterior view: Pictured here are the autonomic centers as well as the spinal (not autonomic)
lumbar and sacral plexi. The autonomic nervous
system organizes and directs visceral economy
through a complicated chain of nerve ganglia lying
on the anterior aspect of the spinal structure. In
turn, these autonomic ganglia send communicating
branches to the central nervous system, enclosed
within the brain, and the vertebral canal. Develop-
mentally, the autonomic is the older of the two
nervous systems. It seems to function completely
outside voluntary monitoring (although recent
experiments have cast a certain doubt on this).
Distortion of spinal structure through myofascial
incompetence and/or disorganization can transmit
structural stress to these plexi and ganglia and interfere with adequate nutrition and, therefore, performance. The next time someone says to you
about some physical misery, "It's just your
nerves," realize that the physical reality he is
talking about looks like the illustration.

12
Function as a Relationship

Lecomte du Nuoy in his *Road to Reason* said, "As long as we ignore the relations that unite a physico-chemical phenomenon to the vital and psychic phenomena that can accompany it in a living organism, we cannot say that we thoroughly understand its significance." This inspired worker spent much of his life searching for the whole man. In these words, he registered his recognition that the summation of separate parts or even separate physiological systems accepted in the classical tradition does not constitute a human being.

Something more than an aggregate of discrete parts is needed to see function, to see meaning. Nevertheless, individual constituent parts must first be known and appreciated. One important clue to this riddle of synthesis is available. Gaston Bachelard discussed it in his epistemological profile *La Philosophie du Non*. In this remarkable insight, he presents five epistemological keys by which a gradient universe of phenomena may be understood. Each of these yields meaning in accordance with the mental sophistication of the observer. In an expanding universe of understanding, the classical linear world explored by Aristotle (the linear world of a cause linked to an effect) gives way to a more subtle spiral universe; here, all parts relate multidimensionally. It is the universe of Einstein, of modern physics. It is the world of biology and physiology. It is a process world, the world of life. The central reality of this universe is relationship. This is the world in which Structural Integration has its place. Our problem in communication has been that this world does not readily submit to logical exposition.

In the linear world, where a specific effect is linked to a specific cause, vital psychic function has usually been attributed specifically to the nervous system rather than to other somatic components (some workers have included the glandular system in this world of affect and psychic quality).

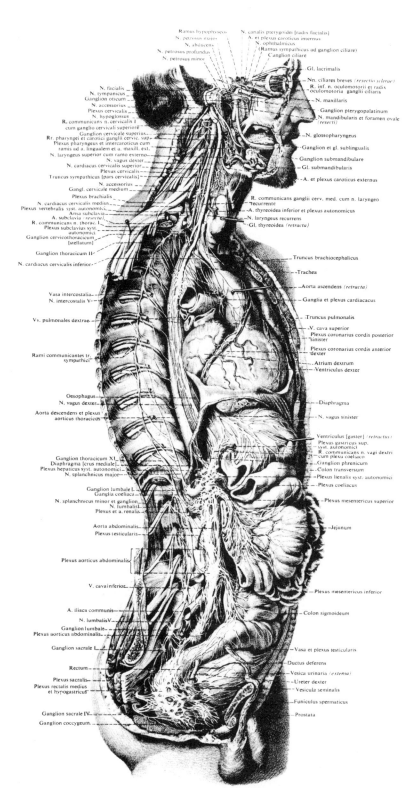

Ramus hypophyseos
N. petrosus major
N. abducens
N. petrosus profundus
N. petrosus minor
N. canalis pterygoidei [radix facialis]
A. et plexus caroticus internus
N. ophthalmicus
(Ramus sympathicus ad ganglion ciliare)
Ganglion ciliare

N. facialis
N. tympanicus
Ganglion oticum
N. accessorius
Plexus cervicalis
N. hypoglossus
R. communicans n. cervicalis I
cum ganglio cervicali superiore
Ganglion cervicale superius
Rr. pharyngei et carotici ganglii cervic. sup.
Plexus pharyngeus et intercaroticus cum
ramis ad a. lingualem et a. maxill. ext.
N. laryngeus superior cum ramo externo
N. vagus dexter
N. cardiacus cervicalis superior
Plexus cervicalis
Truncus sympathicus [pars cervicalis]
N. accessorius
Gangl. cervicale medium
Plexus brachialis
N. cardiacus cervicalis medius
Plexus vertebralis syst. autonomici
Ansa subclavia
A. subclavia (resecta)
R. communicans n. thorac. I
Plexus subclavius syst.
autonomici
Ganglion cervicothoracicum
[stellatum]

Ganglion thoracicum II

N. cardiacus cervicalis inferior

Vasa intercostalia
N. intercostalis V

Vv. pulmonales dextrae

Rami communicantes tr.
sympathici

Oesophagus
N. vagus dexter
Aorta descendens et plexus
aorticus thoracicus

Ganglion thoracicum XI
Diaphragma [crus mediale]
Plexus hepaticus syst. autonomici
N. splanchnicus major
Ganglion lumbale L
Ganglia coeliaca
N. splanchnicus minor et ganglion
N. lumbalis
Plexus et a. renalis
Aorta abdominalis
Plexus testicularis

Plexus aorticus abdominalis

V. cava inferior

A. iliaca communis
N. lumbalis V
Ganglion lumbale
Plexus aorticus abdominalis
Ganglion sacrale L

Rectum
Plexus sacralis
Plexus rectalis medius
et hypogastricus

Ganglion sacrale IV
Ganglion coccygeum

Gl. lacrimalis
Nn. ciliares breves (resectio sclerae)
R. inf. n. oculomotorii et radix
oculomotoria ganglii ciliaris
N. maxillaris
Ganglion pterygopalatinum
N. mandibularis et foramen ovale
(resecti)
N. glossopharyngeus
Ganglion et gl. sublingualis
Ganglion submandibulare
Gl. submandibularis
A. et plexus caroticus externus
R. communicans ganglii cerv. med. cum n. laryngeo
recurrente
A. thyreoidea inferior et plexus autonomicus
N. laryngeus recurrens
Gl. thyreoidea (retracta)

Truncus brachiocephalicus
Trachea
Aorta ascendens (retracta)
Ganglia et plexus cardiacacus
Truncus pulmonalis
V. cava superior
Plexus coronarius cordis posterior
sinister
Plexus coronarius cordis anterior
dexter
Atrium dextrum
Ventriculus dexter

Diaphragma
N. vagus sinister

Ventriculus [gaster] (retractus)
Plexus gastricus sup.
syst. autonomici
R. communicans n. vagi dextri
cum plexu coeliaco
Ganglion phrenicum
Colon transversum
Plexus lienalis syst. autonomici
Plexus coeliacus

Plexus mesentericus superior

Jejunum

Plexus mesentericus inferior

Colon sigmoideum

Vasa et plexus testicularis
Ductus deferens
Vesica urinaria (extensa)
Ureter dexter
Vesicula seminalis
Funiculus spermaticus
Prostata

1511. The sympathetic, parasympathetic, and cranial and spinal nerves, with their ganglia, plexuses, and connections

Dissection by Ludowik. Cf. fig. 1510. Terms see overleaf. (Leveillé-Hirschfeld, 1853.)

12-2 Lateral view: There can be no question that any consideration of the whole man must include some understanding of the physical realities of nerves —— their relative physical size, their paths through the body, their universal distribution, their wide-reaching effects. The nervous networks, central and autonomic, have long been known, and their roles have been investigated in great detail. While basic, this system is not the only mechanism for communication within the body. In this book, we introduce a new point of view, that the myofascial system functions as a means of communication. This system is qualitatively different from the neural, for it is mechanical rather than electrochemical. It is nevertheless a transmitter of information throughout the body. We postulate that lines of strain within the myofascia (i.e., deviation from the horizontal-vertical relation) alter the informational content of the system. (From Spalteholz, ATLAS OF HUMAN ANATOMY, Fig. 1511)

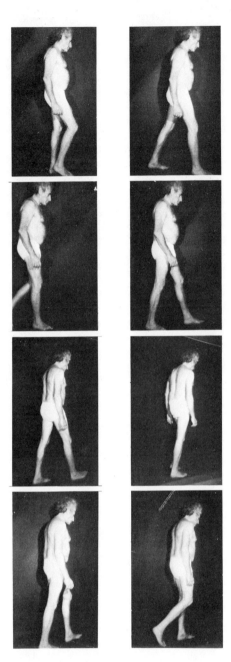

12-3 The world is full of heavy, earth-bound people whose walk dramatizes their misery and is an outward expression of their burden of grief. This would be a psychological description from the appearance of this man as he walks. A physical assay carries a different evaluation; it reports that in his walk this man is the victim of a badly rotated pelvis with compensatory limitations in upper spine and shoulders. The anteriority of his neck and head are balancing his anterior lumbar spine. All these distortions interfere with the psoas-rectus balance necessary for a light, free gait.

In Structural Integration, it becomes increasingly apparent that appropriate interaction of the several systems rather than optimal function of any one is the key. This means that a man's over-all vital or psychic competence is determined not by the individual energy level of any one component system (e.g., the head, the nerves) but by the functioning of all as they interrelate in the total somatic individual. It means specifically that training the nervous system in an effort to produce a superior person cannot be successful. On the contrary, his nervous system must somehow be brought into balance with his other somatic potentials, even though it may demand downgrading the apparent competence of the nervous system.

Such reasoning has startling implications. A lesser nervous system paired with other body systems approximately matching its own relatively lower level would make for a more balanced, more viable life pattern than a very highly intellectual nervous competence paired with a lower general somatic capacity. In our experience, this revolutionary conclusion is warranted. Part of the general malaise of our culture is overstimulation of the nervous system. If the nervous system is successfully to survive the educational, nutritional, and other demands made on it in our current culture, it must be supported from other quarters. Structural somatic balance can add this support. To train our young people for high nervous output, we must give thought to developing a method of raising the energy level of their other somatic systems, to think in terms of the man-as-a-whole.

The human nervous system, in its physical bulk and complexity, has been generally accepted as the vital element distinguishing humans from animals. It has been logical to assume that training and developing this system is properly the primary goal of educational procedures. This may have been an appropriate assumption at an earlier date. The informational burden consigned to the nervous system was less in the days of such universal geniuses as Thomas Jefferson, to take one example. There was less to be known and less to be learned, and the number of people trained for learning was proportionately smaller. In the first quarter of this century, a smaller percentage of the population was exposed to the intensive intellectual training demanded in the best classical colleges. In today's pattern, we try to spread intellectual training so widely that many individuals are faced with nervous demands that their general somatic component cannot support. In this kind of imbalance, vigor (here a synonym for over-all tone level) is consistently drained. The body gives no balanced support to the highly stimulated nervous system. In this sense, the demands on many of our young people are completely unrealistic. They

201

cannot meet them, and in increasing numbers they are electing not to try.

Mainstream research on the nervous system has shed great light on its anatomy and physiology. Nerves transmit electrical currents; these currents can be measured, their rates of transmission and paths studied and recorded. The happenings at the synapse (the junction of one nerve with another), chemical and physical events that together spell the passage of the message, have been worked out in detail. But the study of nerves per se is not the province of Structural Integration. Our work deals primarily with systems derived from the mesoderm. More than any other, these heretofore neglected, seemingly unimportant systems now offer help to achieve a harmonious wholeness of man.

A "whole man" can evolve only when his nervous system is supported internally by his myofascial web and externally by his gravitational field. It is this combination that supports the nervous system, as is evidenced by the increased security of the personality when this system comes into balance with gravity. More than any specific nerve therapy or vitamin, myofascial integration gives buoyancy and strength. Many times this change seems almost instantaneous. Such speed is difficult to interpret. Probably this spontaneity relates to the myofascial ground substance rather than to the collagen fibers, since the fibers are characterized by slow reactions, slow changes.

In Structural Integration, reactions occur that are outward evidence of changes in the nervous system itself. For example, electroencephalographic (EEG) measurements have shown fundamental rhythm changes in brain waves long after actual manipulative work has been completed. Occurrence of such obvious basic change tends to generate an undiscriminating optimism with respect to the breadth of the potential of this method. Where relatively superficial behavior patterns are involved, optimism has been justified. For example, as we have worked with young people in acute schizophrenic breakdown, the stress they manifested was lessened, and their behavior pattern changed. After any structural processing, generalized stress is lessened. We have made studies of the chemical content of the blood that show this, but we may still ask whether this changed blood chemistry is the cause or the result of the improvement.

There are many changes following Structural Integration that involve the nervous system. Significant functional improvement, seemingly of nervous origin, can be brought about. For example, the long-term functional effect of the paralysis that follows polio or cerebral hemorrhage can be greatly lessened. Sometimes hemiplegia or paraplegia can be helped. But close observation of these changes shows unmistakably that damaged nerve tissue has not been restored, but that deep-lying shortened muscle, which is the scaffolding for the nerve tissue, has been lengthened. In this way, the muscular bridging has been repaired and function improved. The picture of the immobilized patient, the so-called paralytic, is primarily a picture of chronic contraction of myofascia, usually relating to deep intrinsic structures rather than to more superficial structures. Their rigid spasm is such that agonist-antagonist balance is lost, partly through local constriction, partly through general compensatory interferences. Such muscular spasm can be relieved at least to a degree, and this can be rated as improvement. But the nerve in itself does not mend. The nerve message does not go through.

Relieving rigidity and improving in some measure support from the gravity field gives a degree of restoration reaching beyond local myofascial improvement. Compensatory movement paths are established more quickly and more surely. Often a subject is no longer as consciously aware of his limitations. The objective observer, however, will still see a residual lack of function—the failure of the nerve itself and the persisting damage in individual nerve pathways. Sometimes, movement is so improved that it is difficult to assume (with consensus physiology) that damaged nervous tissue cannot regenerate. Is nervous tissue, once destroyed, irreparable, as has been assumed? We have no answer. This question can finally be decided only through the measurements possible in newer technology. Damage to a nerve through crushing or tearing (as in an automobile accident) is another area where we find ourselves frustrated and unhappy. Once again, we can evoke improvement in function, but we cannot completely erase damage.

Consolidating these data makes the picture more definite: the nervous system per se is not within the domain of Structural Integration; we do not directly work with it. But we have come to believe that the observable improvement in nervous function demonstrates the wide-ranging effects of the myofascial system. Reinforcements between the energy fields of man and earth, resulting in the greater competence of man's function, depend on myofascial, not nervous, chemistry. As we have said, the chemical responsiveness of the ground substance and the elasticity within the helical collagen fibers seem to be mechanisms that implement myofascial regeneration.

As the structure improves, what accounts for the new competence? Various possibilities suggest themselves. Some nerve trunks are embedded in the surface of the fascial framework (for example, the autonomic nervous system); some are protectively enclosed within the skeletal armor of spinal vertebrae (as is the case with the central nervous system). As the fascial framework shifts its span and position for the better, spatial relations of the embedded or encased nerves must also change. This offers an opportunity for improved nutrition and may be a mechanism by which the nervous system profits. Evidence for this conclusion is offered in better physical coordination and more serene, balanced emotional behavior in the individual.

These behavioral indices have long been accepted as signatures of the health of the nervous system. What is going on in our process of balancing that gives this beneficial result? We must admit that we do not know. It may be that a changed ratio between chemical elements contributes, or that unknowns yet unmeasured are responsible. Up to this point, we can evoke improvement, but we can only begin to define and describe the mechanisms through which it comes about. Metaphorically, but only metaphorically, we can say that integration seems to deal with functional levels of energy, of being. Perhaps this last statement really points to the activation of different spatial levels at which nervous tissue is delivering its charge to the central monitoring system. The work of Dr. Valerie Hunt at the Movement Behavior Laboratory of the University of California at Los Angeles suggests that some of the control of movement originally rather laboriously under the charge of the cerebral cortex is passed on to lower levels (the thalamus, perhaps) as they become more competent. Cortex function and energy are thus freed from mechanical demands.

Researchers under the direction of Dr. Hunt have measured electrical output in various muscle groups through the use of electromyographic (EMG) techniques. Dr. Hunt's measurements of people whose myofascial systems have approached better balance through Structural Integration reinforce our visual observations that balanced usage gives rise to more efficient movement and dissipates less energy. This more efficient movement involves a changed pattern; in the new, only such muscles are in action as directly contribute. (For example, all too many people walk with neck and shoulders initiating the movement, as evidenced not only by visual observation but also by the presence of a myographically recorded interference pattern from muscles in the area. In the body performing efficiently, walking is limited to structures below the twelfth dorsal vertebra. Above this level, the muscular pattern should be one of rest.) Dr. Hunt's measurements show unmistakably the energy economy of this more efficient walk.

A body whose components are symmetrically distributed around a vertical line dissipates less of its energy in meaningless movement and meaningless tensions. Therefore, the electromagnetic energy field that such a body generates around itself remains of necessity greater and more consistent. In such bodies the reservoirs of available energy must stand at a higher level. This may be a component (or a reflection) of the abstraction *energy body.* At least one definite claim may be made: the balanced body is capable of much better perception, much wider awareness. Such enhanced functions may well bridge the levels at which these different energy manifestations take place.

The energy body sought by students of psychic phenomena is defined by them as operating at great distances without loss of intensity or time; this implies that this type of phenomenon is nonelectromagnetic. Ordinary radiant electromagnetic energy disappears with distance —it lessens according to the square of the distance from its source and the time of its radiation. This rate can be measured. Thus we must be dealing with two different kinds of phenomena, semantically confused by the ambiguity inherent in the word *energy* as we use it. We have seen some evidence indicating a relationship between the two. We believe the integrated body to be a more efficient radiator of its electromagnetic energy. It may well be that this has implications for psychic energy as well. This is something only time and better technology can demonstrate. Perhaps there is another, or several other, realities. Is "balancing" actually the placing of the body of flesh upon an energy pattern that activates it. The pattern of this fine energy would not be as easily disorganized and might well survive, relatively intact, traumatic episodes that ordinarily distort flesh.

The pattern of flesh called for by balanced structure is very definite and is essential for economy of function. Departure from this map gives rise to energy confusion and waste—in other words, to inadequate performance. This is what electromyographic assays on twelve unprocessed bodies have shown. In the human energy complex, perception, evaluation, and intervention are simplest at the most dense level, the physical body, where confusion shows as malfunction.

This in no way invalidates our hypothesis that the basic villain is gravity. Any energy system can function in the abstract; our real world demands a patterned system. It is real gravity in the real world that drags down the unbalanced material body and displaces it. By then, distortion of the whole is well under way. Material particles, wherever found, are the expressions of a force field generated by the relationship between their moving molecules. (These may or may not be the only energy patterns in a body.) As the body loses equipoise and therefore integrity, this basic set of relations is disturbed (although the mechanism of the disturbance is still undefined). Disruption at this level will show in personal behavior, both physical and psychological.

At an earlier date, speculation about force fields of matter might have seemed fanciful. Today, scientists both overseas and in this country are speculating on a basic world of nonelectromagnetic, causational energy underlying material manifestation. To date, such speculation has been verbal and limited to workers in the field of ESP. The task of demonstrating and measuring such a field will not be simple; adequate assaying instrumentation has yet to be devised. Indications are that this is a new and different type of energy requiring new measuring devices. Since so many highly qualified investigators are now addressing themselves to this problem, its solution cannot be far off. With this solution will come new insights answering the question, What is man?

If the balance that offers a man so much greater well-being is really a more precise superimposing of a coarse body on an energy element, many physical and psychical phenomena can be understood. If such an hypothesis approximates reality, the remarkable speed at which man changes and perceives his own change for the better (as seen also by any onlooker) would be understandable. Answers and the measurements that establish them cannot be far away. Our concern, however, is less with the speculative question than it is with the more practical related query: How can man be changed so that his energy—his capacity for creativity—may be greater?

13
The Bipolar Unit

Real answers to the question What is life? are limited by the possibilities of a real world. Whatever pure theory may have to offer about man's primary motivations or operational causes—three-dimensional material chemistry, psychological personality, or "energy body"—pragmatic experience grants to some hypotheses more substance than to others. Any theory can be tested only by experience, by how it translates into real life. Does it produce better human beings in a practical way? Structural Integration of a body can and does create a whole man who is greater and more competent than the man embodying the sum of random parts. Having reached this conclusion, we need another hypothesis along which to project a further understanding of the life in which we are manifesting ourselves. Thus at this point we may observe that man is a bipolar set, or system, of elements.

Equipoise of the material body within the gravitational field powerfully and vitally determines function. In body terms, balance denotes a very real, very factual, complex equilibrium in the span and tone of myofascial planes. Within the body-as-a-whole, directional pulls in muscles and fasciae must counter one another with some precision before this can be established. Since we feel that the pelvis is one pole of the energy axis and thus a most important factor, we have in this book tried to point out conditions necessary for local balance in and around it.

Pelvic balance can be assayed by the horizontals joining femoral heads and/or anterior superior iliac spines. Total body balance manifests itself through a series of bipolar axes relating to the three planes of space, in which the pelvic horizontal, though basic, is only a part. These directional axes are not mystical entities; they are equilibrium lines; they define the body in three-dimensional space. They express dynamic physical resultants of directional fields. When their algebraic sum is zero, the body is in a position of maximum energy potential. None of its energy is being wasted in maintaining aberrant positions; it is in a state of dynamic rest.

Practical integration of the body and its energy calls for a primary central line, or axis, within the body, a vertical at right angles to the earth's horizontal. Manifestly, around this vertical, body mass and energy must be substantially symmetrical. The lower terminus of the vertical is the point about which the pelvis balances. The pull of the pelvis, the lower pole, is toward the earth. Span is established by the directional factor of the opposite pole; its pull must be skyward, a lifting away from the earth. Thus if the pelvis is one pole, the upper body (head) must be the other.

Clearly a vertical can exist only if the flexor-extensor system of the trunk is competent. This system is of primary importance to vertical balance of the body. It underlies ease and appropriate span within the entire headward end (upper dorsals, cervicals, and the uppermost segment, the cranium). This is a structural matter involving the myofascial system and related spinal placement and span. Myofascial function in turn affects the nervous tissue it supports. Reciprocally, nervous tissue of the brain and spinal cord is involved in maintaining myofascial balance. Specific performance of the nervous component, cellular nutrition, and communication, both ingoing and outgoing, all are affected by change in the upper pole. Again we emphasize that only in this indirect fashion are the nervous system as well as the glandular dealt with in our integration of structure.

What does this location of the upper pole of the energy field involve? In the accompanying illustrations (Fig. 13-1), the spine is that of average poor structure. To function better, the lumbar section must be straighter, therefore further back. Cervicals as well must be nearer the vertical; dorsals will then necessarily be straighter.

Within average random spinal structure, almost limitless variations are possible. This is emphasized by Fig. 13-2, which Spalteholz-Spanner captioned "Diagram of eight *normal* vertebral columns" (italics ours). These eight spines represent findings from X-rays of random bodies. Visualize the internal compensations in soft tissue inevitable in these spinal pictures. The placement of individual vertebrae or local spinal areas is not accidental; rather, it is rigidly determined by the rest of the structure. Note, for example, in No. 7, the position of sacrum and coccyx as they balance the very anterior cervical section. The inevitable consequence of this combination is the level at which the lower dorsal kyphosis peaks. In No. 8, the exaggerated sacrococcygeal position is made necessary by the posteriority of the overlying dorsal spine.

Spine No. 4, though still highly aberrant, comes the nearest of these eight to meeting our qualification for a

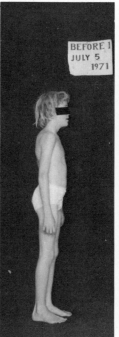
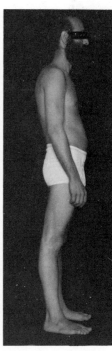

13-1 Average poor structure is a phenomenon appearing in the child as well as the man. Although these two bodies are quite different from each other in age and conformation, their underlying spinal aberrations are similar.

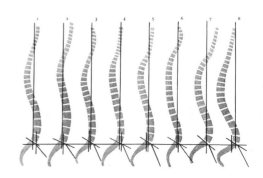

13-2 Lateral views, facing right: These eight spines were labeled as normal by Spalteholz-Spaner. Up to this time, there has been no criterion for judging the normal in spines; in common parlance, structures lacking in pathological symptoms are called normal. More properly, they might be called average. Confusion of pattern has blurred the concept of true normality throughout the body. Until there emerges a spine that relates myofascial structures meaningfully, the imagination remains lost in this confusion. (From Spalteholz, ATLAS OF HUMAN ANATOMY, Fig. 150)

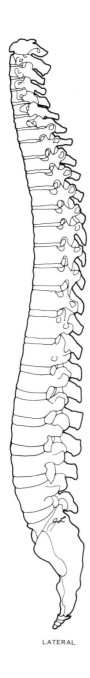

LATERAL

13-3 We offer this ninth spine as a key that unlocks the meaning of body structure. It can appear in the real world only as related myofascial structures from head to foot allow its pattern to surface. This integrated spine can properly be called normal. Like so many structural considerations, this problem of creating a meaningful patterned spinal structure is a circular question. The solution appears only as the circularity is recognized and dealt with.

vertebral column balanced around a vertical. In our terminology, No. 4 is closest to an approximately normal spine. Here, the vertical axis runs through the lumbar vertebrae and traverses the entire cervical group. The balance in this spine allows a better relaxation of the sacrum; the overlying buttock area will carry an easier tone. Common sense says that of these eight spines, No. 4 may be better supported by the gravitational field, less torn down by it.

To project our own idea of a normal spine, we offer illustration 13-3. Here, we can recognize the unit as bipolar. Here, normal span between pelvis and head becomes possible; intervening tissue has tone, it is not merely occupying space. While No. 4 approaches what we think of as a well-functioning normal spine, our projection comes closer to the ideal. We do admit that total attainment of this goal is probably not feasible for the average individual. It involves too much time and, therefore, is too costly. A good approximation is practical, however, and is worth doing in terms of general well-being.

Unbalanced, asymmetric, toneless tissue distributed around an off-vertical manifests itself in displeasing contours and restricted, aberrated body movement. In alignment of spine No. 2, for example, the erector spinae group would counterbalance rectus abdominis. As we have said, grace and efficiency in movement, in walking, requires the psoas, not the erector spinae, as primary antagonist of the rectus abdominis. In this second illustration in Fig. 13-2, it is apparent that as a result of the spinal position and pelvic rotation, the lower half of the trunk cannot offer free movement.

To maintain stability in any anterior lumbar, the posterior erector group must chronically shorten, thus becoming rigid. Then the pelvis cannot rotate around its horizontal axis, cannot adjust as required to "contain" the abdominal contents. The bony pelvic basin no longer acts as container; the role is taken over by the soft tissue of the abdominal wall. At best, this is vulnerable support; at worst, such a soft-tissue container tears under stress—a hernia forms at its weakest point.

The assumption of this book is that incompetent, ineffectual spines are unable to accept their physiological responsibilities and that their failure is centered not in the bony structure, but in the surrounding soft tissue. (This discussion refers to spines that have not suffered organic deterioration.) Spinal weaknesses, then, are basically myofascial problems, lying within cartilaginous components, not bony units. Such tissue can be regenerated quickly and surely. Such spines can become effective, given appropriate support and assistance from the myofascial system.

209

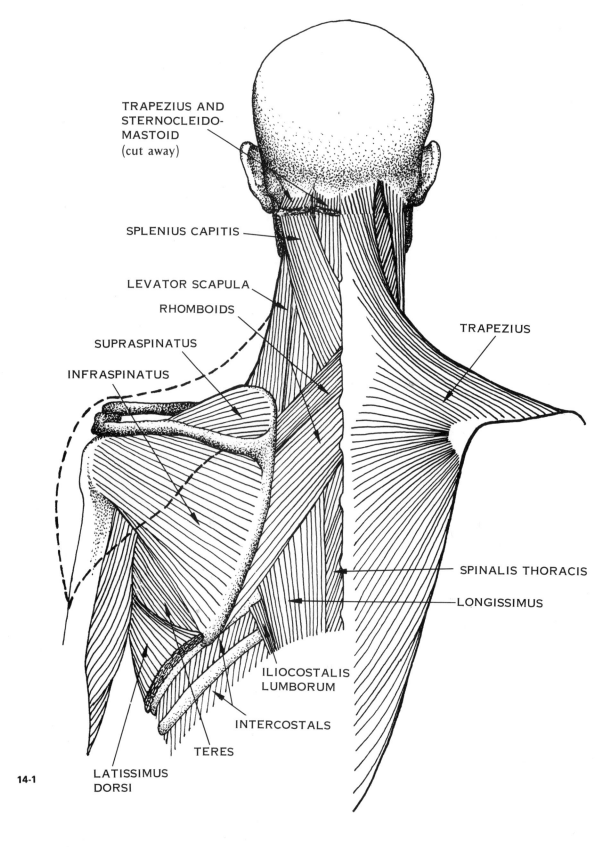

TRAPEZIUS AND
STERNOCLEIDO-
MASTOID
(cut away)

SPLENIUS CAPITIS

LEVATOR SCAPULA

RHOMBOIDS

SUPRASPINATUS

INFRASPINATUS

TRAPEZIUS

SPINALIS THORACIS

LONGISSIMUS

ILIOCOSTALIS
LUMBORUM

INTERCOSTALS

TERES

LATISSIMUS
DORSI

14-1

210

14
The Upper Movement System

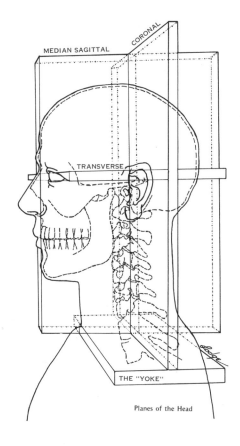

MEDIAN SAGITTAL
CORONAL
TRANSVERSE
THE "YOKE"

Planes of the Head

14-2 It is clear that if a head is to show the vertical and horizontal planes of equipoise, it must be poised over a sturdy, balanced shoulder yoke. Note the contour of the chin and the back of the neck when these conditions are met. Note, too, that the "top of the head" is the point where the plane bisecting the ear intersects the plane bisecting the nose.

It is said that the great French physiologist Claude Bernard, in accepting the citation of the Legion of Honor, opened his discussion by saying, "A man is a something built around a gut." Certainly this statement was justified at the body levels under observation in the late nineteenth century, when systems deriving from the entoderm were subjected to extensive scrutiny. But in our electronic, energy-oriented age, the statement might be that a man is a something built around a polarized line. In order that his energy field may be efficient, the position of the two poles of this vertical, and the physical structures that create and define them is of prime importance. We have not yet discussed the upper pole—what defines it, what it contributes to equipoise.

The pattern of the upper pole is determined by three factors:

1. The position of the upper dorsal spine with respect to the vertical.

2. The balance of the shoulder girdle as it distributes the physical work of the body (unbalanced work effort exerted by arms and shoulders tends to overwhelm and displace a weak dorsal spine).

3. Finally, the alignment of the cervical spine with respect to the vertical. This is particularly important because placement and thereby function and nutrition of the brain, greatest of the nerve plexi (aggregates), are determined by the curve of the cervical spine.

To a certain extent, shoulder (pectoral) girdle, upper dorsal spine, and cervical spine form a single movement system. At every moment, each element of this complex reciprocally influences all other elements. The shoulder girdle is more vulnerable to deformation than the pelvic: it is lighter and bound to the body in only one place, without firm support. Being farther from the ground, it offers gravity greater

211

leverage for its destruction. Consequently, structural deviation from the vertical sets in more easily, whether as a result of chronic dramatizing of negative emotion (fear, worry, grief, aggression) or of habitual poor muscle usage or traumatic impact.

The two girdles, pectoral and pelvic, determine the motor competence of the body. They implement the desire of the individual for movement and offer him the opportunity to exert a physical effect on his material environment. To some extent, they are structurally homologous. However, the differences in primary function—motility in the arms versus weight support in the legs—have blurred the similarity.

The psoas (prevertebrally) and the rhomboids (postvertebrally) connect the two girdles to the spinal vertical. The connection must be stable, yet sufficiently flexible to allow movement by the girdles while retaining a substantially undisturbed vertical. Rhomboids are central to the activity of the shoulder girdle, psoas to adequate functioning of the pelvic girdle. The focus of rhomboid-psoas balance is at the lumbodorsal junction, which is what gives this area its unique importance in body mechanics.

The pectoral girdle consists of two paired bony units, right and left scapula and right and left clavicle, together with related myofascial components. The scapula rides on the upper part of the dorsal rib cage; the clavicle is its ventral partner. The excursions of both are restrained by attaching and ensheathing muscles. The clavicle is a bar of bone lying over the ventral surface of the rib cage. By its thrust, it prevents the dorsal scapula from slipping too far forward. An articular disc on the clavicle and two prominences of the scapula (coracoid and acromial processes) create a semispherical cup, the glenoid fossa. The bone of the upper arm, the humerus, fits into this cup. It is protected and held in place by overlying ligaments and a cartilaginous collar.

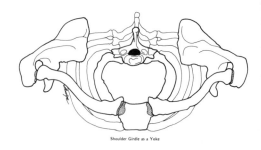

Shoulder Girdle as a Yoke

14-3 This view of the shoulder girdle from above makes its function as a yoke more real. It also points up that lack of balance of the underlying ribs, be it on the right or left side, in the front or the back, can easily destroy the symmetry of the yoke and, in consequence, its strength.

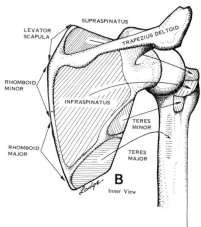

SUPRASPINATUS
LEVATOR SCAPULA
TRAPEZIUS DELTOID
RHOMBOID MINOR
INFRASPINATUS
TERES MINOR
RHOMBOID MAJOR
TERES MAJOR
B Inner View

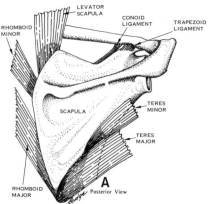

LEVATOR SCAPULA
CONOID LIGAMENT
TRAPEZOID LIGAMENT
RHOMBOID MINOR
SCAPULA
TERES MINOR
TERES MAJOR
RHOMBOID MAJOR
A Posterior View

14-4 This is the right scapula (shoulder blade) seen from the back and from its inner side. The schema points out the muscular balances around this bony focus. It emphasizes that the focus must be appropriately placed with respect to both arm and thorax; the encircling muscles must be similar in tone level and competence. Only then can the energy field that is the upper pole reach equipoise.

212

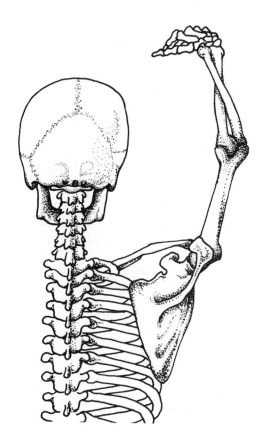

There is only one firm cartilaginous attachment fastening the girdle to the trunk; it is on the ventral surface (the front of the rib cage) at the junction of first rib and sternum. Because of the relative vulnerability of this attachment, the balance of the scapulae is easily modified by aberrated movement in the rib cage. Sometimes, such habits of movement result from traumatic impact of some sort. They may also be behavioral patterns: normal laughter, for example, throws the shoulders back and expands the rib cage. But we all know people who laugh by thrusting their shoulders forward and contracting. This may have originated in some physical damage to the individual's ventral structure, but it is reinforced and perpetuated in his behavior whenever he laughs.

14-5   Posterior view: This illustrates the shoulder girdle with the arm raised. The pectoral girdle must be loosely attached to the ribcage in order that free extention of the arm may be possible. When an arm is raised, the scapula follows it laterally. In a resilient, balanced shoulder, however, the excursion of the scapula is limited by the balance between rhomboids, serrati anterior, and teres. As a result, the scapula maintains its vertical pattern and the arm moves by appropriate adjustment of other important muscles (pectorales and latissimus, for example).

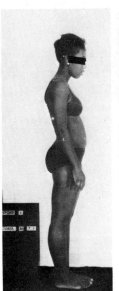
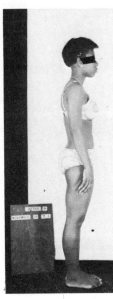
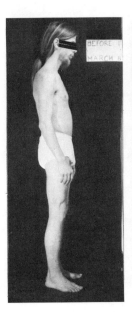
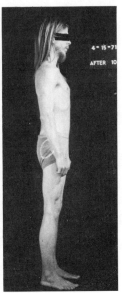

14-6   The shoulder girdle determines the position and competence of the upper spine and head; the spine, in turn, dictates the placement of the girdle. This is the circular relation to be found in so many biological phenomena. For any given placement of the spine, only one position of the shoulder girdle is possible; balancing the spine gives tone to the shoulder girdle; more appropriate fitting of the girdle allows a greater competence in the spine. This is what is meant by <u>reciprocal</u>.

213

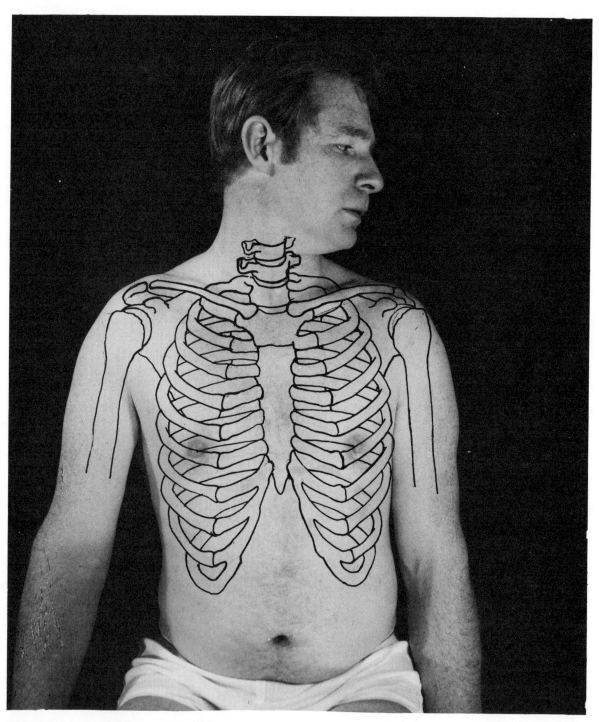

14-7 Deep muscles of a balanced body permit a specified movement without disturbing other areas. This sort of movement relies on a degree of resilient adjustment that permits independent activation. Only as the bones are balanced is this independence available.

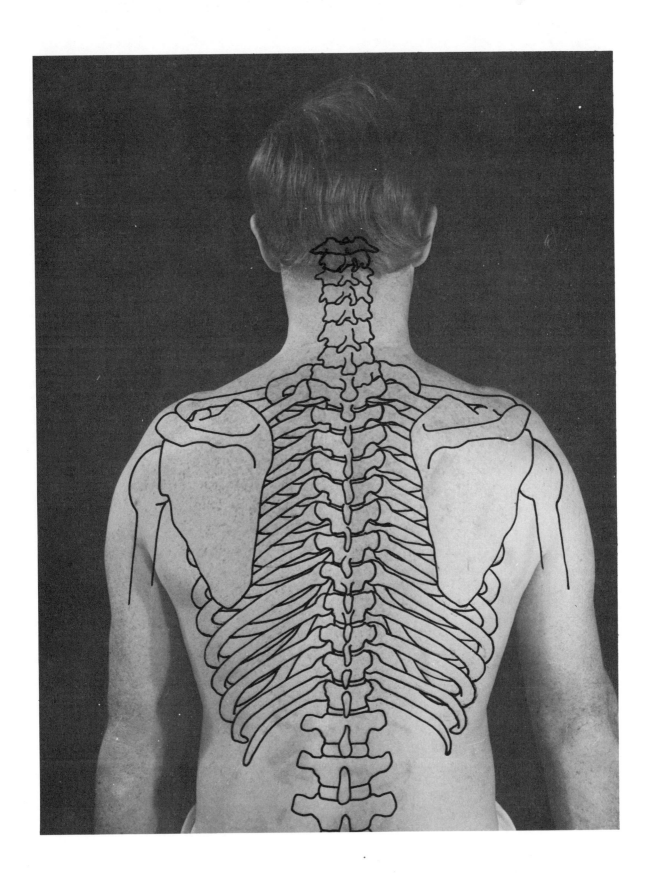

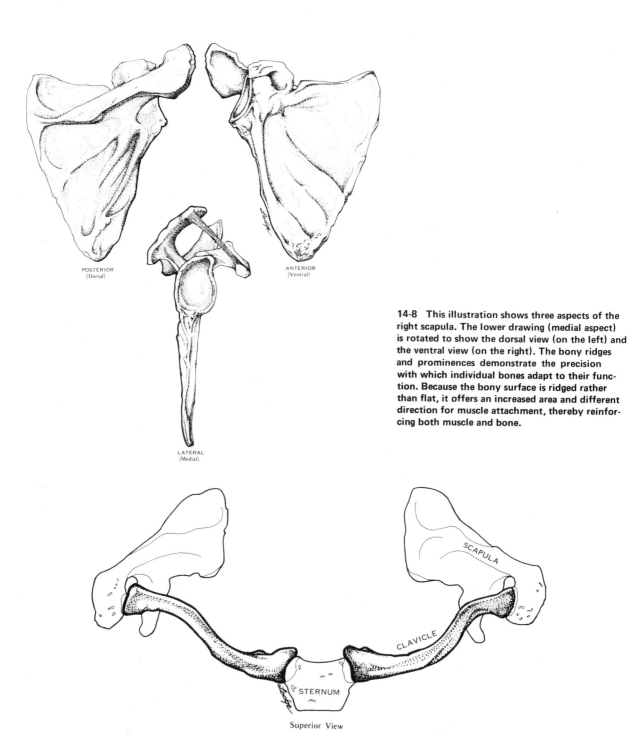

POSTERIOR
(Dorsal)

ANTERIOR
(Ventral)

LATERAL
(Medial)

14-8 This illustration shows three aspects of the right scapula. The lower drawing (medial aspect) is rotated to show the dorsal view (on the left) and the ventral view (on the right). The bony ridges and prominences demonstrate the precision with which individual bones adapt to their function. Because the bony surface is ridged rather than flat, it offers an increased area and different direction for muscle attachment, thereby reinforcing both muscle and bone.

SCAPULA

CLAVICLE

STERNUM

Superior View

14-9 Superior view, facing down: A sturdy, resilient clavicle is needed to maintain the appropriate width between acromial processes of the scapulae. Scapulae that are properly placed and maintained by a competent clavicular structure are not "winged". when humeral heads are too far forward or too close together, arms cannot exert the strength inherent in their structure. If the clavicle is not lifted by a well-placed first and second rib and a balanced sternum, the scapulae wander too far from the spine. The contour characteristic of the well-balanced shoulder disappears.

216

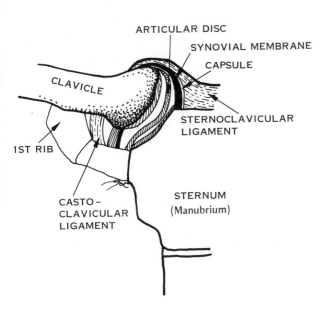

14-10 Anterior view: Detail of a sternoclavicular joint.

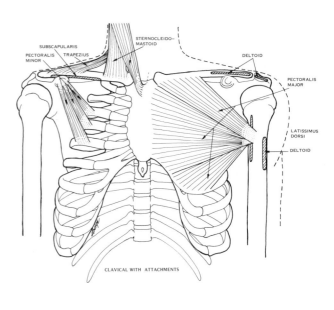

14-11 The anterior contour of a man's chest and shoulder overlies a construction that makes the work of the shoulder possible. This diagram of the clavicle with attachments and the next schema offer a blueprint of the working parts. Note particularly the design that balances the directional pull and the way these balancing pulls determine the position and security of the clavicle and sternum.

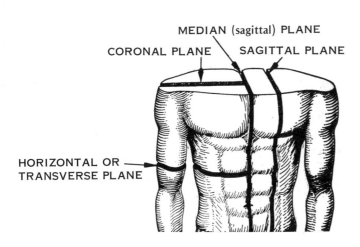

14-12 The coronal section of humerus and glenoid fossa limn some of the directional potential of arm movement. (B from Basmajian, GRANT'S METHOD OF ANATOMY, Fig. 8)

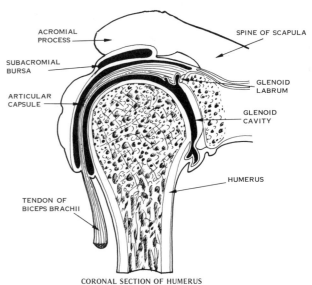

CORONAL SECTION OF HUMERUS

The consequences of any aberrant shoulder pattern are the "winged" scapulae characteristic of the maladjusted girdle of poor posture (Fig. 14-13). These wings are visible indications that the rhomboid muscles have failed. Normally, the job of the rhomboids (together with the serrati anterior) is to hold the scapulae in an appropriate relationship to the spine and to balance the teres. Muscles attaching to a spatially disorganized scapula have lost their span. The girdle as a whole loses competence and destroys the effective interaction of shoulder and spine.

The seemingly innocuous clavicle is central to the balance of the girdle and very important to the structure of the body as a whole. Because of the many important attachments to the clavicle, aberration in its position disorganizes other components of the upper body. The clavicle is joined to first rib and sternum by a disc of tough fibrocartilage and ligamentous bands (the interclavicular ligaments). As we have implied, the home location of the arms is determined by the out-thrusting clavicle. Is the arm habitually too high on the shoulder? Does its attachment at the shoulder form a hook to hang a hat on? If so, the position of the clavicle, not the arm, must be examined.

The location of the scapula, as well as that of the humerus, is determined by the clavicle. Is the scapula an unsightly wing? Then, of necessity, this affects superficial ventral trunk muscles attaching to the clavicle: in the trunk, it is the pectoralis major that is the principal victim; in the neck, it is the sternocleidomastoid. The pectorals, which are muscles of the trunk, and deltoids, muscles of the arm, bridge between upper arm and clavicle. One muscle, the subclavius, together with the costoclavicular ligament, holds the clavicle to the first rib and prevents excessive upward displacement of its median end.

When aberrated, the clavicle tends to be displaced downward in space rather than upward. In habitual poor posture, instead of being able to adjust headward freely, all too often it rests directly on the first rib, immobilized there by a deteriorated subclavius. The two bones, clavicle and rib, become "glued" together; the muscle becomes fibrous, and the mobility that should allow the shoulder girdle to adjust as a horizontal and "easy" yoke is permanently gone. Generally, this tissue deterioration starts after the ventral rib cage has sagged as a result of chronic shortening of the recti abdominis. Such unfortunate sequelae frequently follow assiduous athletic training—too many push-ups, too many sit-ups, all of them shortening the recti abdominis. By the widespread compensations and restrictions it imposes, displacement of the clavicle often gives rise to chronic pain and many shoulder problems.

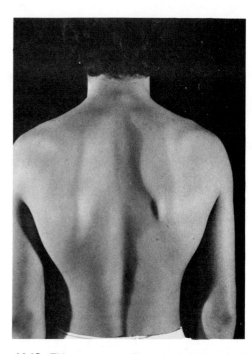

14-13 This young man offers a typical example of the disorganized structure characteristic of many of our young people. Toneless rhomboids have allowed the scapulae to swing away from the body so that the lower margin wings out. He is probably right-handed, and this has contributed to the asymmetrical rotation of the shoulders and arms. This back is a classic example of toneless, ineffective rhomboids. (Note that his waistline, although very slender, is not as narrow as it seems. At first glance the depth of shadow under his left arm exaggerates his contracted lumbars; their true contour must be inferred from the faint line defining the top of his pants.)

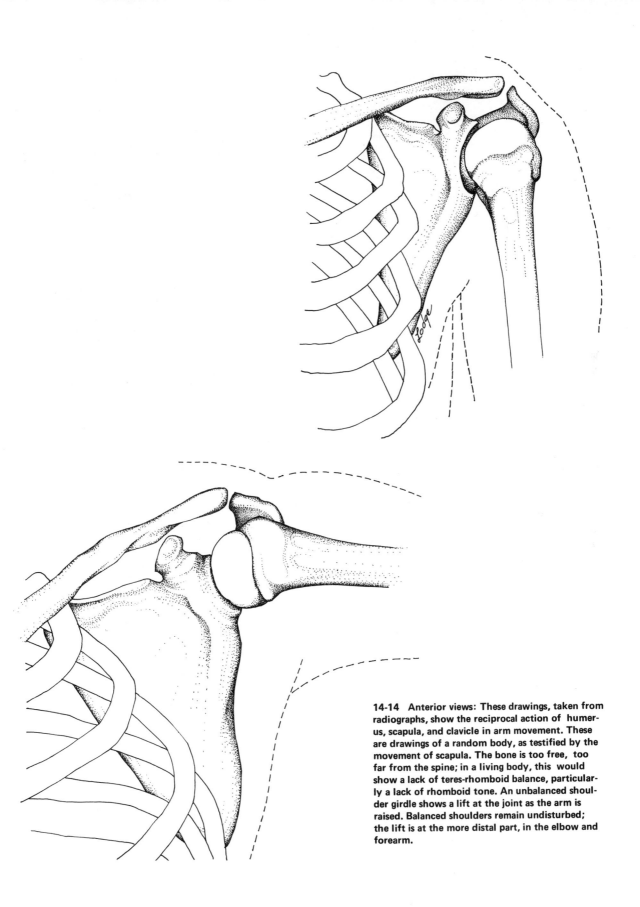

14-14 Anterior views: These drawings, taken from radiographs, show the reciprocal action of humerus, scapula, and clavicle in arm movement. These are drawings of a random body, as testified by the movement of scapula. The bone is too free, too far from the spine; in a living body, this would show a lack of teres-rhomboid balance, particularly a lack of rhomboid tone. An unbalanced shoulder girdle shows a lift at the joint as the arm is raised. Balanced shoulders remain undisturbed; the lift is at the more distal part, in the elbow and forearm.

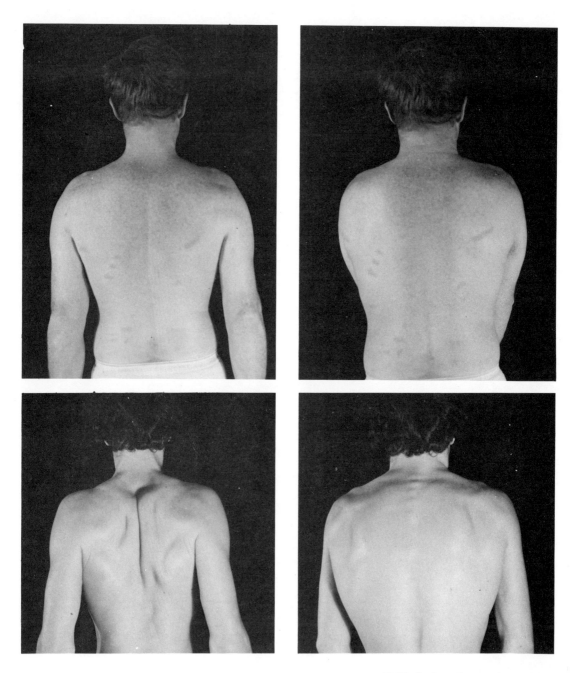

14-15 In the unbalanced shoulder girdle, the scapulae seem to slide independently, without relation to the superficial muscles of the upper back (3 and 4). Balanced shoulder structure limits the excursion of the scapulae; the bones are clearly a part of a unified complex. The difference between these two men is largely a difference in competence of the rhomboid group, the outstanding stabilizer of the shoulder girdle. The balanced girdle (1 and 2) has limited excursion; the unbalanced girdle (3 and 4) moves too far and too freely.

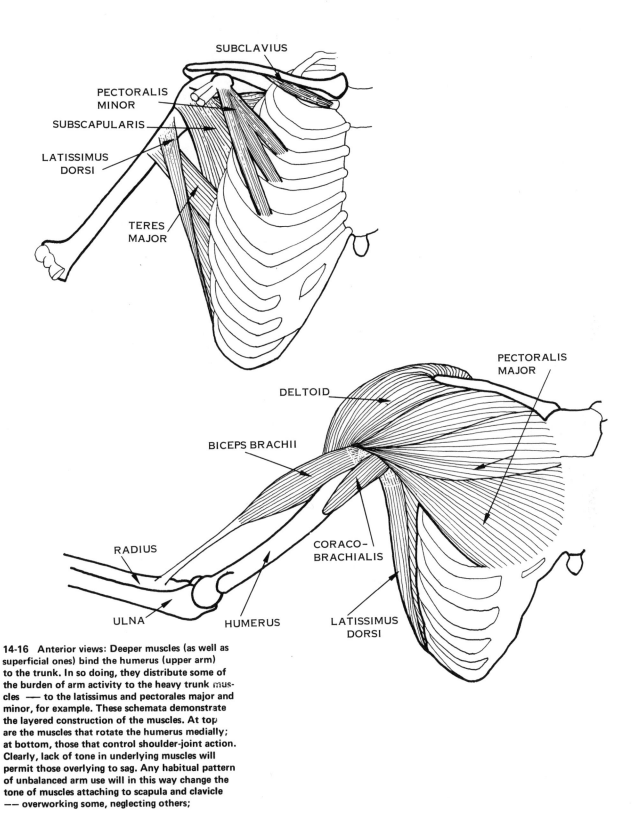

SUBCLAVIUS

PECTORALIS
MINOR

SUBSCAPULARIS

LATISSIMUS
DORSI

TERES
MAJOR

PECTORALIS
MAJOR

DELTOID

BICEPS BRACHII

RADIUS

CORACO-
BRACHIALIS

ULNA

HUMERUS

LATISSIMUS
DORSI

14-16 Anterior views: Deeper muscles (as well as
superficial ones) bind the humerus (upper arm)
to the trunk. In so doing, they distribute some of
the burden of arm activity to the heavy trunk muscles — to the latissimus and pectorales major and
minor, for example. These schemata demonstrate
the layered construction of the muscles. At top
are the muscles that rotate the humerus medially;
at bottom, those that control shoulder-joint action.
Clearly, lack of tone in underlying muscles will
permit those overlying to sag. Any habitual pattern
of unbalanced arm use will in this way change the
tone of muscles attaching to scapula and clavicle
—— overworking some, neglecting others;

221

The dorsal element of the shoulder girdle, the scapula, is equally important. This thin blade of bone lying on the dorsal surface of the rib cage has two protuberances (processes), acromial and coracoid. Along with the lateral end of the clavicle, they make up the cup of the shoulder joint, the glenoid fossa. They overhang and protect the ball-and-socket articulation of humerus with scapula and limit the upward excursion of the humerus. The mobility of the normal scapula allows an almost unlimited freedom of movement in the arms, for the scapula is joined only to the bony shoulder end of the clavicle. Unfortunately, overfree scapulae are "normal."

The bonds uniting the scapula to the dorsal surface of trunk and arm, being muscular rather than cartilaginous, are capable of wide resilient adjustment; therefore, their balance is easily disorganized. In many unbalanced shoulders, the scapula acts as though the superficial trapezius and latissimus were slings rather than participating members of a muscular complex. The bone then rides too freely under these superficial muscles. More than most bones, the scapula needs support and direction from well-toned myofascial tissue. Without it, excessive unbalanced girdle movement disturbs the structure of the ribcage. In turn, associated respiratory and cardiac function suffers.

It is not necessary to know the precise origins and insertions, or even the names, of all the muscles that together form the shoulder. What is important is to see the structural patterns and realize their compact order. Muscles arising from ventral (subscapularis) as well as dorsal surface of the scapula bridge between the shoulder girdle and upper arm. Should the bridge be rickety, or its attachments displaced or inadequate, faulty function must result. No balance is possible.

Muscles from the trunk as well as from the girdle, by inserting into the humerus, form part of the bridge. From the ventral surface (pectoralis major), from the dorsal (latissimus), they make possible and control arm movement. Of this bridging web, two paired sets of muscles attaching to the scapula warrant especial attention—the rhomboids (major and minor) and the teres (major and minor). The respective tone of these two groups, together with the anterior serrati, determines the location of the lower angle of the scapula. Rhomboids major and minor play a vital part in the local structure and function of the shoulder girdle. These flat, oblique muscles are intermediate in depth, lying deep to the trapezius but superficial to the serratus posterior superior. They originate at the spines of the vertebrae and insert along the entire medial border of the scapulae. Because they unite the shoulder girdle with the spine, they

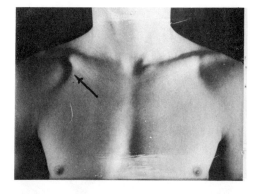

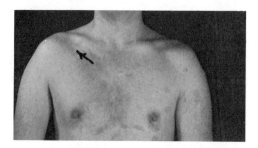

14-17 Here, the degree of tension in underlying muscles is demonstrated by the hollows above and below the clavicle (1). The position of the nipples is another key to the downdrag of the pectorals. Deep construction of this chest is so poor that the ribcage itself has sagged, as have the overlying muscles. Photo 2 demonstrates the greater lift in the ribcage of an integrated body, which "fills in" these hollows.

determine counterbalance in the complex. Without their appropriate interplay, scapulae ride too high on the torso; the body is "round-shouldered." The rhomboid group's tone and span maintain appropriate sturdy verticality of the upper dorsal spine.

When the rhomboids lose their tone and are no longer able to balance the teres or to hold the scapulae in place, their function of supporting the shoulder girdle passes to spinal muscles. The latter are basically extensors, and have not been designed for the new job of supporting structures so far lateral. Thus overburdened, they proclaim their misery loud and clear. Lack of tone in the rhomboids also allows the scapulae to wander too far from the vertebral column; the bones are no longer flat—they "wing" out. In turn, the head of the humerus is permanently turned in the glenoid fossa, and the home position of the arm is changed. Toneless rhomboids distort the underlying serratus groups that maintain space and distance between ribs. Presently, chronic distortions appear in the rib cage and later in the spine. This is often a factor in the compression leading to the painful syndrome called shoulder bursitis.

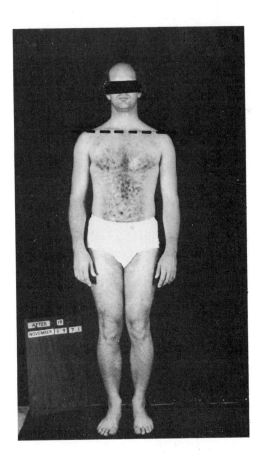

14-18 As a body approaches balance, the shoulder girdle rides snugly but freely over the ribs. It is truly an "easy yoke."

223

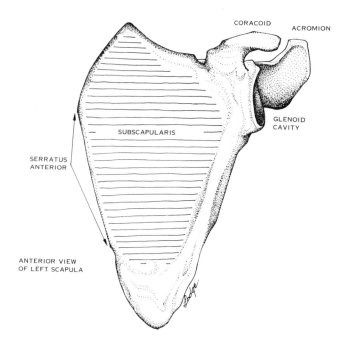

CORACOID ACROMION

SUBSCAPULARIS

GLENOID CAVITY

SERRATUS ANTERIOR

ANTERIOR VIEW OF LEFT SCAPULA

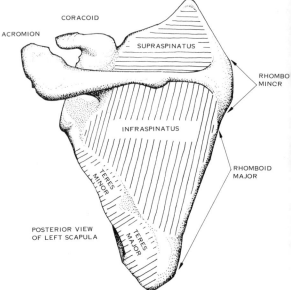

CORACOID

ACROMION

SUPRASPINATUS

RHOMBO MINCR

INFRASPINATUS

RHOMBOID MAJOR

TERES MINOR

TERES MAJOR

POSTERIOR VIEW OF LEFT SCAPULA

14-19 These schemata of the left scapula indicate the patterns of the muscles clothing the bony scapulae. A view of underlying ridges emphasizes the potential of scapular design in a balanced body.

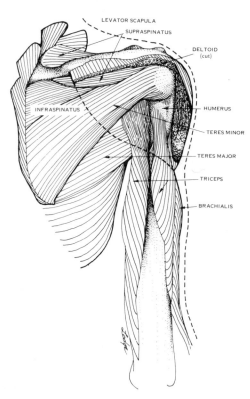

LEVATOR SCAPULA

SUPRASPINATUS

DELTOID (cut)

INFRASPINATUS

HUMERUS

TERES MINOR

TERES MAJOR

TRICEPS

BRACHIALIS

14-20 Clothed in its more superficial muscular layer, the right shoulder looks like this from the back. It is apparent here that muscular pulls of rhomboids, levator, and trapezius must balance if the shoulder structure is to permit the most economical movement of the arm.

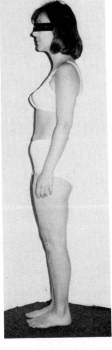
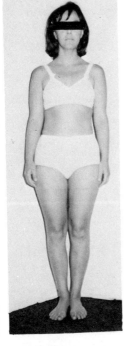

The shoulder girdle guides and controls arm movement, requiring that each member contribute. Deviation from pattern by any one member results in aberrant function for all and modifies the functional efficiency of the energy field that is the upper body. Clearly, if our goal is to create a more efficient man, the reorganization of the shoulder girdle is of prime importance. The practitioner in Structural Integration accomplishes this by manually restraining the muscle, bringing it toward its "normal" position and then demanding specific directional movement of the part. Suddenly, the restricted joint moves; it moves more normally. The constituent myofascia is permanently in a new position, nearer that demanded by pattern.

At this point, we may ask certain basic questions to evaluate progress:

1. Does the shoulder girdle show horizontal lines of balance both anteriorly and posteriorly?

2. Does the shoulder girdle fit as a free and balanced yoke above the ribs?

3. In raising the arms, are the shoulders independent? Do they remain down unless specifically directed to rise?

4. Is it clearly apparent that arms and shoulders move with little participation of the spine? If so, arms and shoulders can work without fatiguing the spinal structure or adversely affecting the viscera innervated by the spine.

5. Can the spine move independently of arms and shoulders? Can it stretch upward while the shoulder yoke, particularly the scapulae, moves lower? If so, the rhomboids are drawing scapulae downward and medially, and the extensors of the back are functioning as they should.

If the answers are "yes" to all these questions, the upper pole is coming to life. The body is exploring and exerting its upward thrust.

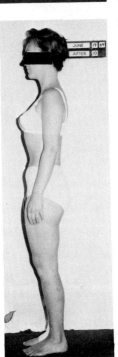
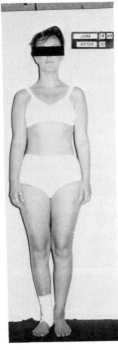

14-21 The progression of a typical endomorph through ten hours of processing is shown in these photographs. The lack of tissue tone, which allows the scapulae to drop into a sling formed by the trapezius, is apparent, as is the improvement in this structure after Structural Integration.

Ten hours of processing give better myofascial tone and balance, but this does not change an endomorph into a mesomorph. The terms endomorph, mesomorph, and ectomorph refer to a quality of body that is genetic, independent of and unrelated to the sequelae of accident and trauma in the life of the individual, which have only accentuated the basic morphic pattern (For further information on morphological types, see Sheldon's classic, PSYCHOLOGICAL TYPES). The work of Structural Integration deals with these sequelae.

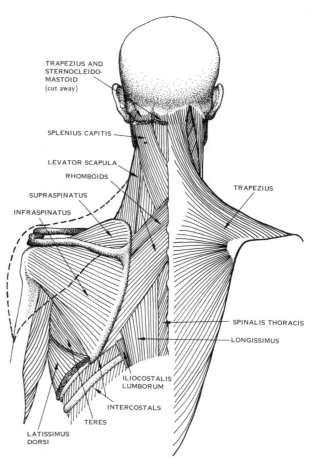

TRAPEZIUS AND
STERNOCLEIDO-
MASTOID
(cut away)

SPLENIUS CAPITIS

LEVATOR SCAPULA

RHOMBOIDS

SUPRASPINATUS

INFRASPINATUS

TRAPEZIUS

SPINALIS THORACIS

LONGISSIMUS

ILIOCOSTALIS
LUMBORUM

INTERCOSTALS

TERES

LATISSIMUS
DORSI

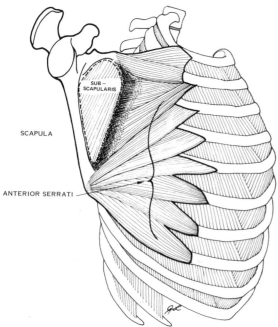

SUB –
SCAPULARIS

SCAPULA

ANTERIOR SERRATI

14-22 The anterior serrati arise from the upper eight ribs and pass between the ribcage and scapulae. Thus they partly encircle the trunk, inserting into the vertebral margin of the scapulae. In the drawing showing the serrati, the shoulder blade has been drawn away from the ribcage (much as a book cover opens away from its contents). It is apparent that unless the tone of the serrati is maintained by the opposing pull of the dorsal rhomboids, the scapulae will become chronically displaced. Both serrati and rhomboids participate in any movement of raising the arms above the head or pushing the shoulders forward.

The drawings are a most graphic demonstration of levels of reciprocity, showing the circular interplay of anterior and posterior muscles. As the arm moves, different movements will call on interchanging balances.

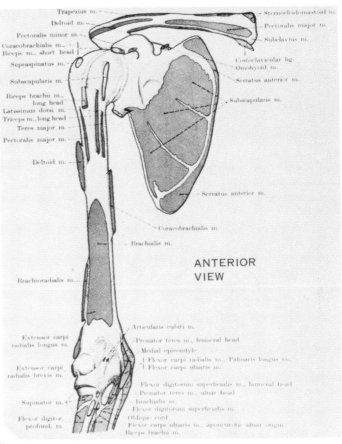

ANTERIOR
VIEW

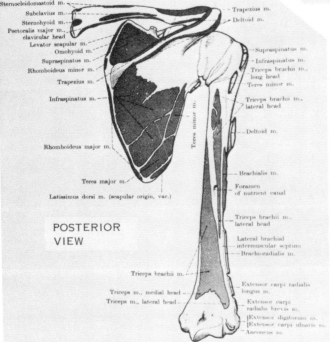

POSTERIOR
VIEW

14-23 The direction and quality of arm movement is determined by muscles that form a bridge
between shoulder and humerus, as is clear from
these schemata showing insertions of shoulder and
arm muscles. In the anterior view (1), it is apparent that if the pectoralis major is too tight, the
head of the humerus will be rotated medially.
This will disturb the balance of other muscles
around the head, and the joint will project sharply
forward, "winging" the scapulae.

Pectoralis major and latissimus dorsi act reciprocally, moving the arm (medially and laterally,
respectively). Chronic shortening in either will
change the home position of the head of the
humerus in the glenoid fossa. It thus changes
muscular relations at the elbow and influences
over-all strength and coordination of arm movement.

This complicated interplay can just as well
originate in the arm and reflect into the torso. Thus
chronic shortening in the pectorals (manifest in
thick, gristled insertions) puts a continual strain
on the latissimus and teres (and thereby on the
rhomboids). Subjectively, this is felt as discomfort in the shoulders and spine (From Sobotta,
ATLAS OF HUMAN ANATOMY, Vol. 1, Figs.
301 and 302

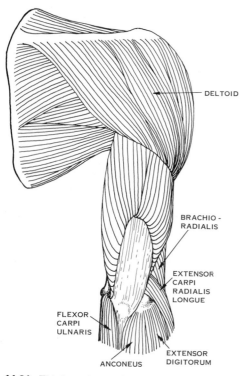

DELTOID

BRACHIO-
RADIALIS

EXTENSOR
CARPI
RADIALIS
LONGUE

FLEXOR
CARPI
ULNARIS

ANCONEUS

EXTENSOR
DIGITORUM

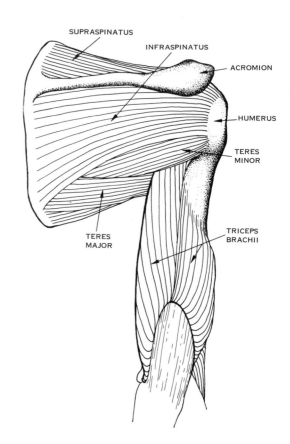

SUPRASPINATUS

INFRASPINATUS

ACROMION

HUMERUS

TERES
MINOR

TERES
MAJOR

TRICEPS
BRACHII

14-24 This is a schema of the right shoulder. If
the shoulder is to show the surface horizontals of
balance, the deeper structure must be patterned.

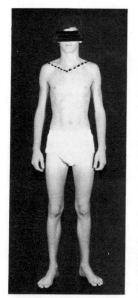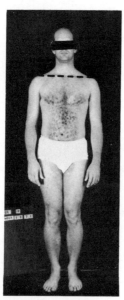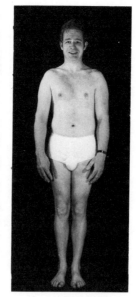

14-25 Here are three of the shoulder girdles you
have already observed. Look at them in terms of
horizontal construction lines. Now leaf through
the other photographs in this book. How many of
them display the proud badge of horizontals?

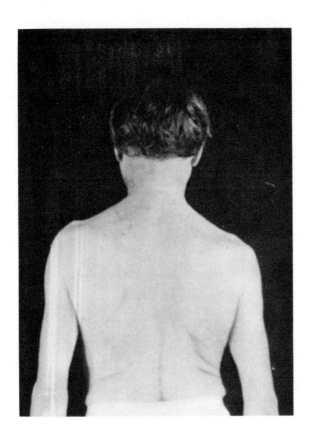 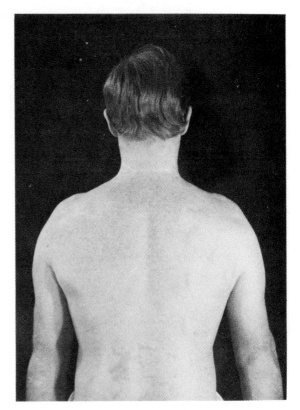

14-26 It is impossible to construct a toned, competent shoulder girdle before the rhomboids are able to maintain the scapulae in appropriate balance. Rhomboids such as those in the man at left cannot be consciously "found" by the individual. At this stage, any attempt to draw his shoulders back will be initiated in the arms, not in the rhomboids. Because of the fact that these insert into the spines of the second to fifth thoracic vertebrae, persistent evasion of rhomboid responsibility allows deterioration of the upper spinal structure. As a body approaches equipoise (the man at right) the scapulae begin to show structural horizontals.

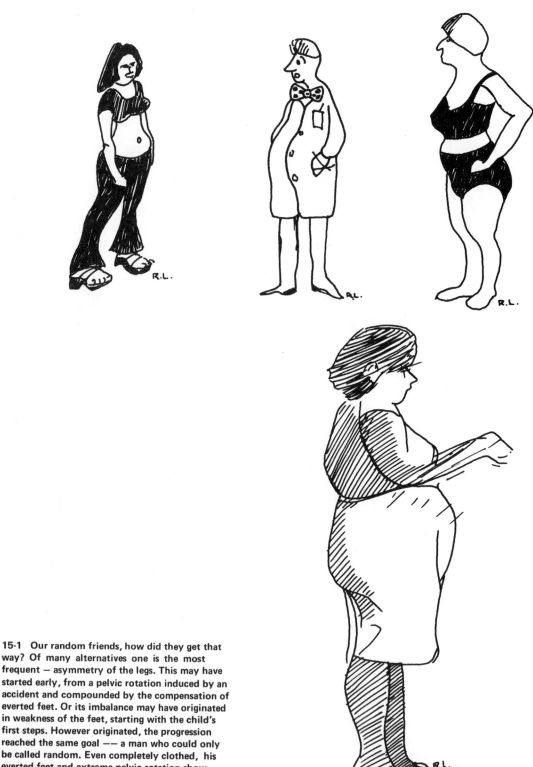

15-1 Our random friends, how did they get that way? Of many alternatives one is the most frequent — asymmetry of the legs. This may have started early, from a pelvic rotation induced by an accident and compounded by the compensation of everted feet. Or its imbalance may have originated in weakness of the feet, starting with the child's first steps. However originated, the progression reached the same goal —— a man who could only be called random. Even completely clothed, his everted feet and extreme pelvic rotation show through. The shape of the clothes is a giveaway, along with the position of the neck.

15
The Vertical Thrust

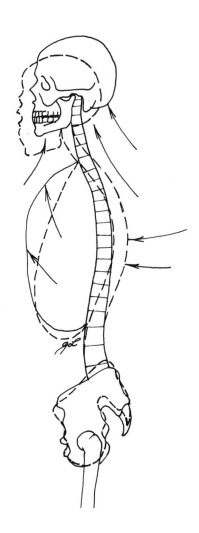

15-2 This schema shows movement of the tenth thoracic vertebra forward, lifting the thorax. In this transformation of the random body (dotted lines) to the integrated body (solid lines) note that the apparent change in height is the result of the new relation among pelvis, thorax, and cervical spine.

All schools of body mechanics agree that good posture calls for a vertical alignment of five significant body landmarks —the midpoints of ear, shoulder joint, hip joint, knee, and ankle. A body so constructed is in a static alignment. Random people cannot show even this static pattern. This vertical design is basic to the dynamic state in which an upward thrust counters gravity. To this goal there is no shortcut. The one road is through the stacking, the vertical alignment we have been building so methodically. At the evolutionary level at which humans now function, progress occurs through a maddeningly slow synthesis. We live in a process world in which the laws of mechanics are insurmountable.

In answer to the question of what is balance, the vertical pattern proclaims its own importance loud and clear. Here, the message *is* the medium, the body itself. Each part calls up the image of a whole, the only whole in which it could possibly be a part. Like every other body part, the neck tells the story of the whole man. For balance, the neck structure must be spaced midway with respect to the sides of the body, and seem midway with respect to the front and back. Alignment, a satisfying balance, requires that only a vertical cervical spine can form the upper segment of a vertically stacked body. This goal is difficult to attain but infinitely worth while. Arriving at this type of balance in the neck calls for erasing any secondary compensations that originally arose in the torso. The reverse situation may also occur; there may be primary tensions in the neck (the result of impact of some accident) that transmit as compensations to the torso. Either situation must be changed before general equipoise can be elicited.

The chronic position of the shoulder girdle, especially of the scapulae, inexorably indexes general as well as local cervical muscle stress. Therefore, the postural fate of the neck (and through the neck, the head) depends on the pectoral girdle and its efficiency. (The term *neck* as used here is limited to the part of the body that surrounds and includes

231

the cervical spine.) Functionally, the three areas (neck, head, and shoulders) are thus not independent units. Length and well-being (we could as well call these functional resilience and nutrition) of four significant superficial sets of muscles binding neck and girdle—sternocleidomastoid, levator scapulae, trapezius, and to some extent splenius—are in turn clues to balance in deeper complexes. They tell the story of their more intrinsic neighbors. The most superficial muscle of the neck, the platysma, has little to do with balance. Like most superficial muscles, it can be seen as a bandage or splint rather than as a scaffolding. Deep-lying, intrinsic structures serve as scaffolding.

When the neck functions incompetently, movement of the head is initiated and largely executed by the superficial muscles that attach to the shoulder girdle. Thus in the random individual, the head or neck turns with little or no participation of the deep-lying intrinsics. This has physiological significance. Muscular contraction moves plasma and lymph through the ground substance of tissue and fosters metabolic exchange at the cellular level. Consequently, inadequate tissue nutrition follows deficient muscle movement. The four major extrinsic muscles of the neck are shown in Figs. 15-4 and 15-5. It is all too apparent how small a proportion of the cervical tissue is involved in movement when only these muscles are participating. For optimal physiological function, two factors are involved; there must be sufficient myofascial movement to circulate nutrition-bearing fluids, and the nutritional quality of the fluid pumped must be adequate. We are omitting specific discussion of nutrition at this point. Our present interest is in fluid flow, not fluid content.

Only two arteries traverse the neck, the common carotid, and the vertebral. Nutritional supply for the head, brain, and sense organs passes through the neck via the common carotid artery, which lies very near the surface and therefore is vulnerable to injury by violence or accident. Immediate loss of consciousness results if carotid circulation is blocked, even momentarily. A smaller vessel, the vertebral artery, threads its way through the foramina of the bony transverse processes and nourishes immediate spinal structures. This also presents a hazard. As it ascends through the foramina of the vertebrae, the vertebral artery is almost like a rubber tube threaded through a series of spools. As long as the spools lie one directly over the other, the flow through the artery is unimpeded.

When accident or habitual posture displaces the head sharply forward, the arterial lumen is narrowed and cervical circulation is impeded. Although often attributed to chemi-

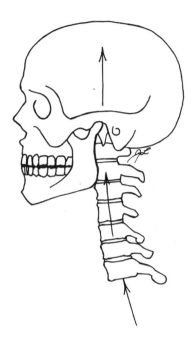

15-3 As the cervical vertebrae move toward vertical alignment, the cranium seems to lift. This is a natural sequel to the greater elasticity of balanced neck muscles.

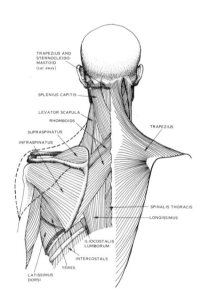

15-4 Four superficial muscles of the neck are important in the flexor extensor system —— sternocleidomastoid, levator scapulae, trapezius, and splenius. Their tone and spatial placement offer information as to the competence and adequacy of shoulder and neck. When these muscles are balanced (as in this illustration), the man's physical tasks are easy, his burden light.

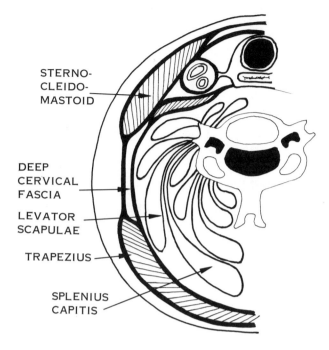

STERNO-
CLEIDO-
MASTOID

DEEP
CERVICAL
FASCIA

LEVATOR
SCAPULAE

TRAPEZIUS

SPLENIUS
CAPITIS

15-5 A schematic cross section of the neck emphasizes how small a proportion of its structure is pre-empted by extrinsic muscles. Extrinsics act as a bandaging and protection to the core structures. They cover and enclose the arterial system, thus conserving the warmth of the head, and overlie and protect the cervical autonomic plexi.

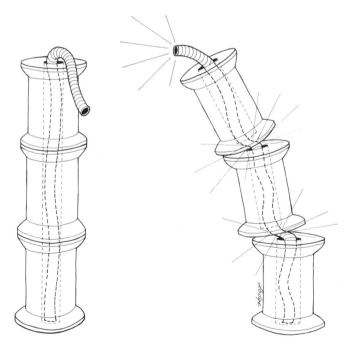

15-6 Cervical vertebrae sit one atop another, in a pattern approaching a vertical. They are reminiscent of stacked spools, which allow free flow of liquid through a tube. Aberrated or unbalanced spools interfere with this free flow. So it is with man's cervical spine. Individual vertebrae, joined by myofascial nets, armor the spinal cord that threads through their central core. Deviation from vertical stacking puts pressure on connecting, enwrapping tissues and on the nervous structures (autonomic plexi and cranial nerves, etc.) that traverse them.

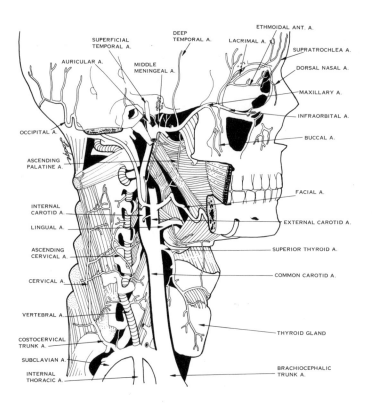

SUPERFICIAL TEMPORAL A.
DEEP TEMPORAL A.
ETHMOIDAL ANT. A.
LACRIMAL A.
SUPRATROCHLEA A.
AURICULAR A.
MIDDLE MENINGEAL A.
DORSAL NASAL A.
MAXILLARY A.
INFRAORBITAL A.
OCCIPITAL A.
BUCCAL A.
ASCENDING PALATINE A.
FACIAL A.
INTERNAL CAROTID A.
EXTERNAL CAROTID A.
LINGUAL A.
SUPERIOR THYROID A.
ASCENDING CERVICAL A.
COMMON CAROTID A.
CERVICAL A.
VERTEBRAL A.
THYROID GLAND
COSTOCERVICAL TRUNK A.
SUBCLAVIAN A.
BRACHIOCEPHALIC TRUNK A.
INTERNAL THORACIC A.

15-7 Lateral views: Two arteries supply the head, the common cartoid and the vertebral. Their vulnerability is all too apparent in these illustrations. The common carotid and its branches are the principal source of nutrition to the brain itself. Many headaches typically result from interference with the carotid flow, and may be relieved instantaneously by its restoration. Loss of consciousness associated with knockout blows or pressure on the neck results from interference with flow in the carotid.

The vertebral artery, on which so much of the nutrition of head and neck structures depends, threads a hazardous path through the cervical vertebrae. Chronic shifting of any of these can seriously cut down on the rate as well as the volume of the flow of blood.

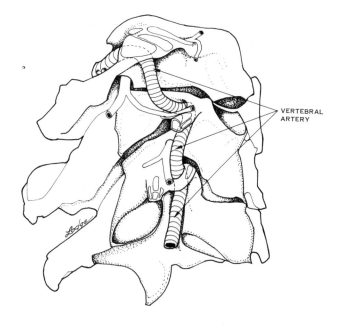

VERTEBRAL ARTERY

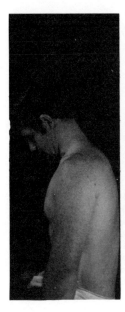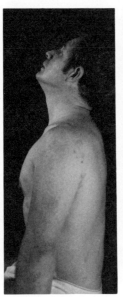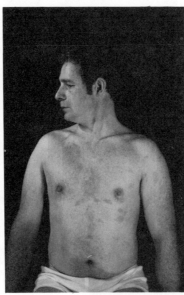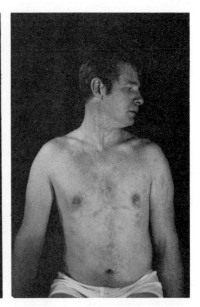

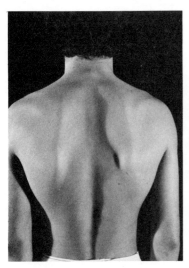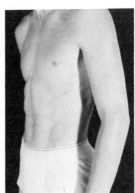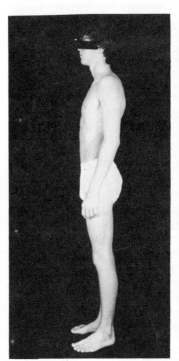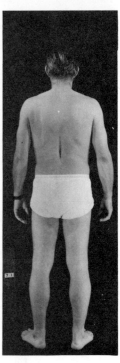

15-8 Lower-lying structure relates to cervical ab-erration. It is impossible (barring history of a specific accident) to determine whether the com-pensation of the lower body resulted from its at-tempt to balance the displaced head, or whether the head is being held forward to counterpoise the very distorted lower body.

As integration progresses, pre- and postver-tebral structures of the neck shift into a position where they can assume their agonist-antagonist roles. The semispinalis group, especially, gains a new tone and contributes to bringing the head back, thus centering its contour on the shoulder girdle.

(The overwide shoulders seen in Mr. B above are a mark, not of superior masculinity, but of distorted relations of shoulder girdle and neck muscles supporting the cervical spine.)

235

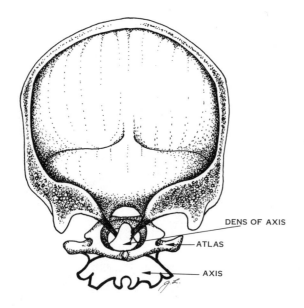

DENS OF AXIS

ATLAS

AXIS

15-9 This is a schema of the cranium, coronal section. The keystone to the position of the cranium is the dens of the axis (second cervical vertebra). To the extent that cervical flexors and extensors maintain alignment reciprocally, the cranium is able to balance around this upward extension of the axis. This precision depends on the ligaments by which the cranium attaches to the dens, which in turn is modified by the enwrapping myofascial "bandage."

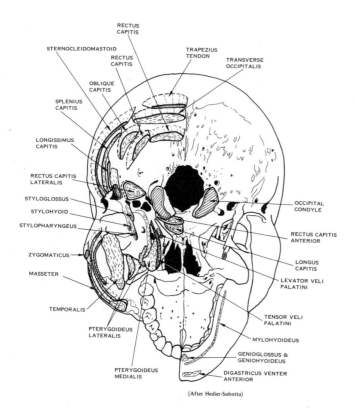

RECTUS CAPITIS

STERNOCLEIDOMASTOID

RECTUS CAPITIS

TRAPEZIUS TENDON

TRANSVERSE OCCIPITALIS

OBLIQUE CAPITIS

SPLENIUS CAPITIS

LONGISSIMUS CAPITIS

RECTUS CAPITIS LATERALIS

STYLOGLOSSUS

STYLOHYOID

STYLOPHARYNGEUS

ZYGOMATICUS

MASSETER

TEMPORALIS

PTERYGOIDEUS LATERALIS

PTERYGOIDEUS MEDIALIS

OCCIPITAL CONDYLE

RECTUS CAPITIS ANTERIOR

LONGUS CAPITIS

LEVATOR VELI PALATINI

TENSOR VELI PALATINI

MYLOHYOIDEUS

GENIOGLOSSUS & GENIOHYOIDEUS

DIGASTRICUS VENTER ANTERIOR

(After Hedier-Sobotta)

15-10 This schema, an inferior view of the skull, represents the complex patterns of muscular attachments that determine the position of the cranium above the spine. It is apparent here how many possibilities exist for interfering with equipoise. (After Sobotta, ATLAS OF HUMAN ANATOMY, Vol. 1, Fig. 357)

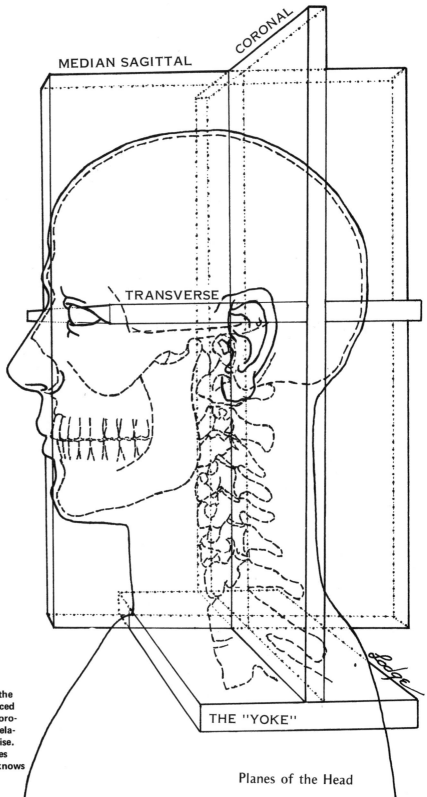

MEDIAN SAGITTAL

CORONAL

TRANSVERSE

THE "YOKE"

Planes of the Head

15-11 A body in equipoise from the soles of the feet to the shoulders will support a head balanced with respect to the three planes of space —— coronal, sagittal, and horizontal. The right-angled relation of these planes is the definition of equipoise. The top of the head is up. As a man experiences this relation of head, shoulders, and neck, he knows where up really is, perhaps for the first time.

cal breakdown, to a hardening of the arteries, and/or to deposition of calcareous matter on blood vessel walls, the sleepiness of senility can result from this type of mechanical blockage. When the blood flows fast and free, arteries do not harden and deposits do not form in vessels. The shortened neck so frequent in the elderly is often compensating for aberrations lower in the structure. Whatever its genesis, it immobilizes and crowds the vertebrae and impedes muscular movement and consequently the flow of both blood and lymph. The slowed responses characteristic of age are among the chronic symptoms that ensue. The younger person more often becomes aware of neck blockages through pain. The garden-variety headache, the one that follows "a hard day at the office," is in fact a report by the nerves of restricted circulation.

The neck, after all, bridges vertically between head and shoulders (perhaps an elevator, not a bridge, would be a more appropriate metaphor). Of necessity, the location of both ends determines the stresses under which it functions. If the bridgeheads deviate, the structure is no longer vertical and is under strain; the precarious supply of fluid to the head is constricted, the metabolic rate in head and brain lowered. (In general, the flow of fluids to parts of the body is amply provided for. Thus it is noteworthy that circulation to the brain is so vulnerable.) These limitations, inherent in structure and unchangeable, underscore the necessity for doing everything possible to keep the bridging free and balanced; if, voluntarily or involuntarily, the top of the head seeks its highest point, extension of the cervical vertebrae aligns them automatically.

Body structure in itself suggests certain other assumptions: the first is that the cranium, a bony container for an essentially hydrostatic system (the brain), will be balanced only if the plane through the occipital condyles is horizontal. To meet this requirement, an axis bisecting the ear must be vertical and centered above the shoulders. Again, random bodies do not fulfill these conditions—the average head is tipped forward and the entire upper cervical structure is displaced anteriorly. The angle of the head defines the degree of misalignment that the cervical spine has had to accept.

Superficial myofascial wrappings reinforce the cervical spine, giving rise to characteristic contours of the neck and offering clues to underlying strain. In many necks, the sternocleidomastoid stands out like a rope (Figs. 15-12 and 15-13); this muscle is countered by the levator scapulae as well as the splenius. No "rope" is apparent when balance exists among these three.

The levator scapulae has its own characteristic problems.

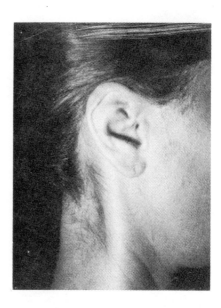

15-12　When the intrinsic muscles of the neck lack tone for proper support of the cranium, the extrinsics try to substitute. In this photograph, the sternocleidomastoid is trying to substitute for an underlying complex. The ligaments uniting dens and occiput should be giving this support at a deeper level.

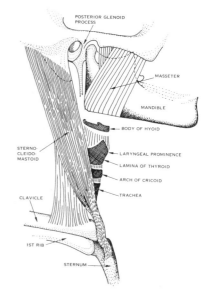

15-13　Lateral view: Each part evokes the whole pattern. A neck like the one in this schema —— its vertebrae in vertical alignment, the occiput poised above them, the mandible defining a horizontal —— gives clear intimation of the body below it. For the neck to look like this, the body below must be giving balanced support. (After Basmajian, GRANT'S METHOD OF ANATOMY, Fig. 715)

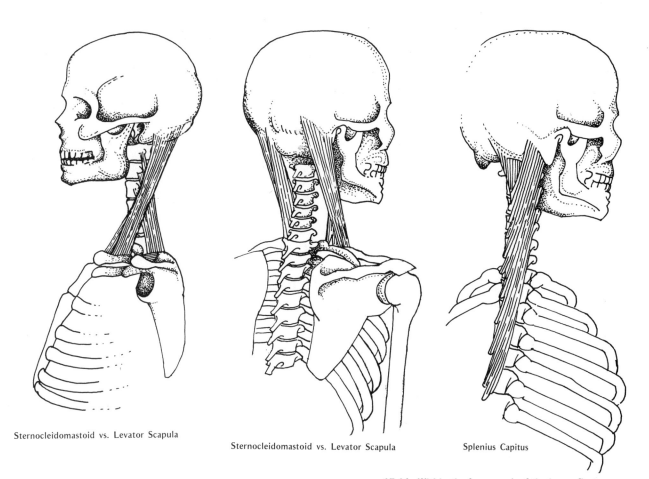

Sternocleidomastoid vs. Levator Scapula

Sternocleidomastoid vs. Levator Scapula

Splenius Capitus

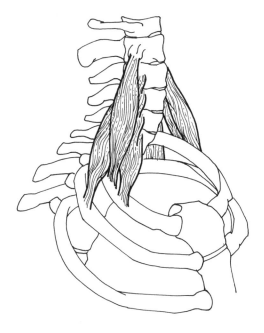

15-14 Within the framework of the larger flexor-extensor reciprocity in neck and shoulders, there are many smaller balances. Though dealing with smaller elements, they are nevertheless vitally important to the whole. The relation among sternocleidomastoid, splenius, and levator scapulae is such a reciprocal. If the balance between true flexors and extensors is destroyed, secondary relations also collapse and verticality in the cervicals deteriorates.

15-15 Three-quarter anterior view: The three scalenes (anterior, medius, and posterior), together with the longus colli and longus capitis, are prevertebral muscles. That is, they attach to the anterior tubercle of the transverse processes of cervical vertebrae; by definition, they are flexors. When extensor postvertebral muscles lose tone, flexors (including the scalenes) shorten and thicken. This schema is of aberrated scalenes. The head is then displaced forward, and the contour of the neck is permanently modified. Since the appropriate length of these muscles contributes to lifting of the two upper ribs, the contour of the ribcage is also influenced. As is apparent in Fig. 15 - 8 g , this is the anterior structure maintaining the dowager's hump.

239

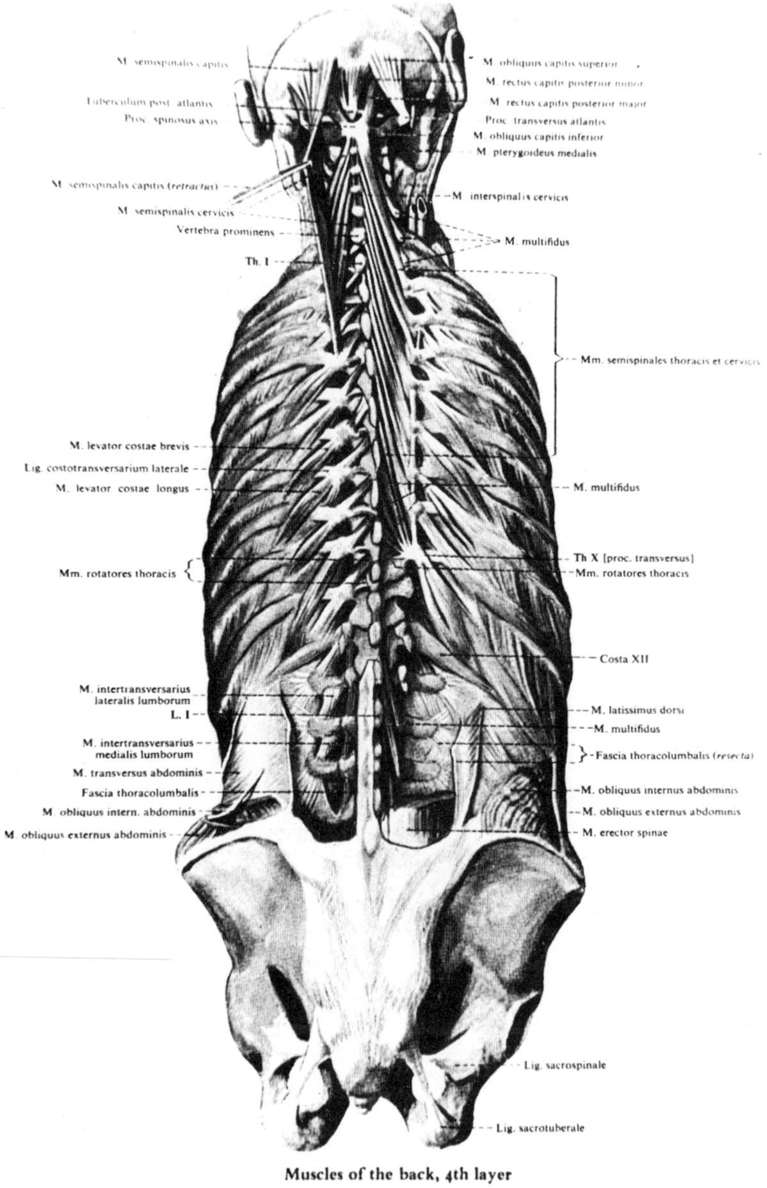

M. semispinalis capitis
Tuberculum post. atlantis
Proc. spinosus axis
M. semispinalis capitis (*retractus*)
M. semispinalis cervicis
Vertebra prominens
Th. I
M. obliquus capitis superior
M. rectus capitis posterior minor
M. rectus capitis posterior major
Proc. transversus atlantis
M. obliquus capitis inferior
M. pterygoideus medialis
M. interspinalis cervicis
M. multifidus
Mm. semispinales thoracis et cervicis
M. levator costae brevis
Lig. costotransversarium laterale
M. levator costae longus
M. multifidus
Mm. rotatores thoracis
Th X [proc. transversus]
Mm. rotatores thoracis
Costa XII
M. intertransversarius lateralis lumborum
L. I
M. intertransversarius medialis lumborum
M. transversus abdominis
Fascia thoracolumbalis
M. obliquus intern. abdominis
M. obliquus externus abdominis
M. latissimus dorsi
M. multifidus
Fascia thoracolumbalis (*resecta*)
M. obliquus internus abdominis
M. obliquus externus abdominis
M. erector spinae
Lig. sacrospinale
Lig. sacrotuberale

Muscles of the back, 4th layer

Intrinsic muscles of the back.
Transversospinalis and short muscles of the neck and back.

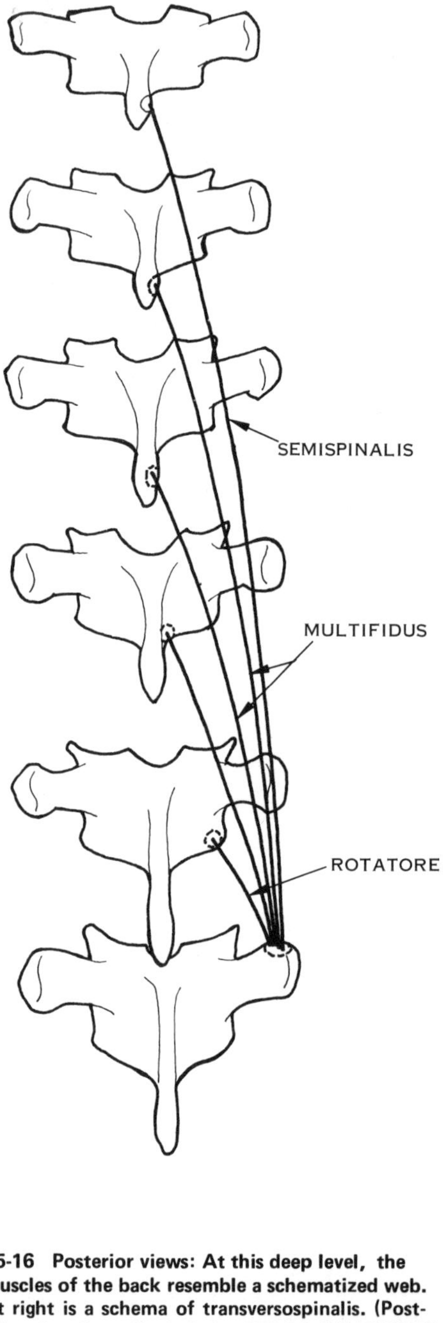

SEMISPINALIS
MULTIFIDUS
ROTATORE

15-16 Posterior views: At this deep level, the muscles of the back resemble a schematized web. At right is a schema of transversospinalis. (Posterior view from Spalteholz, ATLAS OF HUMAN ANATOMY, Fig. 188)

Arising from the transverse processes of the first four cervical vertebrae and inserting into the medial border of the scapula, it raises the shoulders in a shrug or a gesture of protection. Thus, a body dramatizing habitual fear or defense permanently shortens the muscle, which then deteriorates: patches of gristle at its insertion on the scapula bear witness to its lessened mobility. Sometimes, deterioration glues one or both shoulder blades to the trapezius, which then is a new trapezius-levator complex, no longer capable of independent reciprocal movement. It forms the basis for the characteristic ineffectual rounded shoulders, with their manifest loss of structural competence. As trapezius and levator fuse into a single complex, the teres-rhomboid balance is threatened, outwardly apparent in too much width between the two scapulae and in a headward displacement and bunching of dorsal vertebrae and ribs. This contour was once considered a hallmark of advancing age—now, sadly enough, it is all too apparent in the vast majority of teen-agers as well. It bears witness to tissue deterioration, loss of tone, and therefore loss of function. In addition, chronic flexion anywhere in the spine destroys the potential polarity of the body.

The depressions, the "salt cellars" appearing above (or, rather, behind) the clavicle, are the outward and visible sign of shortened scalenes. Originally, round shoulders are formed by lifting and shortening the trapezius, levators, and sternocleidomastoid. The resultant stresses are transmitted to anterior and middle scalenes and distort the ribs into which they insert. Freeing the scalenes allows ribcage and scapulae to fall into a more appropriate girdle pattern, thus lessening tension in the neck. Muscles of the neck and shoulders are part of the mechanics of respiration. In normal breathing, the shoulders *widen* with every inspiration. The relaxation accompanying this widening allows the shoulders to drop appreciably. In random bodies, this respiratory pattern can appear only through substantial reorganizing of shoulders and neck.

Myofascial organization in upper dorsal and cervical spines also clearly reveals the neck's bridging function. In the context of the spine as a whole, we called attention to the supporting lattice offered by the deep longitudinal muscles, the erector spinae: illiocostalis, longissimus, and spinalis. The supporting tissue adjacent to spinal vertebrae is a more complex tapestry than we have suggested. The transverse and articular processes of cervical vertebrae serve to distribute arrangements of myofascial tissues so complex as to seem schematized (Fig. 15-16). Many of these are continuations of structures immediately below; the transverse processes of dorsal vertebrae obviously are scaffolding and support for higher cervical structures. Here muscular structures are truly interweavings.

Deep in the neck is a complex myofascial tapestry. At this deepest level of intrinsic structure, each of the rotators bridges only one interspace of the spine, connecting the root of one transverse process with that of the spinous process above. At a more superficial level, muscular units—for example, the multifidus and semispinalis—may traverse as many as five segments in the course of connecting thoracic with cervical transverse processes. Of the several parts of the semispinalis group, which as a whole runs from lower thoracic vertebrae (the tenth) to the occiput, the massive semispinalis capitis, supporting the head, is almost vertical. (In general, muscles that traverse longer distances are more nearly vertical, whereas muscles running obliquely are, of course, shorter in length.) Even when they appear unitary, long muscles are not single; they are interdigitating aggregates. For example, the multifidus, arising from the dorsal aspect of the sacrum, inserts surprisingly high, at the lower border of spinous process C3. This apparently thick, fleshy mass is, however, an aggregation of fibers, each spanning about three to five spinal segments.

Reinforced fascial webbings like this should offer a design of sturdy flexibility throughout the length of the spine, particularly in the neck. But the real world is full of people who are bewailing their headaches, their neckaches, their backaches, which are all symptoms of lack of appropriate sturdy patterns, lack of flexibility. The flesh overlying the spine gives you a tactile clue to this contradiction. Palpation tells you that these muscle masses are amorphous, solid, unyielding. As you can feel, their inelasticity crowds the cervical vertebrae into a shortened arc. Some of the segments are forced into spaces anterior or posterior to the position of good function; disc deterioration may develop through this displacement. Without help, the subject then is headed toward a lifetime of the miseries he so loudly bewails.

Many deviations from normal muscular tone are to be found in the neck. A cervical or upper dorsal area will be thick and wooden when it is short. By contrast, over-lengthened muscles lack tone and are stringy and flaccid. Poor muscular tone can show in the spacing of ribs; vertebrae or upper ribs may seem too widely spaced. Occasionally, the palpating finger seems to find its way into a hole where tissue seems lacking. None of these situations is necessarily final. The live vital unit, the body, can with appropriate help rehabilitate most of the miseries to which it is heir, particularly if they are local and structural.

Appropriate help comes from applying the primary, vital first principle of Structural Integration: tissue, be it too short

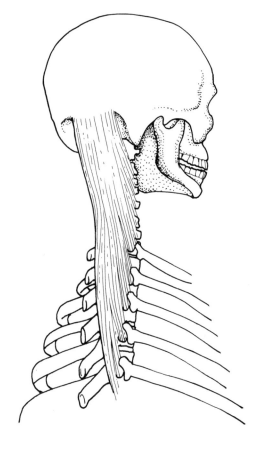

15-17 The posterior contour of the neck defines the quality and tone of the semispinalis group (postvertebral). In the preceding photographs of an integrated subject, this is clearly evident (Fig. 15 — 8a, b, c, d).

242

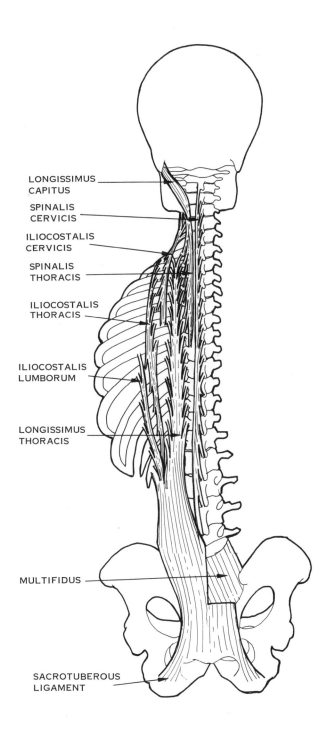

LONGISSIMUS
CAPITUS

SPINALIS
CERVICIS

ILIOCOSTALIS
CERVICIS

SPINALIS
THORACIS

ILIOCOSTALIS
THORACIS

ILIOCOSTALIS
LUMBORUM

LONGISSIMUS
THORACIS

MULTIFIDUS

SACROTUBEROUS
LIGAMENT

15-18 Posterior view: Schema of semispinalis cap-
itis. The action of the deep intrinsic erector spinae
muscle mass establishes and maintains appropriate
extension in the vertebral column. In this sense,
it is the most obvious connecting link between upper and lower pole. It is of interest here to note
how the heavy, dense fibers of the lumbar and sacral ligamentous tissue branch and thin into the relatively delicate structures of the neck. The extension that these muscles can establish must be appropriate to the tone and elasticity of the ventral
flexors.

In the sacral area, the extensor mass consists
largely of tendinous and fascial components. At
the lumbar level, it is a thick muscular mass, which
divides into columns in the dorsal region. The iliocostalis and longissimus are the longest of these;
muscle slips from the longissimus insert into the
cranium deep to the sternocleidomastoid.

or so lengthened and toneless that it seems virtually nonexistent, must be brought nearer to the position it was designed to occupy in the normal pattern. In the technique of Structural Integration, this is done by the hand of the processor. Then a demand for normal movement can and does evoke the rehabilitating response.

In the neck, normal movement calls for response from both extrinsic and intrinsic levels, i.e., from the superficial muscles attaching to the shoulder structure (trapezius, levator, sternocleidomastoid) and from the deeper intrinsic scaffolding (semispinalis, multifidus, and longissimus capitis) of the neck itself. Rotation of a balanced neck activates the longer muscles, as well as the very short, almost ligamentous layers (rotatores, interspinales, and intertransversales) and the short oblique and straight muscles of the suboccipital region. This is a coordination of many levels. Activating this pattern calls forth movement that differs radically from average neck rotation in a random body. Its stability and grace evoke aesthetic appreciation; they also suggest effective interaction of the individual with his environment.

Extension (lengthening of vertebral joints) requires activation of the deep muscles of neck and back. Therefore, the well-being of these deep muscles is essential if the powerful flexors constituting the anterior body (recti abdominis, pectorales, psoas, etc.) are to be balanced appropriately by the extensors of the back. The short, ligamentous scaffolding is not able to extend joints unless a reasonable amount of verticality pre-exists in the spine. This happens only when the excessive compulsive flexion of habitual stooping has been released. The neck, which is the least stable part of the segmented spine, is particularly vulnerable to unbalanced flexion. Chronic flexion in any part of the body, even though as distant as the legs, will reflect in anteriority in the head and neck. Lordosis (anteriority of the lumbar spine) is a primary contributor to the subjective and objective weakness that accompanies cervical anteriority. Conversely, gross cervical displacement makes it impossible to reorganize a lower back. The situation is once again circular; any satisfactory remedy must deal with these circular interplays.

The vertical thrust of the bipolar unit is the expression of a competent spinal structure—lumbar, thoracic, and cervical. This is a spine that moves independently of pelvic and shoulder girdles. The vital core is free of the working sleeve and is characterized by a vertical thrust.

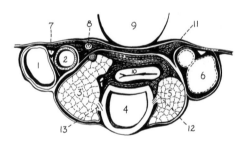

15-20 Superior view, facing down: Cross sections at different levels of the neck show quite different pictures. This one, at one of the lower cervical levels (C 7), pictures an area largely pre-empted by nonmuscular structures. Key: 1. Internal jugular vein 2. Common carotid artery 3. Thyroid gland 4. Trachea 5. Thyroid gland 6. Carotid sheath 7. Vagus nerve 8. Vertebral artery 9. Vertebral body 10. Oesophagus 11. Prevertebral fasciae 12. Left recurrent nerve 13. Anchoring band (After Basmajian, GRANT'S METHOD OF ANATOMY, Fig. 714)

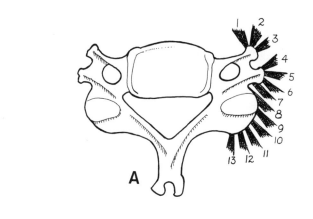

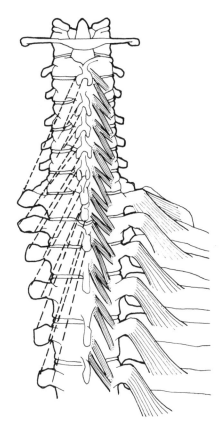

Schema of Rotatores, Multifidus (dotted lines),
and Levator Costae Brevis.

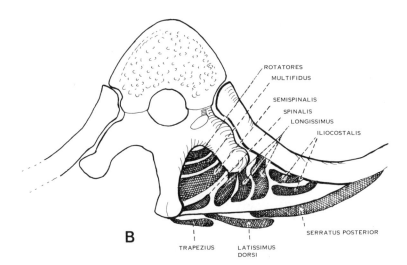

ROTATORES

MULTIFIDUS

SEMISPINALIS

SPINALIS

LONGISSIMUS

ILIOCOSTALIS

SERRATUS POSTERIOR

TRAPEZIUS

LATISSIMUS
DORSI

15-19 A cross section of the cervical spine reveals the patterns of the attached muscular webs. Schematic A (superior view) shows attachments to a cervical vertebra; B (superior view) shows those attaching to a mid-thoracic vertebra; C (posterior view) pictures the deep intrinsic supporting tissues of the dorsal extensors (rotatores and multifidi). Note that of the erector spinae group, only columns of the longissimus reach the skull, where they attach on the mastoid process deep to splenius and sternocleidomastoid. Muscles attached to the articular and transverse processes of a mid-cervical vertebra are: 1. Longus colli 2. Longus capitis 3. Scalenus anterior 4. Scalenus medius 5. Scalenus posterior 6. Levator scapulae 7. Splenius cervicis 8. Iliocostalis cervicis 9;. Longissimus cervicis 10. Longissumus capitis 11. Semispinalis capitis 12. Semispinalis cervicis 13. Multifidus (A and B after Basmajian, GRANT'S METHOD OF ANATOMY, Figs. 673 and 564)

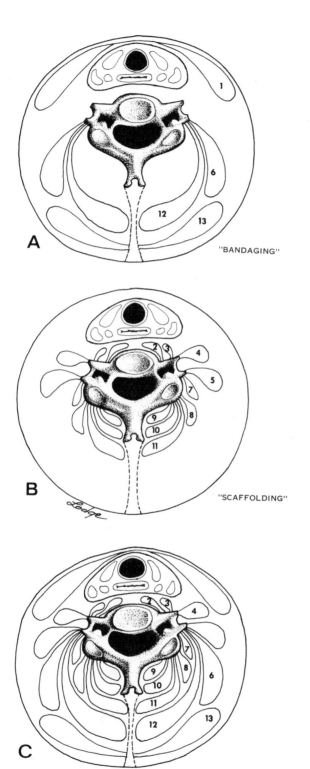

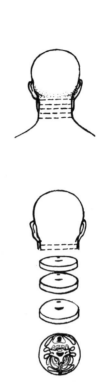

A

"BANDAGING"

B

"SCAFFOLDING"

C

15-21 All three of these schemata are cross sections through the same upper cervical vertebra. A pictures muscles of the superficial level (in our terms, the extrinsic level), which act as bandaging and protection. B is the deeper level (in our terms, intrinsic), which as scaffolding maintains the position and spacing of vital cervical structures — autonomic nervous plexi, glandular units (thyroid, parathyroid), etc. And C is a combining of A and B. These muscles, attached horizontally to the bony vertebral structure at one end only, are directionally oriented by planes of fascia. Like all fascial planes, they are plastic and by slight elongation or shortening can change the tone of the related muscle. In so doing, they lessen or exaggerate pressure on vital structures. This changing pressure is the clue to migraine headaches — in fact, to all headaches. Key: 1. Sternocleidomastoid 2. Cervicis longus 3. Longus capitis 4. Scalenus anterior 5. Scalenus medius 6. Levator scapulae 7. Costocervicalis 8. Cervicis longissumus 9. Multifidus 10. Semispinalis cervicis 11. Semispinalis capitus 12. Splenius 13. Trapezius.

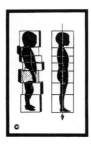

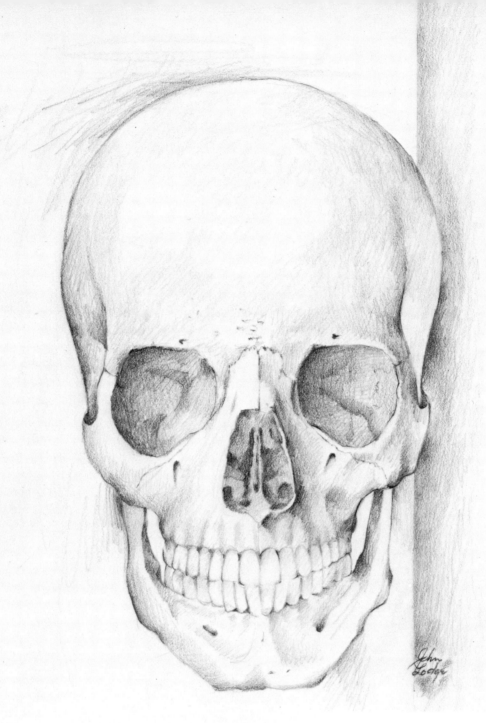

16-1 In the embryo, as mesoderm differentiates into bony core, a complex topmost unit, the skull, develops; like the pelvis, this is a development from the spine. There is evidence indicating that the occipital bone may be a modification and fusion of three vertebral segments. At this stage of development, the resemblance to vertebrae is largely erased. The skull armors and houses the brain and special senses. Among the bones of the body, those of the skull have a unique importance to the creation and re-creation of that special animal, man.

16
The Upper Pole

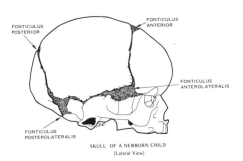

SKULL OF A NEWBORN CHILD
(Lateral View)

FONTICULUS POSTERIOR
FONTICULUS ANTERIOR
FONTICULUS ANTEROLATERALIS
FONTICULUS POSTEROLATERALIS

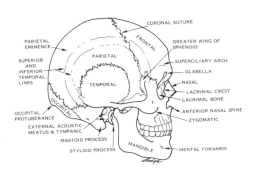

CORONAL SUTURE
FRONTAL
GREATER WING OF SPHENOID
SUPERCILIARY ARCH
GLABELLA
NASAL
LACRIMAL CREST
LACRIMAL BONE
ANTERIOR NASAL SPINE
ZYGOMATIC
MENTAL FORAMEN
MANDIBLE
STYLOID PROCESS
MASTOID PROCESS
EXTERNAL ACOUSTIC MEATUS & TYMPANIC
OCCIPITAL PROTUBERANCE
OCCIPITAL
TEMPORAL
PARIETAL
SUPERIOR AND INFERIOR TEMPORAL LINES
PARIETAL EMINENCE

16-2 At top is a schema of a newborn child's skull — lateral view. At bottom is an adult skull. They are designed to remind you of the way some bones differentiate from nuclei laid down in the embryonic membrane (especially the bones of the cranial vault). They unite as the individual grows older, forming the familiar adult skull. Within this skull are to be found the structures housing and protecting the special senses. It is of interest that the basilar part of the skull and the jaw differentiate from cartilage rather than from membrane.

Thanks to the fasciae and the physical properties of its collagen, we have been able to shift one unit atop another —pelvis above legs, thorax over pelvis, and neck and head on the top. In so doing, we have greatly improved the mechanical stacking of these structural units, but this is not basically a mechanical system. It is a living system within a gravitational field; therefore, it is an electrical system, a polar system.

We must look to this electrical system for the positive, vital qualities of man. It has been postulated that the inferior pole is located within the pelvis. The superior pole of our bipolar vertical quite apparently must be located within the head. But what is the head? The cranium (brain case) is the highest segment of our pile of blocks. It houses the most important of the nervous plexi, the brain. We consider the human organism to be a system of energies, an aggregate of energy segments. Of necessity, the topmost unit, the head, must be unique. All living nervous tissue gives rise to electric currents. Such a massive nervous aggregation as the brain might be expected to generate as well as focus very considerable electrical phenomena, an expectation borne out by modern measurements (electroencephalograms, for example).

We sense the pre-eminence of this great plexus: when we think of "I," invariably, naïvely, we assume that "I" lives in our head. Any practitioner of Structural Integration has facts that belie this assumption—he knows that all points of the body house the "I." (Even an eight-year-old senses this after Structural Integration. Asked how she was feeling, a little girl replied, "Oh, fine: I used to live in my head, but now I live all over me.") This is felt dramatically in the pelvis. To the extent that the pelvis expresses its appropriate horizontal orientation, well-being is sensed not solely there but in every part of the body. Our experience further indicates that well-being does not merely manifest the physiological competence of individual parts, but rather indicates relationship among parts and, more important, between the

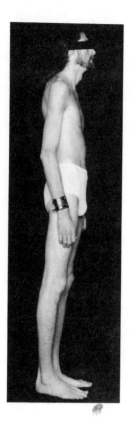
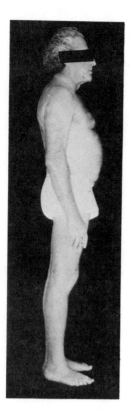

16-3   Certainly, an individual structured like Mr.L could be expected, logically, to manifest an energy field different from the one expressed by Mr. S. Lines connecting the upper and lower poles of these bodies would relate differently to the vertical, and hence to gravity.

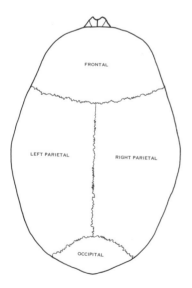
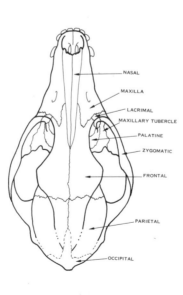

FRONTAL

LEFT PARIETAL

RIGHT PARIETAL

OCCIPITAL

NASAL

MAXILLA

LACRIMAL

MAXILLARY TUBERCLE

PALATINE

ZYGOMATIC

FRONTAL

PARIETAL

OCCIPITAL

16-4   In lower animal species and in primates, a view of the head from above reveals much of the face. In man alone one sees only the crown of the skull, with occasionally the tip of the nose protruding. These skulls, a man's at left and a primate's at right, point up the great structural difference between man and primate. The shape of the head indicates clearly that modern man has evolved to serve a different function in the animal economy. But whereas this beautifully balanced head is labeled _man_, inspection of the humans walking the streets of any city shows all too clearly that few of our fellow citizens conform to this design.

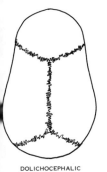

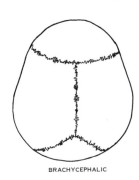

DOLICHOCEPHALIC   BRACHYCEPHALIC

16-5 These are again superior views. Heads differ greatly in the relation of breadth to length (cephalic index). Such differences seem to relate to body structure (ecto-, meso-, or endomorph types). However, cephalic indices seem to have no correlation with the function or intelligence of the enclosed brain.

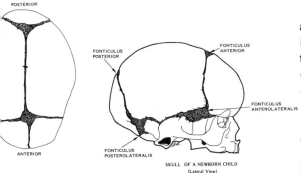

POSTERIOR

FONTICULUS POSTERIOR

FONTICULUS ANTERIOR

FONTICULUS ANTEROLATERALIS

FONTICULUS POSTEROLATERALIS

ANTERIOR

SKULL OF A NEWBORN CHILD
(Lateral View)

16-6 At birth, the various individual bones that have developed from centers of ossification during fetal life are joined only by membranes. Proportional relations of the individual bones are markedly different from what they will be in adult life.

man and the earth's energy field. The position of the head and pelvis in three-dimensional space determines verticality in the bipolar unit. This is again a circular situation. Reciprocal relations of head and pelvis determine how the individual as a whole fits into the gravity field.

The relationship of parts called verticality seems to affect the capacity of man as a species, as many other types of body relationships do not. It is of interest to note the increased intellectual and cultural capacity of the animal we now call man as he has structurally approached a more vertical stance. Examination shows that human skulls, the housing for the upper poles, vary widely in volume capacity as well as in external contour. Physical anthropologists have attempted to find a connection between intelligence and craniometric measurements. This would seem a logical correlation, but it has not been proved. So-called cephalic indices vary with head shape, but such variations are not specific to the different races of humans, nor are they immutable (over the generations). Apparently, nutritional environment as well as genetic inheritance does influence them.

The body type of the individual as well as his basic racial family has a greater correlation with cephalic indices and tends to determine whether he is broad-headed (dolichocephalic), middle-width (mesaticephalic), or long-headed (brachiocephalic)—endomorphic, mesomorphic, or ectomorphic body type, respectively (Fig. 16-5). If the ratio of maximum width to maximum length is less than 75 per cent, the type is dolichocephalic; a ratio greater than 80 per cent classifies the skull as brachycephalic. It is tempting to think that Structural Integration, applied to the very young, may change these indices, but the fact is that the head, although changing to a marked degree, retains its cephalic ratio.

Most people realize that the cranium, which is thought of as a single bone in adult life, is in fact an aggregate of individual segments. The lines that mark the junctions of these parts are called "sutures" (as bony unions, they are classified as syndesmoses). Early in fetal life, centers of calcification appear within the developing membranes. These nuclei grow and expand, but are not fully or finally joined until adult life. At birth, this process is still very incomplete, and the angles (called fontanelles) at which the bones approach one another are still open. At that stage, the brain in these local areas is protected only by a covering membrane. Most parents have experienced this in their children and recognize it as the "soft spot."

The growth pattern of these bones is not necessarily uniform. We all recognize this as we watch the facial changes in children resulting from bony growth. The formation of

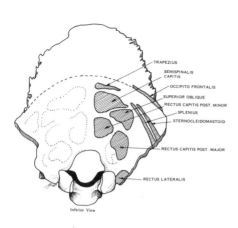

Inferior View

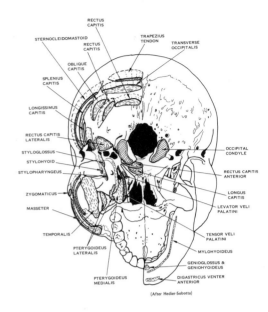

(After Hedier-Sobotta)

16-7 If balance of all muscles joining skull and trunk is a prerequisite for equipoise in the head, these schemata will indicate the complexity of the task. Clearly, balance around the occipital junction (and therefore competence at the atlanto-occilital joint) will be related to muscular

attachments on the base of the skull. This is again a circular situation; the precision of the atlanto-occipital junction influences ease and balance in related muscular components of the joint. (A after Sobotta, ATLAS OF HUMAN ANATOMY, Fig. 357)

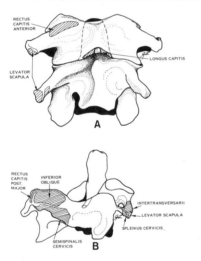

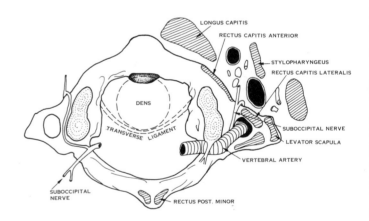

16-8 These three schemata show (A) anterior view of the atlas and axis; (B) posterolateral view of the axis; (C) superior view of the atlas. The mechanism by which they interlock, and the details of the atlanto-occipital junction, are of practical importance to each of us. The mechanics of the aftermath of a " hard day at the office " are clear here. Even a slight congestion caused by immobilizing and shortening the muscles of the upper neck can prevent free blood flow in the vertebral artery (see Chapter Fifteen). In turn, this puts pressure on the underlying suboccipital

nerve and so completes the preparation for a "tension headache." The more arterial congestion, the more nerve pressure; the more nerve pressure, the more rigid the vertebral artery becomes. Only movement of the head on the neck, inducing a lifting of occiput on atlas, restores flow. On the other hand, if the body has been integrated, the various muscles connecting cranium and torso will have developed a degree of elasticity that makes the constriction (and the headache) unlikely. (C after FRAZER'S ANATOMY OF THE HUMAN SKELETON, Fig. 24)

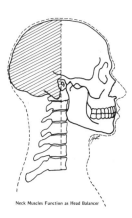

Neck Muscles Function as Head Balancer

16-9 The neck muscles function to balance the head. This schema gives aome idea of the structural relations necessary for a head that is free to rotate easily. It can extend and/or flex competently. Structurally, it is balanced midway between the shoulders as well as midway between anterior and posterior contours. It is apparent that an imaginary axis transversing the bodies of the cervicals must bisect the skull, with substantially equal weight falling before and behind it. In this pattern, and only in this pattern, can the weight of the head balance spontaneously over the atlanto-occipital junction.

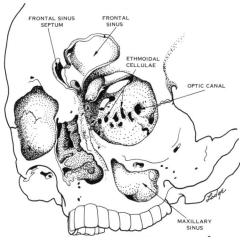

FRONTAL SINUS SEPTUM

FRONTAL SINUS

ETHMOIDAL CELLULAE

OPTIC CANAL

MAXILLARY SINUS

16-10 In the earlier years of this century, a favorite insult of affection was to refer to the other fellow's head as "solid ivory." Any close-up of a skull shows the fallacy of the idea. Bone in any part of the body, but especially in the head, is neither ivory nor solid. Instead, it is reminiscent of a sponge. Its appearance bears witness to its development: inorganic salts deposited within an organic matrix. Like most other bones, the skull has differentiated from the mesoderm.

new cartilage allows bones to increase in size and change in shape. New bone may be deposited on an outer surface as older bone erodes from the inner. This process can not only increase the size of the unit, it can reposition it. Change in structure follows physiological demand. Growth of brain and eye function may demand and develop a larger cranial volume, just as the greater activity of the growing child and adolescent may stimulate change of the upper face to accommodate greater respiratory needs.

The growth of the cranial vault correlates with the growth of the underlying brain. Both reach maximum size around puberty. The chemical and structural qualities that have permitted this drastic shift from infant to adult are not obliterated suddenly. Different structures fuse at different periods: sagittal and coronal sutures may be undergoing this process from the mid-twenties to the early forties. Fusion of the temporal bone with its neighbors may not be final before old age.

Such structural flexibility, although slight, does allow the skull to adapt during the life of the individual to the mechanical demands of an increasingly erect posture. Physiologic function systems (respiratory, perceptive, dentitional, etc.) evoke anatomical adaptation of the cranium. So, too, the myofascial system in its turn plays upon the skull and calls forth appropriate response. The focus of mechanical balance is in the atlanto-occipital junction, where the two condyles of the occiput are designed to slide on related condyles of the atlas. Just below this point, muscles of the back and neck, by their focus, counterbalance the weight of the head as it nods, restraining it from falling forward. Precise nodding motion of the head is lost if this equipoise is interfered with. As the nod is restored through balancing muscles of head and neck, the opening of the condyles can be palpated with the fingertips.

Many misconceptions and oversimplifications interfere with our appreciation of the head, its structure and function. The head is not merely a simple bony bowl containing a semifluid brain, as too many people tacitly believe. Like the pelvis, it is a bony basin, at once divided and reinforced by complicated, sophisticated thrusting bars. What we think of as solid bone is bone that is not solid at all (Fig. 16-10). Like a sponge, it is interspersed with air cavities (sinuses) (Fig. 16-11). A few of these sinuses (those that drain into the nose) are lined with mucous membrane that secretes a mucous fluid. In its normal flow, this latter moistens the passages of the nose, lubricates nasal structures, picks up dust, washes it to the surface, and so forth. Possibly the basic purpose of interpenetrating air spaces in the skull is to reduce the weight of the head. Valuable as this may be to

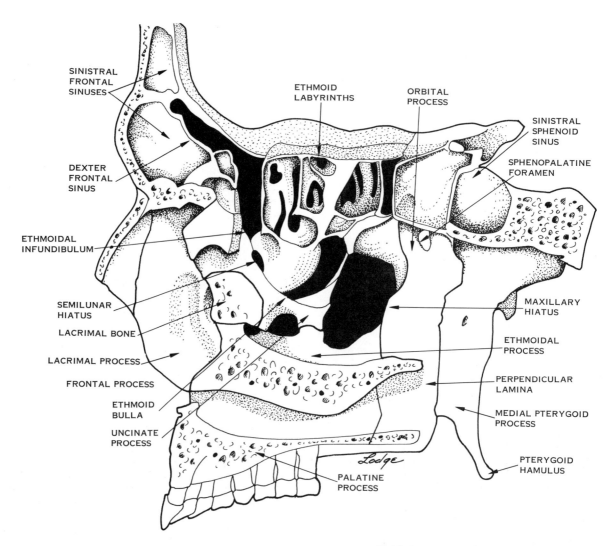

SINISTRAL
FRONTAL
SINUSES

ETHMOID
LABYRINTHS

ORBITAL
PROCESS

SINISTRAL
SPHENOID
SINUS

DEXTER
FRONTAL
SINUS

SPHENOPALATINE
FORAMEN

ETHMOIDAL
INFUNDIBULUM

SEMILUNAR
HIATUS

MAXILLARY
HIATUS

LACRIMAL BONE

ETHMOIDAL
PROCESS

LACRIMAL PROCESS

FRONTAL PROCESS

PERPENDICULAR
LAMINA

ETHMOID
BULLA

MEDIAL PTERYGOID
PROCESS

UNCINATE
PROCESS

PTERYGOID
HAMULUS

Lodge

PALATINE
PROCESS

16-11 Lateral view, facing left: The amount of pneumatization within the bones forming the skull is a complete surprise to most people. This illustration, a schema of the nasal cavity and paranasal sinuses, shows the paranasal sinuses within the bone. Sinuses that are provided with a drainage duct into the nasal structure (the sinus fontalis, for example) are the ones that tend to become infected after a cold or an attack of the flu. Inflammation of tissue closes the drainage duct. Pressure builds up within the sinus, and the misery of congested sinuses is with us, sometimes for a long time. Relief comes only as the tissues lose their blocked state and normal flow is re-established (After Spalteholz, ATLAS OF HUMAN ANATOMY, Fig. 309)

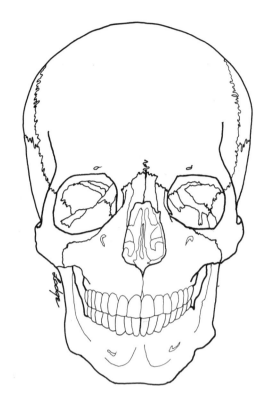

16-12 This anterior view of the skull reveals the intricate pattern of the small bones. They fit together like a picture puzzle. Especially in the orbit of the eye, the zigzag fitting of these many small bones would seem to be less efficient than patterns elsewhere in the body. Seemingly, one or two molded larger bones would absorb the shocks of physical traumata, permit the changes of growth, and allow for the slight expansion and contraction that accompany emotional tension.

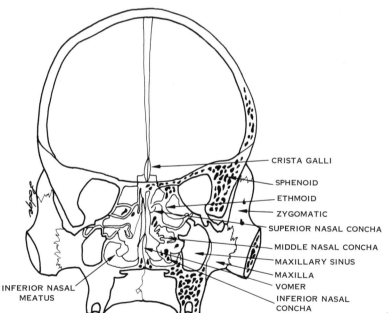

CRISTA GALLI

SPHENOID

ETHMOID

ZYGOMATIC

SUPERIOR NASAL CONCHA

MIDDLE NASAL CONCHA

MAXILLARY SINUS

MAXILLA

VOMER

INFERIOR NASAL CONCHA

INFERIOR NASAL MEATUS

16-13 This coronal section of the skull (posterior view) tells the same story. Pneumatization lightens the actual weight of the skull, and interdigitation of many small bones creates the complex thrusts necessary to adjust to physical and emotional traumata. Thus this complexity provides for ongoing appropriate function.

255

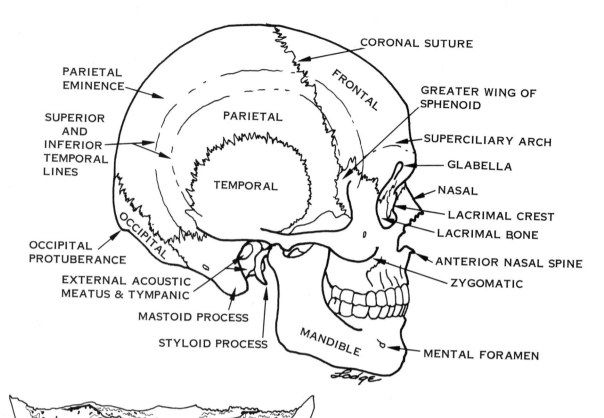

CORONAL SUTURE

FRONTAL

PARIETAL EMINENCE

GREATER WING OF SPHENOID

SUPERCILIARY ARCH

PARIETAL

GLABELLA

SUPERIOR AND INFERIOR TEMPORAL LINES

NASAL

TEMPORAL

LACRIMAL CREST

LACRIMAL BONE

OCCIPITAL

ANTERIOR NASAL SPINE

OCCIPITAL PROTUBERANCE

ZYGOMATIC

EXTERNAL ACOUSTIC MEATUS & TYMPANIC

MASTOID PROCESS

MANDIBLE

STYLOID PROCESS

MENT AL FORAMEN

16-14   The lateral view of an adult skull shows the major bones. Note the ridging of the bones, which thus offer a reinforced surface for attachment of muscles. The sutures have narrowed during post-natal growth of the individual; here, they have reached a state where casual inspection suggests that they are forming a single large container. This assumption of solid immobility is not strictly in accordance with the facts.

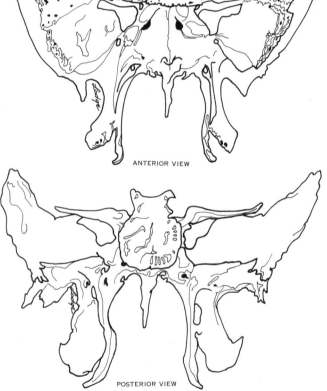

ANTERIOR VIEW

POSTERIOR VIEW

16-15   As an individual separate bone, the sphenoid resembles a butterfly. In position, however, it functions as a wedge that maintains appropiate distance between the lateral walls of the skull (temporal and occipital bones). Its complicated interdigitations allow for many foramina. Thus, the optic canal, orbital fissure, pterygoid canal, and foramen rotundum allow nerves and arteries to traverse the wedge.

the individual, he pays a heavy price for the advantage. These sinuses become a focus for infection and inflammation in the common chronic sinus difficulties so prevalent in our population. Sinus congestion, genesis of the chronic sinus headache, is often the result of blocked ducts. Drainage ducts from sinus to nose are quite small; minimal swelling of the nasal membrane can impede their drainage. It is noteworthy that when the head is appropriately poised on its atlanto-occipital articulation, drainage of the blocked ducts often starts spontaneously, and the chronic sinus problem, even though of years' standing, may disappear.

The skull itself is an aggregation of many bones (Figs. 16-12, 16-13, 16-14). The simple outer surfaces give no suggestion of its complicated internal structuring. Centers of ossification in the fetal head develop into a bony bowl. Eight bones (frontal, right and left parietal, occipital, sphenoid, ethmoid, right and left temporal) enclose the cranial cavity. Their primary function is housing for the brain, cerebrum, cerebellum, etc. Fourteen bones in the head (right and left maxilla, right and left zygomatic, right and left palatine, right and left nasal, right and left lacrimal, right and left inferior concha, vomer, and mandible) are considered to be nasal and facial bones. Bony units forming the nasal cavity function structurally as thrusts holding cranial bones apart. Maxilla and mandible (bones of the jaw) have special functions, not the least important of which is to distribute masticatory pressures through the framework of the skull. The pressures of biting are too great to be completely absorbed locally.

The largest and most important of the thrusting bars separating cranial bones is the sphenoid (Fig. 16-15). This is a complicated, butterfly-shaped unit adjoining and supporting the frontal bone and articulating with the temporal, ethmoid, zygomatic, and occipital bones. It consists of a central body with two paired wings. Structurally, these latter—the greater and lesser wings—play an important part in determining the position of the eyeball. Many other bones (maxilla, zygomatic, lacrimal, and palatine) contribute to the orbit (bony casing) of the eyeball, but the lateral wall, one of the more significant parts of the cavity, is formed by the orbital surface of the greater wing of the sphenoid. The lesser wing contributes to the posterior portion of the roof of the orbit. The body and concha of the sphenoid form its medial wall.

The optic nerve, which conveys visual information from receptors in the eye to interpreters of the brain, passes through the buttressing sphenoid via the optic foramen (as does the ophthalmic artery). Significantly, the optic nerve differs markedly from other nerves connecting the

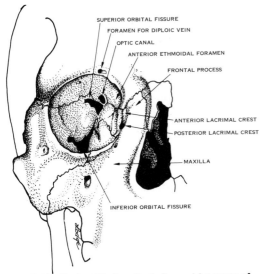

SUPERIOR ORBITAL FISSURE
FORAMEN FOR DIPLOIC VEIN
OPTIC CANAL
ANTERIOR ETHMOIDAL FORAMEN
FRONTAL PROCESS

ANTERIOR LACRIMAL CREST
POSTERIOR LACRIMAL CREST

MAXILLA

INFERIOR ORBITAL FISSURE

16-16 Each orbital cavity is formed by parts of seven bones (temporal, zygomatic, ethmoid, maxillary, sphenoid, lacrimal, palantine). The cavity resembles a cone lying on its side rather than a sphere, At its apex (lying between the body and the "wings" of the sphenoid) is the optic canal, which allows the passage of optic nerve from eye to brain.

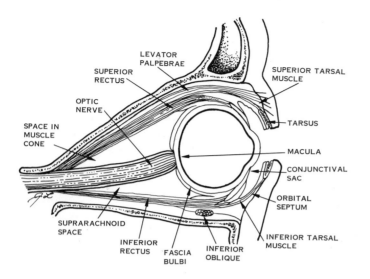

16-17 This schema shows a sagittal section of the orbital cavity. It is apparent here that the eyeball (bulbus oculi) is only about half as long as the orbital cavity. Vision is not distributed randomly over the curved retina, but focuses especially on a very limited spot (macula). The optic nerve, so large in diameter that it is regarded as part of the brain, traverses the orbital cavity. It is capable of considerable adjustment in length and position, hence the eyeball itself is able to withdraw further into the head under emotional stress (grief, for example), or to more closely approach the outer world with curiosity and excitement. This is part of the mechanism underlying the old folklore that the eye is the window of the soul.

Vision in a chronically displaced eye, adjusting to a chronically tipped head, is likely to lose its acuity. Sharp definition requires that light reflected from an object fall on the macula of the retina. (The retina, like the optic nerve, is of nervous origin, developing from ectodermal tissue. It may be considered as a specialized part of the brain.) A chronically unbalanced eye tries to "see" with much larger retinal areas, thereby losing sharp definition.

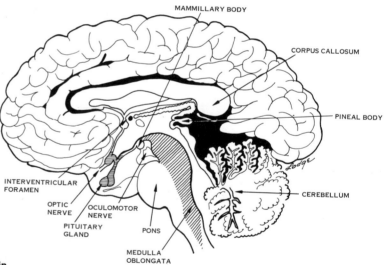

16-18 This schema of the midsection of the brain with the medulla oblongata shows the relation of pituitary to pineal body. Like the pituitary, the pineal body is attached to the roof of the third ventricle. Essentially, it is a framework of connective tissue containing epithelial cells. In humans, it gives the appearance of glandular activity in childhood, then seems later to involute. As is clearly apparent, pituitary and pineal are on different horizontal levels within the skull. In the occult tradition, there is a tendency to relate these two; anatomically, there is no evidence for this.

periphery to the central nervous system. The optic nerve, called the second of the cranial nerves, originates in the brain itself, in the third ventricle. It is a very thick tract, much bulkier than any of the other cranial nerves, almost suggesting that part of the brain itself has penetrated to the periphery to collect information about the environment. To reach the eye, the nerve must traverse the sphenoid; the optic foramen, which connects the orbit and cranial cavity, permits this.

The sphenoid takes to itself additional importance through its function of housing the pituitary, sometimes called the hypophysis cerebri. This endocrine gland attaches by a stalk to the base of the brain at the third ventricle. It is housed in a fossa on the superior surface of the body of the sphenoid. At most, it is half an inch in diameter and a quarter of an inch thick; it weighs less than one gram. Despite its minuscule size, this complex tissue is often called the master gland. It apparently consists of two main lobes; the anterior (adenohypophysis) is only about 20 per cent of the gland by weight; it develops from the third ventricle of the brain, to which it continues to be attached by a stalk. As is apparent in Fig. 18-19, it lies adjacent to the optic nerve and optic chiasma. This last-named is the area of consolidation of the optic tracts from ventral to dorsal.

Both units of the pituitary secrete many hormones, all of them protein in nature. The anterior lobe (adenohypophysis) elaborates at least six biologically distinct substances. The names of most of them indicate their activity: somatotropic (growth promoting), thyrotropic (stimulating thyroid secretion), adrenocorticotropic (ACTH, which specifically stimulates adrenal steroid hormones), two gonadotropic hormones (influencing maturation of ovarian follicles, FSH, and corpora lutea, LH), and prolactin (stimulating activity of mammary glands). The anterior pituitary normally enlarges in pregnancy. Pathologic enlargement, as from a tumor, occasionally causes pressure on the optic chiasma, affecting vision. Oversecretion by this lobe can cause gigantism and may also be linked to hyperglycemia and overactivity of the adrenals and thyroids. Similarly, lowered activity may lead to dwarfism and underdevelopment of the genital system.

The posterior lobe, the neurohypophysis, about one-third the size of its neighbor, the anterior lobe, seems simpler in its functions. Its microscopic structure is uniform and offers no clue as to how or why it elaborates its two hormones: oxytocin stimulates contraction of the uterus (an important part of the delivery of a child); vasopressin raises blood pressure and inhibits diuresis. With this impressive list of

OPTIC CHIASMA
OPTIC NERVE
3RD VENTRICLE
HYPOPHYSEAL STALK
MEDIAN EMINENCE
DIAPHRAGMA SELLAE
INFUNDIBULAR STALK
SPHENOIDAL SINUS
PARS TUBERALIS
PARS INTERMEDIA
INFUNDIBULAR PROCESS
CLEFT
DURA MATER
SPHENOID BONE

16-19 The hypophysis cerebri (pituitary gland), a most important endocrine organ, is attached by a stalk to the third ventricle. The gland itself is housed in its own special fossa on the superior surface of the sphenoid. Its far-reaching hormonal effects are hardly credible in view of its size. Its hormonal secretions are apparently all protein in nature. On dissection of the brain, the area around the pituitary resembles this picture. However, it is impossible in dissection to clearly distinguish glandular boundaries or to differentiate these tissues from those of the neighboring optic tracts.

259

functions, it is understandable that the pituitary is so often called the master gland.

Some controversy exists as to whether the pituitary actually secretes such a variety of hormones. There are, for example, authorities who believe there is evidence that cells in the neighboring hypothalamus elaborate the polypeptide hormones, and that the hypothalamus, usually considered part of the brain itself, is in fact an extension of the posterior pituitary. There is also a certain amount of evidence that the pituitary may elaborate only one hormone, a giant protein molecule with many different attached groups. According to this theory, the specific groups, in dissociating from the giant molecule, activate the different systems.

Because of its far-reaching chemical influence on the emotional as well as the physical body, the pituitary has always been regarded with a certain awe. Occult practices have been designed to stimulate it. In occult thought, it shares the place of prime importance with only one other gland, the pineal, which is also located in the brain. Neither structure nor function of the pineal is clearly understood. In the seventeenth century, Descartes postulated the pineal as the seat of the Rational Soul. In the twentieth century, it is known that the pineal is influenced by certain wave lengths of light and elaborates a secretion, melatonin, which in the young in some way determines the rate of sexual development.

Whatever the importance of these two glands may be, one conclusion is unmistakable: they, like all structures of the brain, are part of a system that in physics is defined as hydrostatic. In anatomy books, we attempt differentiation by isolating and describing the many structures within the skull. Any such separation, of course, subverts physiological reality; there are no definable boundaries within this hydrostatic system. Often, it is not possible to determine structural beginnings and endings, although the over-all change in pattern is apparent. Obviously, as the position in space of such a system alters, pressures within will be redistributed. A chronic shift in the posture of the head away from the horizontal will alter hydrostatic pressures affecting the many significant areas within the brain. So will tensions exerted on the skull by unbalanced overlying muscles or by the cartilages that join the various bony units.

Consistently tipping the skull to front or back or to either side will change internal relationships and pressures in the nervous tissue. Blood, lymph, and spinal fluid will also be affected. It may be that in addition to the relatively simple mechanical factors, there are also magnetic force fields surrounding this great plexus, the patterns of which are disturbed by asymmetric physical flesh. This is not known at

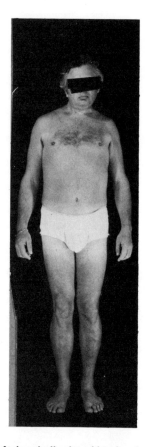

16-20 A chronically tipped head such as this one may result from many causes. Birth injury or genetic misendowment are the most likely if there is not obvious history of major physical accident. Some of this man's neck muscles are not resilient, are incapable of adjustment. To produce this picture, bony cervical structure must be seriously aberrated and incapable of movement. It is quite clear that at no time in the day or night, from one end of the year to another, is it possible for this man to reach equipoise with respect to his head. He is likely to be aware of deficiences in his special senses. But certainly, one could expect that the physical strain within his head and neck would express in his consciousness as emotional strain, a continual sense of depression and inadequacy, a permanent existence at the edge of emotional exhaustion. Can this physical distortion be remedied? To a certain extent, this man can be made more comfortable, physically and emotionally. If his problem is the result of a physical rather than a genetic accident, the outlook is more hopeful. In any event, the road will be long and the going rough.

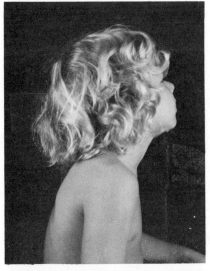 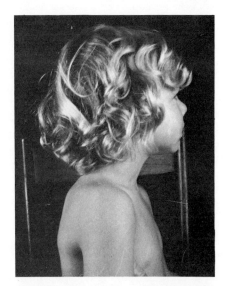

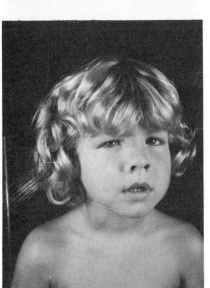 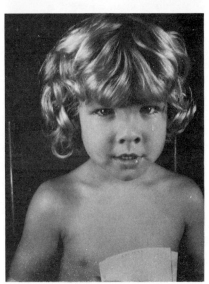

16-21 At a certain time in the Structural Integration of a human, it is necessary to concentrate time and effort on his head and neck. Specifically, the goal is to organize the cervical spine. In our method, this concentrated effort is unprofitable unless there have been six hours of work invested in aligning the body below. When the whole human has been prepared, the results are dramatic, as shown in these photographs. In this four-year-old, note particularly the change in the way the eyes look out of the head. The greater ease in the After 7 picture probably results from the change in the way the cranium sits on the atlas. In the Before picture, the rotation at this junction is very apparent. The pictures of the child were taken before and after the seventh hour of Structural Integration. (See also Centerfold 9 and 10)

the present time. It would seem a likely hypothesis, however, in that so many and so varied physiological functions are improved by establishing equipoise.

Vision is usually changed for the better following Structural Integration. The outward sign is a changed position of the eyes. Eyes looking out from a random body are seldom symmetrical; one eye may seem deeper in the skull or may be slightly higher than its mate. Usually, the position of the eyes calls attention to bony asymmetry of the face and/or head. The sphenoid bones seem peculiarly vulnerable; traumatic blows on the side of the jaw, infections in nasal structures, or inept dental mechanics may cause an altered facial expression. The onlooker tends to see such shifts as expressions of psychological personality. In fact, however, these changes are merely recording a slight shifting of the sphenoid.

The sphenoid articulates with many other facial and cranial bones—zygomatic, frontal, ethmoid, and mandible are among them. Many of these contribute to the orbit of the eye. A very minor displacement of the sphenoid will thus change these bony relationships and alter the setting and expression of the eye. All these bony units are held in place by muscles that, in relaxing, allow the attached bone to be more effective.

The orbit of the eye, which is pyramidal rather than spherical in shape, is only partially filled by the eyeball. Six muscles determine range and direction of the eye, four of them straight and two oblique. It is these muscles, together with fat and nutrient fluids, that fill the posterior orbit. This arrangement offers labile balance. The eye can express its well-being by very apparently projecting its attention to the outer world, thereby stimulating the chemistry and physics of the mechanism. Or it can dramatize its unhappiness by literally withdrawing to a greater depth and lessened mobility; this involves a change of chemistry as well as physics in a negative direction of apathy and lessened mobility. Understandably, persistence in the second behavior pattern shifts the psychic expression and functioning of the eye as well as its physical equipoise.

Glasses or any artificial aids to vision immobilize the eye, thus preventing exercise of the muscles controlling vision. This lack of physical exercise gives the starved, toneless appearance characteristic of eyes that always look through glasses. It is the reversal of this situation—the ceaseless focusing and refocusing of his eye, its continuous muscular movement—that gives the man really interested in the outer objective world his live, vibrant look, witness to his mind's activity. In the eye, as in all other parts of the body, movement translates into vital life; immobility shifts us toward the

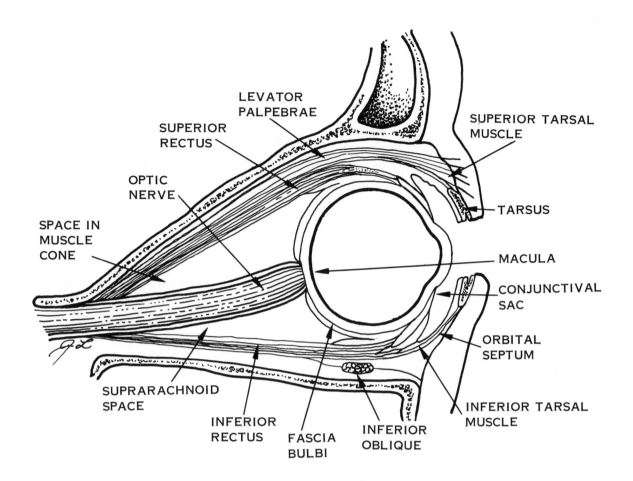

LEVATOR
PALPEBRAE

SUPERIOR
RECTUS

OPTIC
NERVE

SPACE IN
MUSCLE
CONE

SUPERIOR TARSAL
MUSCLE

TARSUS

MACULA

CONJUNCTIVAL
SAC

ORBITAL
SEPTUM

INFERIOR TARSAL
MUSCLE

SUPRARACHNOID
SPACE

INFERIOR
RECTUS

FASCIA
BULBI

INFERIOR
OBLIQUE

16-22 The isolated eyeball is composed of three concentric coats: an outer fibrous protective coat (sclera and corneal), a vascular middle coat supplying nutrition (choroid, ciliary, and iris), and an inner retinal coat. This latter is derived, like the lens of the eye, from the ectoderm. It is, therefore, nervous in origin and related to the brain itself.

Only the retina translates the impinging light into the nervous impulses that activate the appropriate areas of the brain. It is a continuation of the fibers of the optic nerve. Where the fibers spread out to form the inner layer of the retina, there is a small circular area (about 1.5 mm diameter) that cannot "see." This is the so-called blind spot.

Directly behind the cornea and lens is the "yellow spot," the macula lutea. This area of the retina "sees" sharply and precisely. Attempting to force any other area into precision "seeing" is structurally and functionally impossible. Some methods of eye training (the Bates and related systems) attain their excellent results by teaching the individual to use his eye in such a way that the light of the incoming image falls directly on the macula. He then enjoys the sharp acuity of effortless sight.

apathy that eventually becomes death.

Three other sensory systems are housed and protected within the head—those of hearing, smell, and taste. Of these, hearing is second only to vision in reporting his world to the individual. In its relation to communication, the ear has a function that the eye cannot challenge in importance. The ear participates in a two-way system—it hears the outgoing speech as well as the incoming sounds. This two-way communication system is the foundation of human culture.

There are three parts to the physical system of incoming hearing—the external, middle, and internal ear. The external ear is a cartilaginous shell (auricle or pinna) located outside the head and leading to the tubelike meatus, which penetrates the skull. The pinna seems designed to catch a great number of sound vibrations, concentrating and transmitting them to the inner ear. This function and its physical implementation are even more apparent in animals that depend on acute hearing for survival information. Evolutionists see the development of hearing as an important survival mechanism at the time when vertebrates emerged from water into a dark, cluttered environment of dense underbrush and short perspectives, where vision was a very limited asset. At that stage, hearing served them well. Today, under the impact of trucks and motorcycles, many of us wish we heard rather less. Some scientists think this wish may be granted in a few hundred years, for the general sense of hearing is steadily being impaired by the noise pollution in our environment.

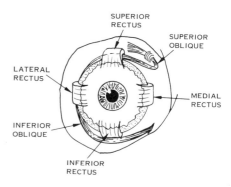

16-23 An anterior view of six eye muscles. For good sight, as we have said, the image must fall on the macula of the retina. To ensure this, the eyeball must be able to turn freely. Six muscles make movement of the eyeball possible around its vertical, horizontal, and sagittal axes: adductors and abductors turn the eye around its vertical axis, elevators and depressors around the horizontal, and rotators around the sagittal. There are, of course, other problems of mechanics. For example, myopia and presbyopia (near- and far-sightedness) and astigmatism are very common and involve more complicated mechanisms. Nevertheless, eyes that look straight forward, eyes that are on a horizontal line, eyes that are both on the same vertical plane (one eye not deeper than the other) spontaneously ease coronal strains arising from deeper levels. Muscular balances controlling vision are monitored by nerves at the third cervical vertebra and by the autonomic plexi lying along the side of the neck (upper, middle and lower cervical ganglia).

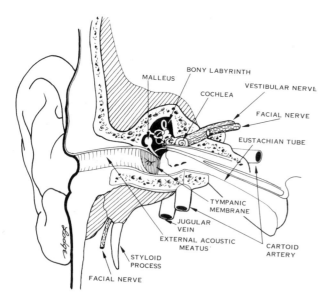

16-24 This is a schema of the deltrous portion of the temporal bone, which houses the organ of hearing, the inner ear. It also houses and protects the vestibular apparatus, which orients the individual within the gravitational field. Phylogenetically, the vestibular seems the older organ; in the simpler organisms (e.g., some fish), it is more important.

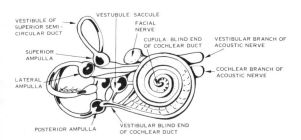

VESTIBULE OF
SUPERIOR SEMI-
CIRCULAR DUCT

VESTIBULE SACCULE
FACIAL
NERVE

SUPERIOR
AMPULLA

CUPULA: BLIND END
OF COCHLEAR DUCT

VESTIBULAR BRANCH OF
ACOUSTIC NERVE

COCHLEAR BRANCH OF
ACOUSTIC NERVE

LATERAL
AMPULLA

POSTERIOR AMPULLA

VESTIBULAR BLIND END
OF COCHLEAR DUCT

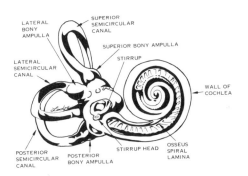

LATERAL
BONY
AMPULLA

SUPERIOR
SEMICIRCULAR
CANAL

SUPERIOR BONY AMPULLA

STIRRUP

LATERAL
SEMICIRCULAR
CANAL

WALL OF
COCHLEA

POSTERIOR
SEMICIRCULAR
CANAL

POSTERIOR
BONY AMPULLA

STIRRUP HEAD

OSSEUS
SPIRAL
LAMINA

16-25 The specific organ of hearing is the membranous labyrinth of the inner ear (top schema). The walls of its fluid-filled canals form the terminus of the fibers of the auditory (eighth cranial) nerve. It is here that the mechanical vibrations of ordinary sound are converted to the electrical currents characteristic of nerves. The disturbance that we call sound is here readied for transmission to the brain for registration and interpretation.

The delicate membranous organ is housed within a similarly shaped bony shell (schema at bottom). The resemblance of the bony labyrinth to a snail shell has given rise to its name — the cochlea. This chambered nautilus is attached to a vestibular apparatus, the semicircular canal, a unique mechanism telling us how we are placed in space, what our relation is to gravity. This biological gyroscope consists of three units placed at right angles to each other (superior, horizontal, and posterior semicircular canals). As in the labyrinth, a bony armor protects the membranous organ. The report that reaches our brain concerning our spatial position actually records fluid movement in the semicircular canal.

The middle ear, a small, bony, air-filled cavity, is separated from the external by the tympanic membrane, commonly called the eardrum. Three tiny bones, malleus, incus, and stirrup, bridge the middle ear from eardrum to oval windows. The malleus is attached to the tympanic membrane. The inner end of this bridge, the third ossicle (stirrup), closes the minute oval window, the very tiny entrance to the internal ear or labyrinth. This bony bridge transmits sound to the inner ear, where mechanical vibrations are transformed to wave impulses. Any thickening or hardening of the minute muscles controlling tension in the tympanic membrane or the ossicle will necessarily be reflected as lessened acuity in hearing.

The middle ear has a second important function: it maintains free passage for air from the cells that honeycomb the mastoid process of the temporal bone to the outer atmosphere. The connection is made through the pharyngotympanic (auditory) tube, which is often called the Eustachian tube in honor of the man who first described it in the sixteenth century. This open tube connects the middle ear directly with the pharyngeal cavity and more distantly with the nasal cavity and mouth. Thickening and thus partial or complete closure of this tube is one of the more common origins of the progressive loss of hearing in older humans. The maddening blocked feeling that sometimes accompanies a cold actually reports partial or total closure of the Eustachian tubes. Infection in the throat may cause a congestion that can spread to involve the Eustachian tubes, blocking the sense of lightness and acuity in hearing.

The smallest ossicle, the stirrup, fits the "oval window," a tiny aperture leading into the bony capsule of the inner ear. This houses the specific organ of hearing, the labyrinth, a complicated system of membranous canals filled with "inner fluid" (endolymph). Within its walls, the fibers of the acoustic (eighth cranial) nerve terminate. These fibers carry the auditory message to the brain itself, at this point no longer by mechanical conduction but by electrical transmission. In turn, the membranous structure is sheltered in a bony labyrinth of similar but simpler design. Because of its resemblance to a snail shell, it is called the cochlea. The delicate nerve structures are further guarded by bathing in a fluid medium, the "outer fluid" (perilymph). The whole organ lodges in the denser petrous portion of the temporal bone. It is rather surprising to find within this specialized organ, located in the depth of bone, both muscular structures and collagenous fibers. The very small tensor muscle controls the tone of the tympanic membrane; it favors high-pitched tones. The stirrup (or stapedial) muscle may act as the reciprocal of the tensor.

A second very important division of the inner ear is referred to as the vestibular apparatus. Its function is not that of hearing but of space orientation; it responds specifically to the forces of gravity. In terms of the long evolutionary history of living structures, the vestibular part of the ear seems to have preceeded the cochlear. In early fishes, only the vestibular part of the organ of hearing is represented. Apparently, it functioned to maintain appropriate balance of the fish in water.

All parts of the ear, superficial as well as deep, are connected via the acoustic, or eighth cranial, nerve with the brain (medulla oblongata and pons of the brain stem as well as some centers located higher in the brain). This is a relatively thick nerve; more than half of it serves the vestibular (equilibrium) apparatus. Estimates of the number of fibers in the nerve differ, but the average is about fifty thousand.

By contrast, the optic nerve seems to consist of more than a million fibers. This apparently reflects the difference in the demands made by modern man on his visual competence as compared with his auditory. The central auditory pathway ends near the Sylvian fossa; the surrounding cortical tissue serves a higher function of hearing—that of understanding the meaning of sounds heard and their relation to practical life. The function of memorizing—from telephone numbers to musical scores to Shakespeare—seems to have a definite location in this cortical area. The specificity of functional impairment when physical damage has been inflicted on this part of the brain supports such a hypothesis. A man is a psychospiritual being as well as a physical flesh-and-blood mechanism. The performance of his psychospiritual potential depends in large part on communication and hence on the physical integrity of the auditory tracts and their adnexa. In wider perspective, his psychospiritual behavior reflects the integrity of head and neck, which in turn involves the integrity of the whole body, the whole man. A vital index of his psychospiritual level is his ability to communicate with his fellow men; the entire social and intellectual culture of modern man rests on his ability to give and receive communications. The mechanism for this is housed in the upper segments of the head and neck.

It is worth noting that the most valued, most relied on of our sensory receptors, the eye, is a reporter only. It perceives and therefore reports only in straight lines, though these are almost limitless in length. The eye can see the far stars but cannot report what is going on around a corner or in the next room. In other words, the eye receives and reports electromagnetic waves of light that travel only in straight lines and can be totally obliterated by a very simple barrier.

266

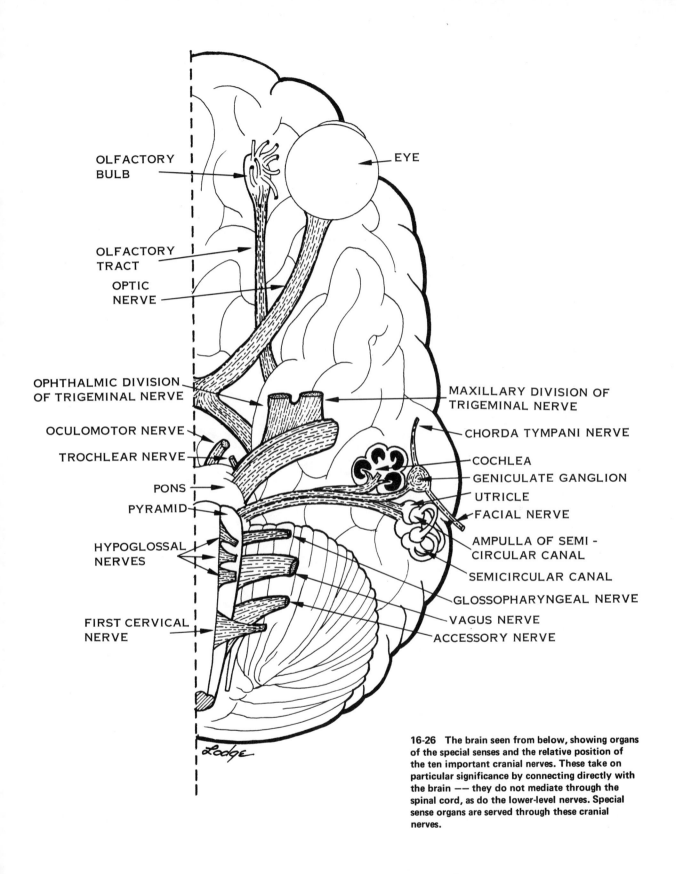

OLFACTORY BULB

EYE

OLFACTORY TRACT

OPTIC NERVE

OPHTHALMIC DIVISION OF TRIGEMINAL NERVE

MAXILLARY DIVISION OF TRIGEMINAL NERVE

OCULOMOTOR NERVE

CHORDA TYMPANI NERVE

TROCHLEAR NERVE

COCHLEA

GENICULATE GANGLION

PONS

UTRICLE

PYRAMID

FACIAL NERVE

HYPOGLOSSAL NERVES

AMPULLA OF SEMI - CIRCULAR CANAL

SEMICIRCULAR CANAL

GLOSSOPHARYNGEAL NERVE

FIRST CERVICAL NERVE

VAGUS NERVE

ACCESSORY NERVE

Lodge

16-26 The brain seen from below, showing organs of the special senses and the relative position of the ten important cranial nerves. These take on particular significance by connecting directly with the brain —— they do not mediate through the spinal cord, as do the lower-level nerves. Special sense organs are served through these cranial nerves.

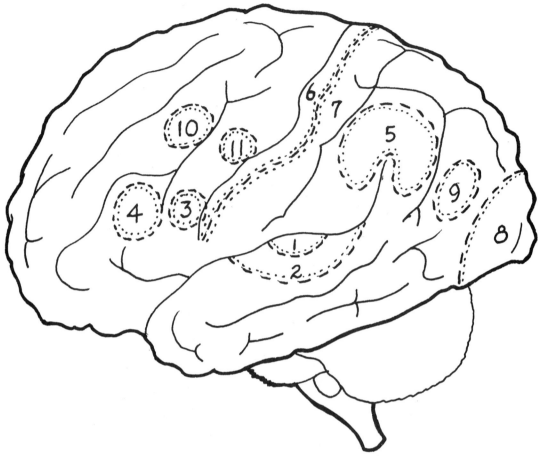

16-27 Lateral view of the brain. Physiological research has shown specific areas of the brain to be associated with particular functions. Some evidence of this has been accumulated by observing functional impairment resulting from localized physical damage, tumors, etc., some by electrical stimulation of specific brain areas and observation of response. Key: 1. Acoustic 2. Acoustic association 3. Motor speech 4. Motor control of larnyx 5. Sensory 6. Sensory association 7. Correlation 8. Visual association 9. Reading center 10. Writing center 11. Motor control of hand.

1. ACOUSTIC

2. ACOUSTIC ASSOCIATION

3. MOTOR SPEECH

4. MOTOR CONTROL OF LARYNX

5. SENSORY

6. SENSORY ASSOCIATION

7. CORRELATION

8. VISUAL ASSOCIATION

9. READING CENTER

10. WRITING CENTER

11. MOTOR CONTROL OF HAND

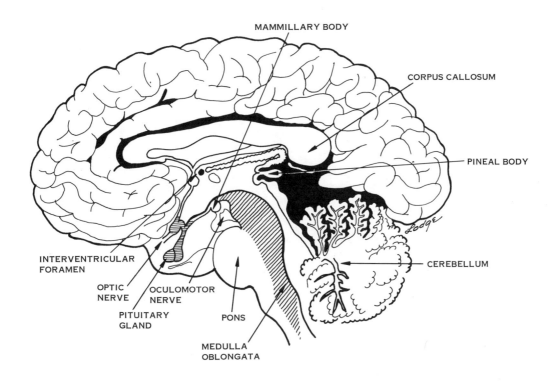

MAMMILLARY BODY

CORPUS CALLOSUM

PINEAL BODY

CEREBELLUM

INTERVENTRICULAR FORAMEN

OPTIC NERVE

OCULOMOTOR NERVE

PITUITARY GLAND

PONS

MEDULLA OBLONGATA

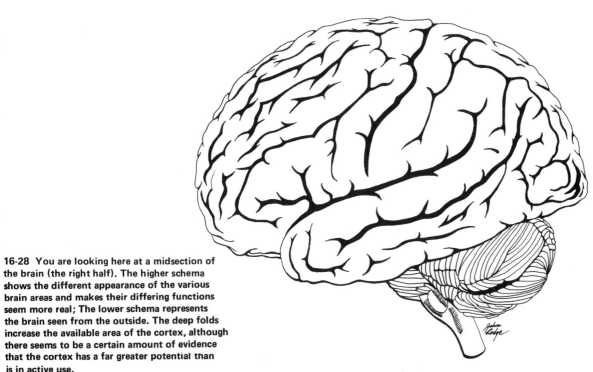

16-28 You are looking here at a midsection of the brain (the right half). The higher schema shows the different appearance of the various brain areas and makes their differing functions seem more real; The lower schema represents the brain seen from the outside. The deep folds increase the available area of the cortex, although there seems to be a certain amount of evidence that the cortex has a far greater potential than is in active use.

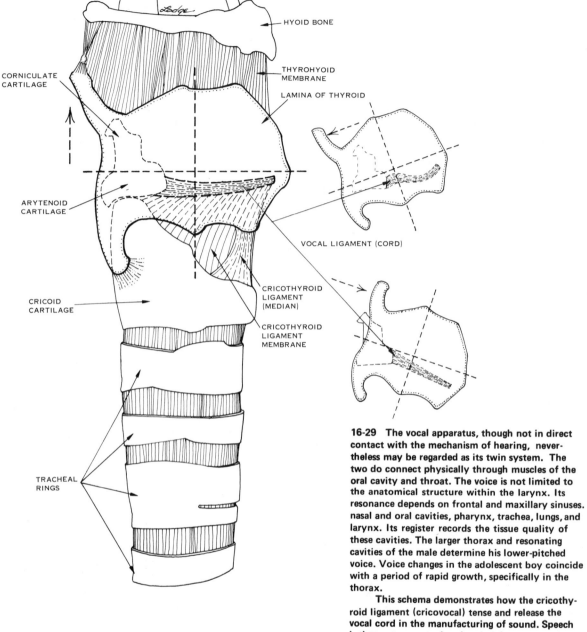

LESSER HORN
OF HYOID BONE

HYOID BONE

CORNICULATE
CARTILAGE

THYROHYOID
MEMBRANE

LAMINA OF THYROID

ARYTENOID
CARTILAGE

VOCAL LIGAMENT (CORD)

CRICOID
CARTILAGE

CRICOTHYROID
LIGAMENT
(MEDIAN)

CRICOTHYROID
LIGAMENT
MEMBRANE

TRACHEAL
RINGS

16-29 The vocal apparatus, though not in direct
contact with the mechanism of hearing, nevertheless may be regarded as its twin system. The
two do connect physically through muscles of the
oral cavity and throat. The voice is not limited to
the anatomical structure within the larynx. Its
resonance depends on frontal and maxillary sinuses.
nasal and oral cavities, pharynx, trachea, lungs, and
larynx. Its register records the tissue quality of
these cavities. The larger thorax and resonating
cavities of the male determine his lower-pitched
voice. Voice changes in the adolescent boy coincide
with a period of rapid growth, specifically in the
thorax.

This schema demonstrates how the cricothyroid ligament (cricovocal) tense and release the
vocal cord in the manufacturing of sound. Speech
is the motor expression, hearing the sensory receptor of communication —— the psychospiritual
function of humans. Well-being in both halves of
this system depends on the tone of local myofascial tissue. Functional improvement of both units
through balancing is noteworthy. As the head approaches an equipoise through integration, marked
vocal changes become apparent. The timbre of the
voice alters, as does the range. This can be understood as change in myofascial restrictions. Usually
a woman's voice extends its range a third of an oc-
tave upward, a man's by a third downward.

Light does not rely on a dense medium (air, for example) for transmission. The ear, on the other hand, reports only occurrences close at hand—a few inches, a few feet, even a few miles. Vibrations that transmit sound travel by way of material media—air, water, etc.—and each vibrating three-dimensional particle becomes a secondary source of disturbance in all directions. Thus sound, in contradistinction to light, does carry its message around corners, and a very different type of barrier is needed to block it. In contributing to two-way communication, hearing with its expressive counterpart, speech, has another great advantage over sight, which has no such counterpart. Only on rare occasions does the eye itself convey outgoing information to another individual, and then only unreliably, seemingly by psychic rather than visual means.

Our cultural pattern calls for a two-way communication system, a sender as well as a receiver, an expressor as well as a receptor. The ear is the receptor, one-half of its own two-way system. Its twin is speech, a motor expression activated by the speech centers of the brain. The mechanism of speech depends on the integrity of neighboring systems —alimentary and respiratory—to implement and express the nervous message.

The basic organ of speech is the larynx, a modification of the upper end of the trachea (windpipe). The larynx uses the principle of a pipe organ to produce sound. A slit, or cleft (the rima glottidis), is set into vibration by air ejected from the lungs, which here function as bellows. The elastic edges of the slit, the so-called vocal cords, are under the control of laryngeal muscles. Interaction of the vocal cords with ejected air determines pitch and intensity of emitted sound. This vibrating air then passes through the resonating chamber of mouth or nose and is further modified by tongue, palate, and lips. Since the size and shape of all these structures is a function of myofascia in the oral cavity, pharynx, and chest, it is axiomatic that a man's voice and speech will offer unmistakable clues to his over-all well-being. The infinite variation of voice and accent depends on oral and pharyngeal muscles, some of which are absent in less vocal animals. The voice also conveys information about the state of the middle ear (Eustachean tube). Hearing and speech are structurally closely linked.

In integrating total structure, alignment of the head, neck, and thorax determines the upper pole of our physical man. In most random bodies, the head compensates lower-lying aberrations by being carried too far forward. Vital re-creation of physical man into a more psychospiritually oriented being demands verticality, that is, it demands equipoise in the "home" position of the head. Anteriority of head and neck can be chronic only if cervical prevertebral flexors are hypertoned with respect to their extensors. These hypertoned flexors—by definition, they lie anterior to the spine—include all facial muscles (oral and nasal) as well as the prevertebral cervicals.

It is easy to overlook one salient fact: the floor of the mouth, its roof, as well as the flesh constituting postnasal linings and pharynx are all structured from latticed muscle. Through the medium of this lattice, they attach directly or indirectly to the spine. Chronically anterior cervical spines are always accompanied by modified facial conformation. Compensations in the neck will show on the face. In turn, myofascial structures inside oral and nasal cavities must be brought toward equipoise before the cervical spine can take its appropriate position.

The cervical spine as upper pole has a special significance. This is understood in its relation to pain or any malaise. If the individual is reporting misery to himself from anywhere in the body, tension and distortion will be apparent in the cervical spine and in turn will be reflected in facial muscles. We say, "John is not looking well today." John's problem may well be a shoe that is too tight. Face and head are the primary reflectors of thought and emotion. These, too, may have their habitual and permanent effect on structure. We have spoken of the relation of lumbar and cervical spine; facial as well as lumbar muscles are related to the cervical spine and determine its "home" position and consequently its competent function.

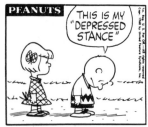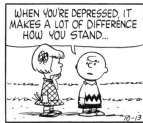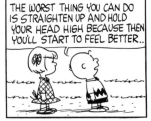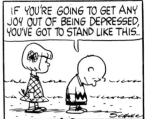

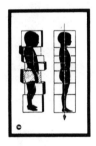

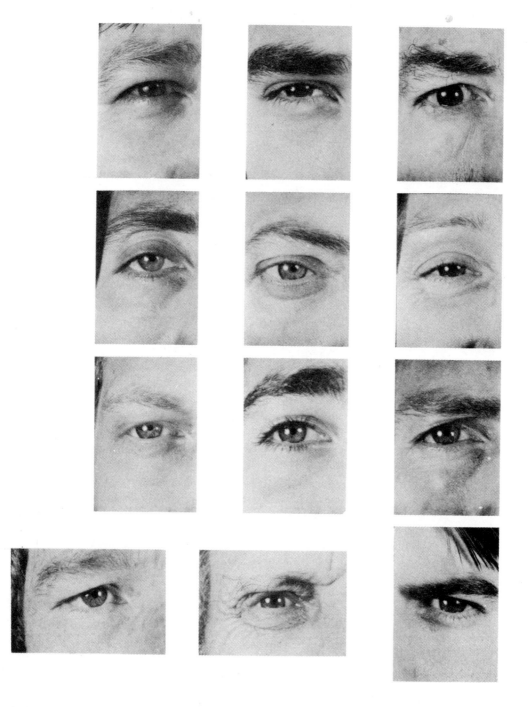

17-1 These pictures show clearly that what our forebears called the "windows of the soul" referred not to the eye itself but to its myofascial framework. They are further evidence of the fashion in which consistent emotional set determines myofascial organization and, in turn, is determined by it. These are not photographs of people under stress; they were taken in a casual, relaxed setting.

17
Many People Refer to This Drama as Pain

"Does that hurt?" ask people who are looking at the profound changes that occur in a demonstration of the first hours of Integration. There are several answers. The first is, "That depends." It depends on you and your attitudes toward pain. It depends on whether the area in question is in serious trouble. In our sense, does it deviate widely from normal (in our sense) tone and position? An "area" hurts in direct relation to its degree of aberration. This means that every human undergoing Integration is aware of and reports his change differently. The answers to another pair of questions should give you greater understanding: What do you mean by pain? What is your attitude toward change?

Humans resist change. Somewhere deep down, they feel that somehow they have "made it" under existing circumstances. What assurance do they have that they'll continue to "make it" given a different set of circumstances? Conservatism, the tendency to maintain and protect the status quo, to avoid the unknown, to avoid change, is universal. It can be seen throughout the animal kingdom. In attempting to label our more superficial conservatisms, we call them habit patterns. Spontaneous movement feeds back the muscular pattern that is easiest. This becomes the "habit," the index of the least effort.

There is no painful experience apart from the motor intent to withdraw from the experience.* The desire for self-preservation, inertia, resistance to change are understandable and predictable. The experience of change to the average man often manifests itself as "pain."**

Sophisticated people recognize that the word *pain* covers a variety of phenomena. Moderns, verbalizing their own

*J. Silverman, 1972, unpublished manuscript.
**An excellent technical review of modern theories of pain and their implications is to be found in J. A. Downey and R. C. Darling, eds., *Physiological Basis of Rehabilitation Medicine* (Phila.: Saunders, 1971), Ch. 19.

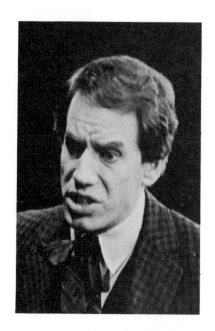
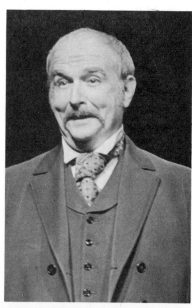
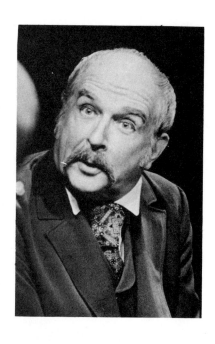
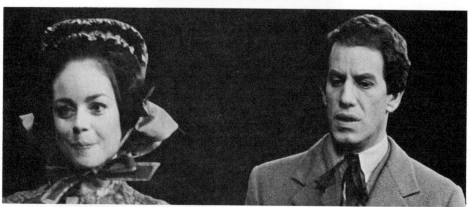
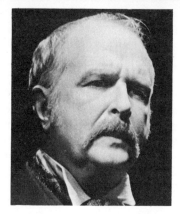
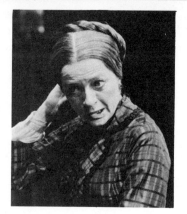

17-2 (Photos by George Connolly)

276

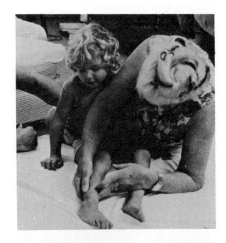

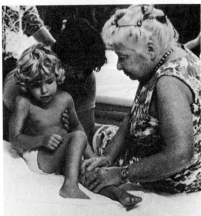

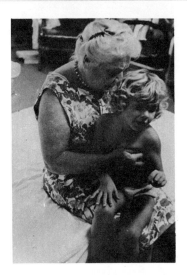

17-3 Pain? What pain?

These three photographs of Toby in the course of processing are one answer to the people who say, " I hear that Structural Integration hurts."

pain, more often than not are describing a response to something going on in their emotional world. They are apt to call any of their negative responses, even a mere report of change, "pain." This "mental" pain can be very intense; it may even initiate significant physiological change. A negative emotional shock can be severe enough to knock out normal physiological functioning, causing loss of consciousness or even death.

The apparent mechanism of response to psychic shock is often myofascial, a neglected fact of life. A soldier who is exposed to the grim reality of battle all too often responds by vomiting—a muscular response dramatizing emotional rejection. Even a child who finds something bitter on his tongue responds by myofascial rejection, expressed through his muscular facial pattern or even ejection. This is the healthy organismic response to unacceptable experience. Deviation from this is part of the toxic pattern of neurosis. Feldenkrais expresses this succinctly: "Force that is not converted into movement does not simply disappear, but is dissipated into damage done to joints, muscles, and other sections of the body."*

The medium through which the individual communicates and influences his outside world is myofascial. Involved in a compelling emotional rejection pattern, his safe and speedy escape is dependent on the resilience of these systems. A man whose myofascial components are in reasonable balance is able to recover emotional equilibrium thanks to this physical elasticity. A man at the edge of physical balance has no margin of safety on which to rely. The average human is not really interested in the verbal abstraction "equipoise"; he *is* vitally concerned in lessening his pain. What he calls pain is usually a perception of his own emotional level. Watching the world around us, especially the facial expressions and behavior of our young people, one sees that the general emotional level seems consistently negative. (There is only one continuum of emotional level, positive-negative; other descriptions and evaluations of feeling states can be seen as points of reference along this spectrum.) All too many people live in a state of this kind of chronic pain, in chronic negative withdrawal.

We may well ask what they are perceiving. What is this pain? What is this bit of awareness that we name a "man" perceiving about the processes going on inside his skin? Pain is inside the skin. It is neither in the sky nor the earth, it is in the man. It must be within his own envelope; no other localization is possible. For an answer, we look to the vital, living substance. Immediately, not one but many clues appear.

*M. Feldenkrais, *Awareness through Movement,* (N.Y.: Harper & Row, 1972), p. 58.

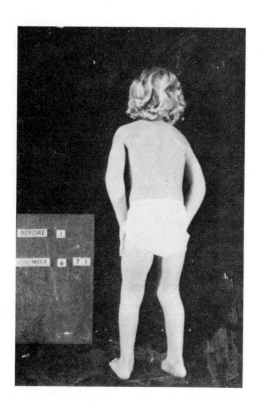

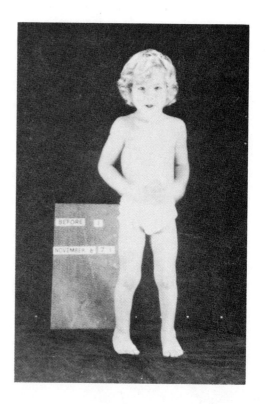

17-4 These pictures of Toby, taken routinely during processing, record the erasure of the psychological pain of a sick child that comes along with the improvement of his physical problem. This four-year-old boy, as we see him before processing, has an extreme pelvic rotation. As a result, he is unable to keep his feet flat on the floor. He runs continuously rather than walks, because in the act of running, he is able to balance on his toes, the only part of his foot that he can control. To us, at this point, the most striking aspect of this child is the emotional pain to be seen in his face. His progression under eight hours of Structural Integration is shown in these pictures. Most significant of all are the photos shown earlier in Chapter Sixteen, depicting what happened to this child in the seventh hour of processing, the hour in which head and neck are balanced above a balanced body. We repeat these photographs here to complete the record.

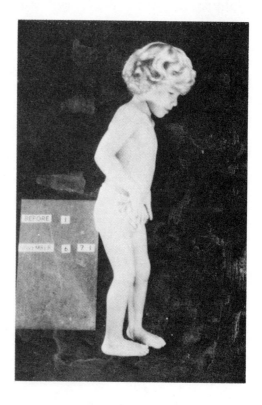

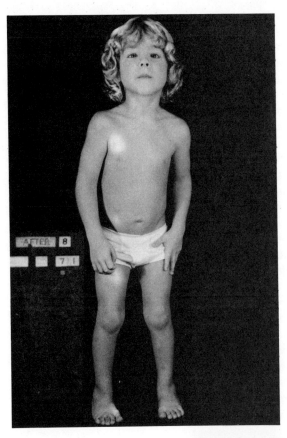
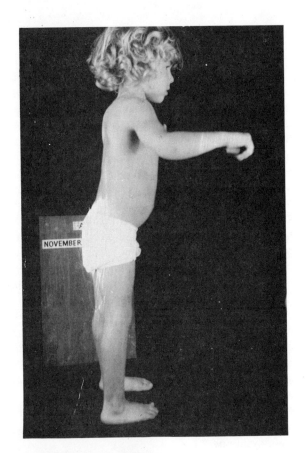
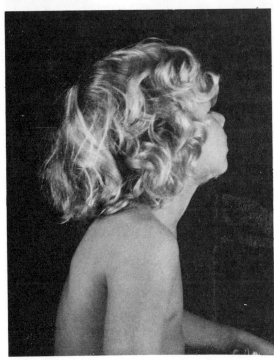

279

First is the surprising discovery that so-called emotion reflects physical material balance or imbalance. Even from the outside, we can perceive that negative response immediately precipitates movement away from myofascial balance, myofascial ease. Visually, it is apparent that one of the most immediate responses to negative emotion is hypertonicity in myofascial flexors. Consequently, a man starting from a seriously distorted physical balance is less able than his more balanced brother to accommodate this movement and recover from emotional shock. We are likely to term the second man more relaxed. Quite obviously, the word *relaxed* here describes a body in a relative myofascial equipoise, where physiological flexors and extensors are not chronically blocked. In a different idiom, this body can recover more immediately from "shocked" glandular function and its myofascial concomitants. An observer becomes aware that any man in an emotional crisis, responding to the emotion he thinks is driving him, is really reacting to chemical and physiological changes inside his skin. At this level, psychology is not the primal force; its place has been taken by physiology. Certainly, this displacement has not banished psychology to an outer darkness, only to a deeper level. This tends to unravel the confusion enclosed in the word *psychology,* which in the lay mind is asked to cover everything from behaviorism to motivation. We emphasize here once again that behavior is usually chemistry, is usually physiology.

At the level of everyday problems, balancing and stabilizing emotion can be immeasurably furthered by any system able to create or restore vital physiological response. Although psychological hang-ups occur, they are maintained only to the extent that free physiological response is impaired at the glandular, visceral, myofascial, and other levels. Restoration of function can be initiated from many levels, but establishment of myofascial equipoise is one of the most obvious, one of the speediest, one of the most powerful of these. To the extent (and at the speed) that restoration of physiological flow occurs, the individual is less "hung up."

All of this, however, is an exploration of "change" and of what "change" is in the experience of a human being. As we have said, humans tend to resist change. They verbalize their resistance as pain, emotional or physical. All too often their emotional pain—their depression, their grief, even their anger—is a perception of physiological imbalance, an awareness of chemical lacks or overloads in blood and tissue. These may be at macro- or micro-levels, down to and including the cellular.

The emotional, affective reflection of this imbalance

—negativity, withdrawal, destructiveness—may be thought of as the façade of pain in the human condition. There is a further dimension to pain, that of the sensory apparatus, which is apparently more precise and more susceptible to scientific exploration and evaluation. But in our belief, the habit of thinking in terms of two dimensions—emotional and sensory—has given rise to a consistent semantic confusion which shows little sign of lessening. In the sensory dimension, specific nerves have commonly been considered the basic element in physical discomfort, reporting directly to the brain. This process evokes in the body chemical change that enters the individual's awareness in the guise of negative emotion—pain. The sensation of discomfort then has a negative emotional component, which pre-empts and drains the vitality of the individual. The man who operates in a narrow margin of chemical safety is rapidly exhausted by such bombardment.

It has long been thought that pain as sensation travels along definite nervous pathways. In this sense, it resembles sight, hearing, and touch; to this extent, it is sensory and presumably is transmitted from sensory to receptor endings just under the skin. Two types of fibers, sheathed and unsheathed, are apparently involved in transmission. Sheathed, or myelinated, fibers transmit very rapidly (100 meters per second), and their activation is felt as "sharp, bright" pain. These are divided into two types; the thicker A fibers and the thinner B fibers. The unmyelinated C fibers are much smaller in dimension and conduct impulses of low amplitude at a rate of about one meter per second.* There has been speculation that these large and small fiber systems have opposite roles. Both A and C fibers transmit through the spinal cord to the thalamus. This seems to act as a relay station, distributing information to various cortical and subcortical levels of the brain. As in other sensory systems, these signals are interpreted in the cortex.

Such straight-through transmission from peripheral receptor to pain center in the brain was the accepted map of pain as late as the middle of the twentieth century. It is known as the specificity theory. Many contradictions challenged it and have caused re-examination of its underlying premises. The decade 1950 to 1960 produced evidence that there were, in fact, very few high-threshold (A) fibers, and

*W. K. Livingston, "What Is Pain?" *Scientific American*, vol. 88, no. 59 (1953), p. 63.

there was no evidence that they always produced pain.* As early as the turn of the century, Charles Scott Sherrington, a master physiologist, defined pain as a "psychical process." Today, more than half a century later, in spite of sophisticated measuring devices, we do not know at what point in the chain of events the physiological process of nerve transmission becomes "psychical."

Physicians as well as psychologists know that pain is modified by the interpretation given to it. What we perceive is not to be equated with reality. The stimulus carried to the brain by individual nerves is "real." The psychical perception of this is a summation of past experiences. A five-year-old boy, lacking experience, may or may not know what his stomachache portends. Cultural assumptions ("pain is warning"), acceptance or rejection of pain, parental attitudes ("Oh, let's get on with it—that little pain is nothing") affect our five-year-old's perception and understanding.

Pain is rarely, if ever, devoid of emotional coloring. Its intensity is all too often dictated by anxiety and related variables. Any theory of pain, to be adequate, must be broad enough to take these variables into consideration. In response to this necessity, modern ideas about pain have advanced. A "pattern theory" postulates that pain impulses are produced by intense stimulation of nonspecific receptors—that there are neither specific fibers nor specific endings for pain. Such an assumption permits the inclusion of Pavlov's classical observations. This investigator subjected dogs to electrical shocks, burns, and cuts, but consistently followed such tissue insult with the presentation of food. Presently, these stimuli were accepted by the animals as a call to food. At this point, the dogs responded with no evidence of pain or withdrawal.

Pain is now generally regarded as a central summation of impulses. Physiologists tend to accept the idea of an input-control mechanism preventing its too great intensity. This mechanism, called by its postulator, R. Melzak, a gate-control system,* has to do with the working relationship of large and small fibers. According to this theory, attention, memory, and emotions monitor sensory input at various levels of the nervous apparatus and alter psychological perception.

The word *pain,* according to Melzak and Wall, is a linguistic label for a rich mixture of experiences and responses. In

*R. Melzack and P. D. Wall, "Pain Mechanisms, a New Theory," *Science,* vol. 150, no. 3699 (1965), p. 972.

*R. Melzak and P. D. Wall, *op. cit.*

Structural Integration we see something of this variety of response and the confusion with which it enters the individual's awareness. It could hardly be expected that the profound tissue changes documented in our photographs (changes in position, changes in tone) could be accomplished without a dramatic report by the tissue to the central awareness we call the man. Many people refer to this drama as pain. Even they are quick to acknowledge, however, that it differs from what they ordinarily call pain—an aching tooth, a bruise, a cut.

Structural Integration involves fascial change. The pain of fascial change is transitory; the minute the pressure is removed, the "pain" is gone. In a majority of people, the quality of the drama changes abruptly and surprisingly into a feeling of physical lightness and joyousness. This is entirely different from the residual "pain" following hurt or damage of some sort. The sensation following nervous bombardment in a headache, for example, is one of exhaustion ("I'll be better after a good night's sleep"). The sensation following fascial integration has none of this quality. It is a "high," a sense of great well-being enveloping the individual totally. The first part of physical integration is felt by the individual as an unknown change; it therefore turns on his anxiety. Change, he remembers subconsciously, is something he resists at all costs. He withdraws, and naturally he names this intense experience "pain." But is it?

Noordenbos, a Dutch authority, defined pain as the label we place on sensation when a rigid system is bombarded by an excessive burden of stimuli with which it cannot cope because of the nature of its rigidity. "Pain is experienced when stimuli, whatever their nature, exceed certain limits. Is it not therefore quantitative and might it not simply be stated that *pain is too much*?"*

Thus we see that any evaluation of a human as a whole requires an understanding of psychophysical response, the rich sensational fabric through which a man perceives his world and the interrelation of psyche and soma. We need to understand their expressions and their interplay. An earlier generation used a psychological orientation. "Faith" was their wonder-worker for spiritual and physical serenity. A modern point of view claims that knowledge can relieve much of the burden once put on faith.

For us, it is less necessary now that faith be available to relieve pain. Pain can be relieved by rendering the system resilient, as Noordenbos points out. This is a proper goal for Structural Integration.

*W. Noordenbos, *Pain* (Amsterdam: Elsevier Publishing Co., 1959), p. 176.

18
Evolution Is the Expression of Internal Events

Our personal evolutionary potential lies within us. Originally, this was the message of mystics and occultists. At this point, it is being documented in the changes brought about by Structural Integration. The practitioner of Structural Integration separates the confusion of random fascial structure and re-relates it around a vertical line with new appropriateness. The result is a spectrum of subjective experiences that throw light on conceptual formulations of earlier cultural ideas. The latter, in turn, offer additional keys to understanding our results.

The physical science of mechanics, in its description of space and material; the chemistry of mesodermal derivatives; the influence of gravity and heliotropic factors on living organisms; the insights of yoga and other ancient methods for physical fitness in theory and practice all throw light on the changes we have observed and documented. Our ability to create these changes predictably and reliably and, by measuring, to validate them widens the scope of the word *evolution*. Evolution is matter moving toward more effective order; in the words of Herbert Spenser, "*Evolution is an Integration of matter and concomitant disposition of motion; during which the matter passes from an indefinite, incoherent homogeneity to a definite, coherent heterogeneity; and during which the related motion undergoes a parallel transformation.*"*

Every mature human has developed from three embryological germ layers: entoderm, ectoderm, and mesoderm. Ideally, these three basic cell types integrate and balance, making possible functional wholeness in the

*As quoted in the definition of *evolution* in the *Oxford English Dictionary* (Oxford: Oxford University Press, 1970), p. 911.

adult human. Clearly disparate in the embryo, they remain differentiated (although not separated) in the adult. Physiological systems deriving from two—entoderm and ectoderm—have been extensively investigated by modern science, but the role of systems proliferating from the mesoderm (bone, blood, and myofascial structures), which contribute to and support their two sister systems, has been less thoroughly explored. In seeking to document the human's functional response to the great energy field in which he lives—gravity—we have found ourselves consistently involved with mesodermal derivatives, particularly in terms of their capacity to register and make structural alterations in response to stress. The potent, all too influential energy envelope of the earth—its gravitational field —although subliminal to man's cerebral consciousness, controls and directs him in its effect on his fascial component (derived from mesoderm). In turn, through controlling and directing his use of this derivative of mesoderm, his fascial system, man is able to use gravitational energy to his advantage.

As practitioners of Structural Integration, we not merely infer but literally see the disorganization of myofascial components in random humans. We can deliberately create a higher degree of myofascial order; as we see it, the implication of this is that however important derivatives of entoderm and ectoderm may be to man's over-all function, the key to his integrity in three-dimensional space lies in the disposition and tone of his collagen tissues, his myofascia. Improved spatial organization has astonishingly wide ramifications in physiological behavior, therefore in psychological behavior as well. Further, it seems that changing any one of the derivatives of a germ-layer affects the whole set: a change in the myofascia affects blood and bone as well, at a different rate.

Humans report the changed awareness induced by Structural Integration with the words "This is different; I feel better." "Better" seems to refer to their subjective sense of a greater vital energy. In point of fact, "better" is the man's feeling-report of a change in relations between his structural element (fascia) and the gravity field. This is the "something new" that has been added—new support for viscera and nervous structures, an improved chemistry. We can speculate that the apparent increase in energy is the feeling-perception of this greater sturdiness that *up*lifts within the gravity field. The disintegrative entropic factor, the *mis*use of gravity resulting from fascial distortions, has been lessened.

The upward development of living organisms is subject to a variety of influences. A seed planted in the earth develops upward apparently in response to an antigravity factor. While a specific heliotropic light factor is also necessary to its chemical maturing, the young plant will try to grow upward even when kept in darkness. In the plant, deprivation of either factor—light or the opportunity for upright stance (gravitational organization)—causes loss of pattern and consequent deterioration. This is equally true of humans; they become less "human"—because less organized—if deprived of either light or the opportunity for upright stance.

His vertical extension relates a man to two separate energies, the energy of the sun and that of gravity, supplying two separate body needs. Bodies "feed" on energy; there are many and varied sources of this basic "food." Exposure to the energy of sunlight demonstrably changes chemical constituents of blood and cells; exposure to the positive effects of gravity (when the vertical is freed and unblocked) changes fluid flow (and thus chemistry) in myofascia and in mesodermal tissue throughout the body. Convincing demonstrations of these hypotheses can be validated only in the idiom and parameters of science. A promising start has been made in this direction. Technical papers offering validation from several viewpoints have been published.*

Man thinks linearly, one thing at a time, but experiences multidimensionally. Philosophically speaking, reality seems unitary and may be delineated in a façade of objective scientific parameters. Its subjective dimension, though less ordered, is equally compelling. In this late twentieth century, the latter even seems the more important to many people. The words "I feel" are pervasive in a way unknown or suppressed in the earlier days of this century. Psychotherapy and the hope it has generated as a universal explanation account for this about-face. Ironically, this situation has changed the emphasis; it has legitimized what Fritz Perls called the "blaming game." What, then, has become of the elegant wholeness of monism, originated by the Aryans and stated in its most superficial terms by the Romans: as "a sound mind in a sound body"? The true dimension and harmony of monism, as well as its apparent boundaries, can be explored as the more orderly physical body offered by Structural Integration emerges. One of the probable causes for the eclipse of monism is no doubt the recognition that it is not precise. There is no exact equivalence between body and psyche; a true one-to-one correspondence cannot be clearly delineated.

*Julian Silverman, Ph.D. and Ida P. Rolf, Ph.D., two papers in *Confinia Psychiatrica* 16:69-79 1973. Julian Silverman, Ph.D. and Valerie Hunt, Ph.D., three untitled papers, to be published.

Ancient Hindu cultures nurtured and tried to exploit monism through yoga techniques. Gatustha yoga (called by moderns hatha yoga) was a system of training that aimed at developing order in the body through freeing joints and thereby encouraging more extensive movement. It is noteworthy that the physical techniques of yoga were not indulged in merely for their own sake or for exercise. Their practice, together with the control of breath, was a means of stimulating the nervous-emotional system in such a way that, among other changes in consciousness, the phenomenon called Kundalini could be evoked. Development of this kind of energy, especially through breath control, brings out another aspect of human personality, normally latent in our time—the psychic. All too often, people who are predominantly interested in their psychic development fail to realize that psychic awareness is best grounded in and supported by a physical body whose sensitivity and sturdiness allow psychic events to occur naturally and with adequate support. The stable structure afforded by an adequate mesodermal system has a much more important role in the channeling of psychic energies than is usually recognized.

Yoga practice recognized this; their development of the individual person was many-sided. Even though the psychic man was the goal of yoga, the physical, material manifestation (body) was included in the ancient schedule. Many yoga schools (earlier equivalents of our human-potential movement) saw this in social as well as personal terms. These teachers recognized that increasing orderliness in the physical body somehow fostered order in the psychological personality. They realized that a true social morality is in general the behavioral expression of people with well-ordered, vital bodies. They saw and took into account that the moral deviants, the thieves, and the criminals were often characterized by bodies lacking in order, in balance and pattern, in energy. Such insights were used in fostering their caste system.

These yoga teachers saw clearly that as people attained the order understood in the yoga body pattern, they were more apt to express themselves in organized (what moderns call *moral*) behavior. The natural expression of physically effective personalities came to be recognized as "good." In fact, they went further, defining as good and acceptable any action that gave rise to enhanced physiological functioning. Emotion (guilt, fear, excessive grief, etc.) that interfered with physiological good function, that slowed blood pressure, that depressed circulation and/or hormonal secretions, automatically became "bad," undesirable, "negative." The yardstick for moral judgment was thus physiol-

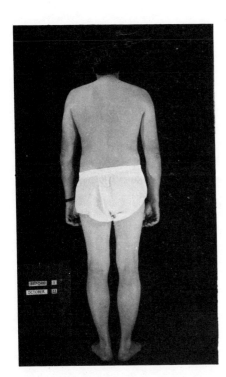

18-1 We repeat here one of the many examples of deviation from the structural vertical in this book. The muscular pattern in the shoulder girdle shows scapulae that have wandered too far from the spine. This favors the downward randomizing entropic disintegration brought on by misuse of gravity. The upward thrust of the antigravity evolutionary vertical has been lost.

When too far lateral, too distant from the antigravity potential of the extensors of the spine, scapulae exert a downward and/or rotational pull on the spine, as can be seen. This effect then may be exaggerated by weight and directional pull from the arms. (In accordance with the elementary law of levers, rotational pull exerted by a weight farther from a fulcrum will be greater in its effect than that of the same weight acting from a nearer point.) Thus the weight of an arm that is too far lateral has an inordinate advantage in disorganizing and randomizing the structures to which it relates. This principle may be seen at work not only in shoulder-arm structures, but also in the lower limb and pelvis.

ogy. These early monists understood that their internal emotional lives reflected physiological balances. In later cultures, as multiplicity has superseded monism, the man-as-a-whole has been forgotten. We have lost this sweet simplicity. It may be that, although it was in the right direction, the pure monistic explanation was too simple.

Why is yoga not a perfect answer for the modern seeker? Although probably the best of the "exercise" systems, yoga as taught today does not go far enough. The body organized through yoga achieves joint mobility but does not consciously recognize and seek out the gravity field as its basic supportive factor. It does not and cannot achieve a true vertical relationship. Photographs in any book showing yoga patterns will illustrate this. As a system of exercises, gatustha (hatha) yoga was a vast improvement over others available at the time of its inception. It is still a superior system of individual development, but it is not a "final revelation." Revelation in any case has never been final, a closed system.

True verticality, the goal of Structural Integration, is more than a figment of the imagination. Indeed, it is very real; it is a functional phenomenon, a line around which the body's energy force fields balance. Again, these energy forces are not abstract; they manifest in real myofascial material structures. Through its vertical stance, the organism is no longer earth-bound; the vertical expresses an energy relation between earth and sun. In its own way, the vegetative world also glorifies the polarized vertical; its upward striving is material evidence of vital polarity. Whenever life differentiates toward a greater, more complex degree of order, the upward thrust becomes more apparent and more significant. As order evolves, a gravity/antigravity structural organization defines itself, and this basic polarity, rooted in the earth, expresses in terms of vertical lift.

A. Drucker* discusses the effects of this on humans from the viewpoint of the physicist. He points out that deviations from symmetrical form distort the living structural vertical. A specific example of this appears in Fig. 18-1. Such mechanical considerations offer significant clues to the mechanisms by which randomizing entropic forces distort the body. Drucker takes these considerations a step further, showing that they imply a difference between biological and chronological time. These are not equivalent in their effect, nor do they necessarily manifest similarly in different humans. Biological time reflects and summarizes the randomizing forces that have distorted organic structures and organic symmetries past their limits of elasticity, hence

*A. Drucker, unpublished manuscript, 1973.

permanently. (It must be remembered here that the word "symmetry" refers to structure in three dimensions of space rather than two. Thus there is a lateral symmetry, an anterior-posterior symmetry, an upper-lower symmetry. Additionally, and most important of all in humans—systems which are vertically organized and move in space—there is the intrinsic-extrinsic symmetry which is concerned with the relations between deep and superficial myofascial structures in the body.) Balance of these in the human framework fosters lightness and resilience in movement and minimizes structural drag. To the extent that its energy fields remain symmetrical, randomizing deterioration of an organic system—physical or chemical—is slowed. Biological time in such a system expresses itself more slowly than chronological time.

Under these conditions, full vigor is prolonged unless and until a major trauma displaces equilibrium. We see this happening in a few of our fellow humans. They not only grow old gracefully, but seemingly they do not age until long past the significant birthday that retires their more random kin. Their bodies and minds over a long sequence of years seem ageless. Oliver Wendell Holmes, George Bernard Shaw, Albert Szent-Gyorgyi, Michelangelo Buonarroti (he was architect of St. Peter's in Rome when he was near eighty), Igor Stravinsky, Carl Gustav Jung—these immediately come to mind as falling into this group of outstanding humans in whom extreme old age did not equate with senility. Somehow, mental order and form seem to manifest themselves through these people regardless of age. Are these unusual characteristics given only to extraordinary individuals, or are they traits toward which we may all not only aspire but consciously work?

It is the consensus that evolution is an almost infinitely long process undergone by a species. But evolution (or some equivalent term) is descriptive of the selective tendency toward desirable order in an individual. In the first case, it is an unconscious group process. In the second, it is more likely to be the result of individual action, susceptible to conscious direction. Within the parameters of modern

290

science, the work of Dr. Neal E. Miller* and his associates has shown the change in nervous function that can result from training. Until the very elegant work of this group, it was generally accepted that the central and autonomic nervous tracts were independent of each other, that the so-called autonomic system could not be voluntarily or consciously directed. However, this modern experimenter demonstrated on animals that with the use of rewards (sensations the animal regarded as pleasurable), he was able to alter functions generally considered autonomic. Blood pressure, body heat, etc., were previously considered entirely beyond conscious control.

Such animal experiments and the development of biofeedback techniques on the human level has altered the premises with which we define functional control. Barbara Brown, an outstanding worker in this field, has been quoted as saying, "Almost any part of an individual's own physiologic functioning can be controlled with biofeedback techniques."* Although this evaluation may be somewhat overoptimistic, it points the way to wider mastery of the human condition by a technique that operates through a pinpointing of awareness, a discrimination of perception.

*For the interested reader, a listing of Dr. Miller's articles is included, since this is not readily available to the layman.
Neal E. Miller, "Learning of visceral and glandular responses," *Science*, vol. 163 (1969), pp. 434-445; and "Psychosomatic effects of specific types of training," *Annals of the New York Academy of Sciences*, vol. 159 (1969), pp. 1025-1040.
——— and A. Banuazizi, "Instrumental learning by cruarized rats of a specific visceral response, intestinal or cardiac." *Journal of Comparative and Physiological Psychology*, vol. 65 (1968), pp. 1-7.
——— and L. DiCara, "Instrumental learning of heart rate changes in cruarized rats: Shaping and specificity to discriminative stimulus," *Journal of Comparative and Physiological Psychology*, vol. 63 (1967), pp. 12-19.
——— and L. DiCara, "Instrumental learning of urine formation by rats; changes in renal blood flow." *American Journal of Physiology*, vol. 215 (1968), pp. 677-683.
———, L. DiCara, and A. Banuazizi, "Instrumental learning of glandular and visceral responses." *Conditional Reflex*, vol. 3 (1968), p. 129.
———, L. DiCara, H. Solomon, J. Weiss, and M. Dworkin, "Learned modifications of autonomic functions: A review and some new data." *Circulation Research* (Supplement 1), vols. 26-27 (1970), pp. 13-111.

*The News, Van Nuys, Calif., February 2, 1970.

Fig. 11-23 and its accompanying caption, repeated here, further illustrate this second, more personal dimension of evolution. The drawings record the drastic and fundamental changes that have occurred in each of us, not in prenatal life but in the slower rhythms of postnatal childhood and adulthood. They show the changes occurring in bone, commonly regarded as a rigid and relatively unalterable tissue. These changes in this most solid of body structures have been brought about by muscular, functional demand. Here function has altered form at its most dense organic level. Here dense tissue evolution has resulted from behavior. Can more such in-depth evolutionary change be induced if order is deliberately made available through an attentional component? The word *evolution* is to most of us a verbal abstraction. The forces it represents seem equally tenuous. In fact and in flesh, they are the daily reality of all of us. This kind of evolution of the material body, accessible to anyone, is a start on the road. There may be other evolutions possible to man—of the "finer body" of the occultists, of the group body, of others yet unsuspected.

It is obvious that this book can serve merely as a directional pointer to a wider realm of fascinating, exciting explorations of the mind and body as they interrelate. Descriptions and conclusive validations of this are only just starting to appear in the objective world of science. In the intimate, meaningful, personal realm of feeling, the report on the integration of structure is summarized in the enthusiastic "It feels so good." Even though the reasons for this feeling have not yet been fully delinated in scientific terms, the feeling itself is of major significance. This is the stuff that, in the history of man, has always prophesied advances in knowledge. As the great Buddha himself admonished us, "Do not believe in anything because it is said . . . nor in the mere authority of your teachers or masters. . . . Believe when the writing, doctrine, or saying is corroborated by your reason and consciousness." For twenty-five hundred years these words have been a touchstone for common sense. In this late twentieth century, as in the days of the Lord Buddha, they still allow each man to separate gold from dross.

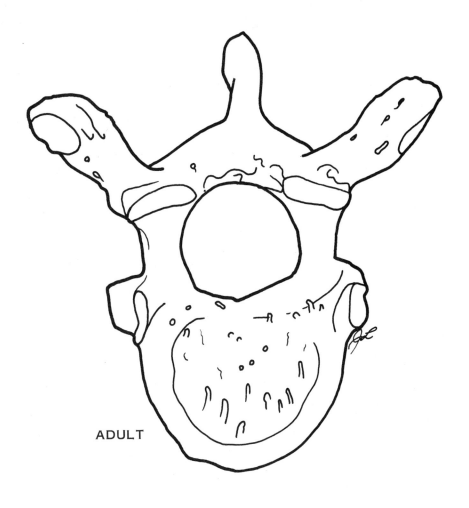

ADULT

18-2 This schema of a thoracic vertebra of a new-born indicates clearly how far development has to proceed before the vertebra of an adult is reached. Note the lack of well-developed bony processes able to contribute leverage to attached muscles. These processes will develop after puberty, in response to the directional demand of muscles. This means that the location and integrity of bone is, in a sense, a direct response to the functional demand of the moving muscles. In turn, this implies that through much (if not all) of life, structural integrity at any level (its direction and, within narrow limits, its pattern) can change over time in response to functional demand. At the present state of our knowledge, it would be highly arbitrary to assign a limit to this change, either in respect to structure or time.

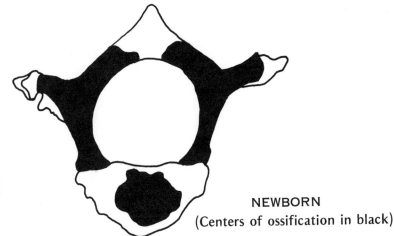

NEWBORN
(Centers of ossification in black)

Index

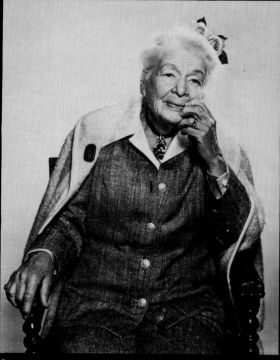

© Karsh, Ottawa

This is Ida P. Rolf's long-awaited book, written over a period of years in time stolen from her full schedule of teaching and lecturing. Here, with the aid of over 600 illustrations, Dr. Rolf explains the theory and practice of the body therapy known as rolfing.

The purpose of rolfing is to put the body into a natural balance, or alignment, with the energy field in which it moves—the field of gravity. This rebalancing is accomplished through ten hour-long sessions of systematic manipulation that loosen and reorganize the myofascia, the connective tissue that surrounds the muscles. After rolfing, not only do you stand taller, look better, and move with greater ease, but you have more vitality and a greater sense of well-being.

The book is intended for two types of readers: the interested but untrained layperson and the professional wanting technical information. In spite of its many illustrations, it makes no pretense of being an anatomy book. Rather, its goal is to establish a new point of view, a new way of looking at the human body.

About the Author

Ida P. Rolf is that rare person with creative insight—one who has the ability to see things in a new way. She came upon the idea of rolfing, or Structural Integration, during her search for solutions to family health problems. Finding available methods inadequate, Dr. Rolf investigated the effect of structure on function. Her technique, primarily designed to relieve painful conditions, improved general functioning as well and contributed to psychological well-being.

Dr. Rolf received her Ph.D. in biochemistry and physiology from Columbia University in 1920. Her work at the Rockefeller Institute in the departments of chemotherapy and organic chemistry provided further study and experience. For the past two decades Dr. Rolf has been teaching practitioners of rolfing through her Institute in Boulder, Colorado. Now in her eighties, Dr. Rolf still teaches advanced classes and oversees the Institute's activities.

HARPER & ROW, PUBLISHERS
COVER DESIGN: FRED CHARLES

ISBN: 0—06—465096—0